Series on Bioengineering & Biomedical Engineering   5

BIOMEDICAL ENGINEERING PRINCIPLES OF THE BIONIC MAN

George K Hung

Rutgers University, USA

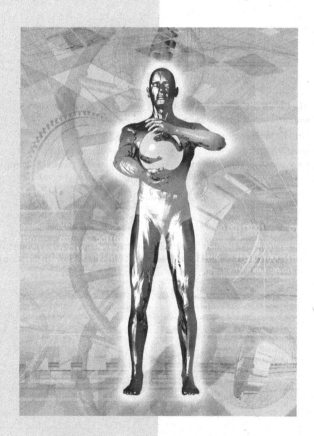

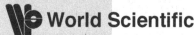 World Scientific

NEW JERSEY · LONDON · SINGAPORE · BEIJING · SHANGHAI · HONG KONG · TAIPEI · CHENNAI

Published by

World Scientific Publishing Co. Pte. Ltd.

5 Toh Tuck Link, Singapore 596224

USA office: 27 Warren Street, Suite 401-402, Hackensack, NJ 07601

UK office: 57 Shelton Street, Covent Garden, London WC2H 9HE

British Library Cataloguing-in-Publication Data
A catalogue record for this book is available from the British Library.

BIOMEDICAL ENGINEERING PRINCIPLES OF THE BIONIC MAN
Series on Bioengineering & Biomedical Engineering — Vol. 5

ISBN-13 978-981-277-977-9
ISBN-10 981-277-977-9
ISBN-13 978-981-277-978-6 (pbk)
ISBN-10 981-277-978-7 (pbk)

Printed in Singapore.

To my close and long-time golfing friend, Mort Reinhart, whose numerous medical procedures inspired this book on the bionic man. His medical procedures included: intraocular lens implants for cataracts, monovision correction, quadruple heart bypass, external beam radiation treatment for prostate cancer, and a total knee replacement.

- G.K.H.

FOREWORD

The inspiration for this book is my father, Mort Reinhart, who also happens to be the golf partner of Dr. George Hung, this book's editor. At 76, my father is still able to pursue an active lifestyle as an avid golfer with multiple replaced, repaired and rejuvenated body parts. He has ocular implants, a knee replacement and has undergone cardiac bypass surgery; George kiddingly refers to him as "the bionic man".

To me as an orthopaedic surgeon, my father seems to be a fairly typical patient who has benefited greatly from the wonderful biomedical devices and techniques widely utilized in many areas of medicine. This textbook describes some of these devices and conveys sense of excitement about the opportunity for further advances as new technologies emerge in Biomedical Engineering.

Golfers like my father and Dr. Hung often look to innovations in equipment design, and materials to improve their performance. The same process works in medicine where physicians, patients, and researchers hope for improved personal "performance" through advances in technology. However, whereas in golf the idea is to improve the external equipment, in medicine the idea is to improve the internal attributes of the player.

New technology alone is not sufficient to drive innovation in medicine. The other factor which continues to push innovation is the increasingly high demands and expectations of patients. Many individuals with a variety of medical conditions expect that their problems can be addressed so that they can continue to pursue all of their activities at a high level and over increasingly extended periods of time. More and more the focus in helping patient is not simply in relieving symptoms, but in truly restoring near normal function.

This book presents a fabulous and fascinating array of technologies which are already well developed, or are currently under development. Advances in materials, design, electronics and biologic techniques all have the potential to enable patients to sense the world around them and move through their daily activities with greater enjoyment and ease.

In my specialty of Orthopaedics, the traditional focus has been on repairing or replacing broken parts with various mechanical devices. However, in Orthopaedics as well as in many other medical specialties as described in this book, the focus is broadening from simple mechanical solutions to biological solutions as well. Various biomedical techniques are described that augment or assist normal structures, that monitor and correct abnormal conditions on an instantaneous basis, and that can stimulate or substitute for impaired bodily symptoms. The new frontiers in biology, including tissue engineering and gene therapy, offer opportunities to regenerate or recreate healthier systems as well.

The concept of a "bionic man" may on the surface seem to imply a mechanical or robotic condition. However, with these new techniques a bionic man is actually a combination of enhanced natural functions as well as substitute or artificial parts. This new bionic man is actually more human in that he has greater ability to enjoy life not only in his required day to day activities but also in the desired activities which bring him pleasure.

This book presents students with basic scientific principles and hopefully also provides the inspiration to pursue new and creative ideas, and visionary thinking about how to continue to improve this bionic man.

Glenn Reinhart, M.D.
Freiberg Orthopaedic & Sports   PH: (513) 221-5500 9825
Kenwood Rd Ste 200   FX: (513) 221-1962
Cincinnati, OH 45242   EM: gareinhart@zoomtown.com

Dr. Reinhart is a specialist in sports medicine and shoulder surgery, and is a member of the American Academy of Orthopaedic Surgeons and the Arthroscopy Association of North America. He currently serves as the medical director of the Kenwood Surgery Center and has provided care as a physician for numerous high schools, collegiate and professional teams. In addition, he has a special interest in pediatric orthopaedics and shoulder reconstruction.

PREFACE

Aging is as inevitable as the change of seasons, from spring to summer, and then winter to fall. As we age, mobility, strength, and stamina all decline. These are the classic signs of aging. The aging process is written in our genes. As the telomere length recedes, the rate of cell division declines, and the fabric of our bones and skin lose their resilience, leading to the loss in vitality.

Yet, remarkable progress has been made in the understanding of the aging process, and in turn how to slow its progress. A vitally important arsenal in anti-aging is the minimization of oxidation, or rusting, of the body. Free radicals that result from oxidation can interfere with the natural repair process in the cells, leading to genetic damage that increases the rate of aging. Proper nutrition and exercise play significant roles in slowing the effects of aging. Nutrients with anti-oxidant properties act at the microscopic level to counteract the damaging effects of free-radicals, and in turn maintain the integrity of the structure of the cells in the body. Exercise act at the macroscopic level to strengthen muscle, joint, and bones as well as increase the functions of the cardiovascular, respiratory, and hormonal systems to better counteract the physical and emotional stresses of daily life.

Nevertheless, there is only so much nutrition and exercise can do to stem the tide of aging. Eventually, some body parts will begin to break down over time. The baby boomers, who have dominated the social, economic, political demographics of the population over the last half century, will now dominate the search for elixirs and remedies to hold back the ravages of time as they age and their body parts begin to malfunction. Repair or replacement of the body parts provides a means in a sense to reverse the aging process. Biomedical engineers have built components or devices to assist and revitalize the aging human body. Indeed, it is now not too extraordinary to find senior persons who have had surgery for cataract, monovision, Lasik, heart bypass, hip, knee, and/or cochlear implants. Thus, the maturing of the baby boomers also heralds the age of the bionic man, who is literally composed of various replacement organs or biomechanical parts.

The purpose of this book is to provide a comprehensive and up-to-date scientific source of biomedical engineering principles of "replacement parts and assist devices" for the bionic man. It covers biomechanical, biochemical, rehabilitation, and tissue engineering, as well as applications in cardiovascular, visual, auditory, and neurological systems. It can serve as a text or reference for students, scientists, and laymen interested in the fundamental underlying principles of biomedical devices and procedures, as well as recent advances in transplant, gene therapy, and stem cell research. The book's emphasis on fundamental principles that are reviewed within relevant chapters ensures the content will remain relevant and useful for years to come.

George K. Hung, Ph.D.
Piscataway, New Jersey

CONTENTS

IV. HEART

V. TISSUE ENGINEERING AND GENE THERAPY

VI. JOINTS

VII. MASTERS ATHLETES

I

BRAIN AND REHABILITATION

Chapter 1

Restoring Limb Function after Paralysis

William Craelius, Ph.D.[1]

[1] Dept. of Biomedical Engineering, Rutgers University
599 Taylor Road, Piscataway, NJ 08854, USA
Tel: 732-445-2369; Fax: 732-445-3753; Email: craelius@rci.rutgers.edu

1.1 Introduction

1.1.1 *Need of the population*

Motor impairments of the limbs commonly accompany many neurological or musculoskeletal conditions and injuries, including stroke, cerebral palsy, Parkinson's, injury to the central nervous system (CNS), rheumatoid arthritis, and many others. Stroke in particular attacks over 700,000 Americans each year and there are over 4.8 million stroke survivors, making it the leading cause of paralysis in the U.S. Stroke affects 5 to 8 people in every 1,000 over the age of 25 years, and 47 in every 1,000 over the age of 55 years. The total estimated economic impact of stroke was $62.7 billion in 2007. Together, stroke and TBI account for over 10 million people in the United States left with long term disabilities. Incidence of stroke is likely to increase, as risk factors for stroke, such as high blood pressure and carotid artery disease, increase in the aging U.S. population. Cerebrovascular events usually affect one side primarily, resulting in hemiplegia, that limit fundamental activities of daily living (ADL) such as walking, eating, dressing, driving a car, writing or typing, telephone usage, equipment operation, and self-care. Beyond functional loss, persons can experience chronic pain and distortion in the affected limb, as well as inexorable musculoskeletal deterioration through learned disuse (Platz et al., 2001).

Hemiplegia, a weakness that primarily affects one side of the body, is seen in the majority of stroke survivors causing severe disability. Cerebrovascular events manifesting as hemiplegia usually result in asymmetric body dysfunction. This can have multiple effects. First, when the leg is involved it may greatly affect an individual's ability to walk. It is a major concern for people surviving a stroke because it may negatively affect the ability to perform activities of daily living and limit overall independence. As a result, improving mobility is one of the main goals of stroke rehabilitation and has relevance throughout the stroke survivors life. A second result of a stroke is that there can be at least partial loss of bodily awareness of the affected side.

Some ambulatory ability can usually be restored by immobilizing or assisting the ankle with an orthosis, but this assistance tends to inhibit neurorehabilitation, that depends on active neuromuscular efforts. Restoration of normal gait and lower-limb (LL) function is thus rare after hemiplegia.   Restoration of upper-limb (UL) function is even more problematic due to its enormous complexity, and the higher priorities given to ambulation, and compensatory strategies learned for ADL that may inhibit recovery. As a result, persons with paralysis of the UL are unlikely to recover much functionality. For example, a study of stroke patients entering rehabilitation with non-functional arms revealed that 61% showed no improvement after 2 years (Turton et al., 2002). Many individuals that do recover significant arm function experience episodic relapses, making it risky for them to carry things.

In general, recovery outlook after central hemiplegia is poor, and most individuals can expect to regain only partial mobility, and very limited UL functionality. Mounting evidence suggests, however, that the central nervous system (CNS) is sufficiently plastic to effect more significant reversals from paralysis, when given the proper stimuli (Edgerton et al., 2001; Krebs et al., 2003; Feys et al., 2004; Reinkensmeyer et al., 2004; Bharadwaj et al., 2005; Riener et al., 2005). It is believed that sensorimotor stimulation provided by repeated voluntary attempts to extend movements of the limbs, or even applied sensory stimulation, can cause the brain to reorganize and re-gain control and coordination. Restoration of at least some functionality may be possible through intensive physical therapy involving repetitive exercising, both passive and active, of the affected limb. We cannot predict, however, the types, amount, and duration of movements, exercise, or stimulation that will be effective, nor can we predict which individuals will respond to given protocols, and whether the outcome of such demanding therapy will be worthwhile. Moreover, there are few tools available to help the process, and only a limited availability of rehabilitation services, since they are costly, constrained by time, practicality, travel distance, and motivation, and are variably applied depending on individual providers.

To summarize, there is much evidence that bionic exploitation of residual sensorimotor functions in persons with hemiplegia can sometimes produce significant recovery.

1.1.2 *Potential for functional restoration*

Fortunately, most individuals with hemiplegia have access to physiotherapy delivered by dedicated professionals, but this access is necessarily limited by time and available technology. Even therapies that employ state-of-the art approaches offer little for neural recovery, since they focus on assistive devices, encouraging compensatory strategies through constraint-induced movement therapy, or on active manipulation of the joints with robotic devices. Except for simple assistive devices, these regimens and devices are generally too impractical for most individuals to use without expert assistance and large expense, and the more advanced approaches are unlikely to be widely available soon. As a result, after termination of regular physiotherapy, neglect-induced declines in function are inevitable, and clients may increasingly depend on medical and pharmacological treatments for spasticity, sores, and pain.

Neglecting the affected muscles and joints is counterproductive, since disuse patterns and associated pathology commence soon after immobilization of limbs. Clearly, this situation could be remedied if scientifically-designed tools were available to encourage clients to implement proven sensorimotor protocols at home. The value of relatively short-term sensorimotor exercise training, within supervised rehabilitation protocols, is well-established (Ouellette et al., 2004; Pang et al., 2006; Lam et al., 2008), and the additive benefits of in-home exercise carried on for 12 weeks beyond the standard post-stroke therapy has been shown in clinical studies (Duncan et al., 2003). Thus there is no reason to believe that progress would not continue indefinitely with proper training tools.

1.2 Rehabilitation Approaches

1.2.1 *General*

A myriad of strategies, devices, and protocols have been developed to help restore function to persons with hemiplegia, each of which may in fact be efficacious for neurorehabilitation, but none of which is a priori superior or indicated for any given client. There are two assumptions commonly held among the emerging and competing therapy options: (1), the CNS is sufficiently plastic to reorganize itself and regain sensorimotor control after injury, and (2), sustained and repetitive movements of the affected limbs can promote re-learning by the CNS, leading to sensorimotor recovery. Beyond these, there is insufficient theory upon which to build a rational treatment plan, due to the enormous complexity of hemiplegia and its sequellae, involving not only the CNS, but the PNS, muscles, joints, metabolism, as well as psychology. For this reason, it has been suggested that the most promising therapy regimens should be open to empirically combining several (Hogan et al., 2006).

While advanced neurorehabilitation strategies differ widely, and often overlap in methods, they generally can be distinguished as those that work on: (1) strengthening or relaxing individual muscles, or (2) promoting functional movements. The first category includes standard physiotherapeutic exercises administered by a professional. The second category includes tools such as constraint-induced movement therapy, biofeedback devices, and movement assistive devices, that generally induce or encourage both passive and active motions. The second category, into which this chapter falls, can also be termed, 'sensorimotor training,' (SMT) whereby the client attempts to move the affected limb while receiving sensory input regarding his success at normal motion. The goal of SMT is thus to coerce re-organization of the damaged motor cortex by helping the client associate his volitions and possible subsequent movements with their sensory consequences, including proprioceptive, tactile, and visual modalities. SMT requires active volition by the client, whether or not he is assisted by mechanical robots.

1.2.2 *Training the affected UL*

Rehabilitative approaches to paralysis of the UL can be categorized as: (1) standard supervised exercise protocols, (2) constraint-induced movements, (3) assistive devices, (4) active devices and (5) biofeedback of movements using EMG and virtual reality. These approaches involve sensorimotor training to various degrees that encourages and/or assists repetitive motions of the affected limbs.

To apply appropriate technology, the rehabilitation engineer should have an understanding of the potential user. The following tables (Table 1.1 and 1.2) are not exhaustive, but is meant to outline specific problems of the target populations, and their potential to use specific technologies.

Encouraging exercise with rigorous protocols or by constraining the sound arm for several hours per week can force clients to use their affected limb, thereby encouraging plastic reorganization within the CNS. Highly motivated clients who constantly use their affected arm for several months, either with exercise regimen or by constraint, have regained considerable function (Page et al., 2005; Wolf, 2007). To provide structure for patients doing constraint-induced therapy, a workstation for directing and recording tasks has been developed (Lum et al., 2004). Unsupervised exercise and constraint therapies have limitations, however, since they may teach compensatory strategies involving the trunk and shoulder, with little impact on the underlying paralysis.

Table 1.1 – Problems of Stroke and TBI and Potential Solutions.

	Residual Abilities	
'Irreparable' damage to areas of the brain that formerly controlled one or more limbs, i.e. Stroke and TBI.	Central nervous system plasticity; sensory perception intact.	Re-learning movements through proper training and sensory feedback to reduce conflict. Repetitive task training and playing in an engaging environment.
Fixed flexure of affected arm and generally stiff joints and co-contraction of agonist and antagonist during movement, i.e. 'synergy'	Usually can be extended by unaffected arm.Proprioception may be intact, but possibly anomalous.	Anti-flexion exercise, stretching, weight bearing.
Loss of wrist and hand dexterity. Poor force control.	Some muscles are usually active, even in early recovery.	Staged protocols that begin with restoring reaching ability and progress to hand grasping.

Table 1.2 – Problems of SCI and Potential Solutions.

	Residual Ability	
C1-C2 All vegetative and motor functions are not controlled.	Brain Cognition intact.	Brain signals, either from EEG or internal electrodes, can control computer for communication with human and robot BCI.
C3-C5 Lost All motor functions below neck	Usually can be extended by unaffected arm. Proprioception may be intact, but possibly anomalous.	Anti-flexion exercise, stretching, weight bearing. Neuroprostheses to restore standing.
C6-C8	Some muscles are usually active, even in early recovery.	Staged protocols that begin with restoring reaching ability and progress to hand grasping, Neuroprostheses for arm and legs.

Functional electrical stimulation (FES) of muscles represents a type of sensorimotor training. The earliest commercial versions were developed at CWRU, such as the FreeHand (Fig. 1.1). The value of FES in the acute phase of stroke was shown in a randomized trial involving 100 patients who were given SMT for 6 weeks shortly following the event. These patients out-performed the controls even after 5 years (Feys et al., 2004). Arm and hand function can be restored to some degree using FES. The Freehand used implanted myoelectrodes to stimulate muscles for grasping and bending the elbow. The electrodes, and subsequent movements of the paralyzed UL, were activated by the movements of contralateral arm.

The freehand system

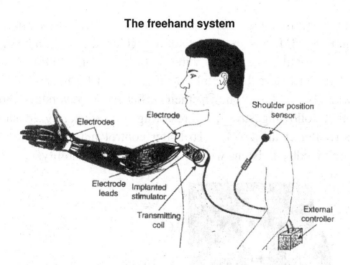

Figure 1.1. The Freehand, showing electrodes implanted into the arm, a transmitting coil to activate them, a shoulder position sensor to indicate volition to grasp, and an external controller.

Variations of the Freehand include a strictly external orthosis that activates the grip muscles using non-invasive EMG electrodes, with activation by buttons, as shown in Figure 1.2.

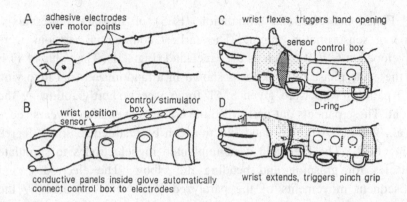

Figure 1.2. Grasp control with surface EMG electrodes. The wrist postion controls opening and closings.

A more sophisticated interface to muscular control is the Bion™, as shown in Fig. 1.3. Bions are the size of a grain of rice and can be injected into muscles, without external wires (Micera et al., 2006). They are activated by an external RF coil that is activated by the user. Clinical trials with Bions have shown their efficacy in reversing shoulder subluxation following stroke, by restoring tone to paralyzed shoulder muscles (Salter et al., 2004). To better control muscle activity, using closed loop feedback, Bions will have muscle sensing ability.

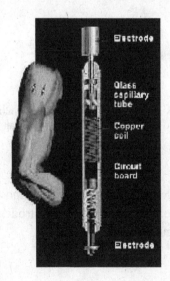

Figure 1.3. Bions can be injected into muscles for external control. The bion consists of a bipolar electrode that can be activated from and external coil.

Advanced assistive devices use FES, either externally applied, or using BIONS™. A depiction of a grasping control system, controlling the extrinsic forearm muscles, is shown in Fig. 1.4.

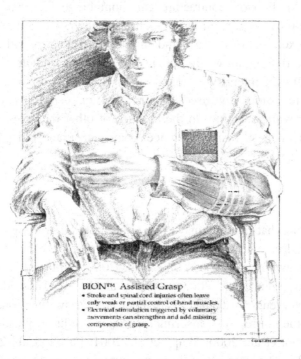

Figure 1.4. Depiction of an external coil controlling an internal array of BIONS™ to program grasping muscles.

1.2.3 *SMT and feedback tools*

Task-oriented sensori-motor training, sometimes aided by constraining the sound arm, is central to promoting neuroplastic rehabilitation of the upper limb (Platz, 2003; Winstein et al., 2004; Goffredo et al., 2008). In comparison to protocols for strengthening specific muscles and joints, a functional task approach was more beneficial in the long-term outcome (Winstein et al., 2004). Some studies, however, concluded that therapies involving repetitions of complex or task-oriented motions and are not superior to those using simpler motions or standard occupational therapies or (Woldag et al., 2003; Fasoli et al., 2005).

There are assistive devices for adapting to ADL and orthotic devices for overcoming the common and troubling complications of contracture and spasticity of both the hand and arm (Kottke et al., 1966; Yasukawa et al., 2003). Flexion contracture can immobilize the arm, impairing hygiene and dressing, resulting in skin breakdown, as well as defeating stretching exercises of the arm and shoulder. To help extend the elbow, wearable orthoses allow the client to perform isometric exercises, helping maintain integrity of muscles and tendons. Similar anti-flexion orthoses are commonly used for the fingers, especially to prevent contracture while sleeping. In the absence of other therapies, prolonged application of these assistive devices may discourage independent use and rehabilitation.

1.2.4 *Robotic arm movers*

Robotic arms that continuously move the affected arm passively, with some back-drive-ability to allow active motions, have been developed (Reinkensmeyer et al., 2000; Volpe et al., 2001; Lum et al., 2002; Fasoli et al., 2003; Flint et al., 2003; Hesse et al., 2003). These devices and physical interventions may help shoulder and elbow function, and have supported the concept of sensorimotor training induced plasticity of the CNS (Scheidt et al., 2000; Volpe et al., 2001; Fasoli et al., 2003; Page et al., 2003). The simplest of these are motorized movers of the affected arm that are controlled by motions of the sound arm. Since the paralyzed arm is often in a highly contracted and stiff state, powerful motors are required to move it. Robotic arms can provide standardized repetitive exercises for joints and muscles, but they work mainly at a biomechanical level and the degree to which this contributes to neurorehabilitation is unclear. Several companies market robotic arms, with one of the earliest being patterned after the MIT-MANUS and marketed by Interactive Motion Technologies, Inc. The T-Wrex is a robotic/orthotic device that is meant to be worn by the user, providing reaching assistance as well as passive motion training (Reinkensmeyer et al., 2000), and is marketed by Hocoma, Inc., Rockland, MA. The WaveFlex and H3 Hand are sold by Orthorehab, Inc.; Smith & Nephew, Inc. market the Kinetic series hand devices. The Rutgers Master II, is a robotic glove that moves the fingers, and is in clinical trials (Bouzit et al., 2002). More sophisticated devices combine robotic motions with FES or with electromyographic (EMG) signals from the affected arm (Popovic and Sinkjaer, 2002). These devices give users some control over their assisted movement through their residual muscle activity. The complexity and expense of robotic machines may limit use at home.

As an inexpensive alternative to custom robotic arm movers, a force feedback joystick has been tried with stroke subjects (Reinkensmeyer et al., 2002). This approach allows the user to manipulate a wide variety of games with the joystick, depending to his ability, and, by interfacing to the computer, it can provide a comprehensive tele-rehabilitation program. The joysticks would be useful for moderately affected arms, to provide a limited range of motion, without isolation of specific joints.

1.2.5 *Biofeedback*

Another category of SMT tools measures motions of relatively unconstrained limbs using accelerometers, goniometers or optical means, and uses the outputs for biofeedback. Accelerometer and goniometer technology has been well established as an accurate and convenient method for registering limb motion in 3D in healthy persons, for athletes (Hung, 2003), as well as those with stroke and other neurological conditions (Green, 2007). For example, the stroke Upper-Limb Activity Monitor (SULAM) applies an accelerometer and goniometer on each wrist and other joints and monitors daily activities and motion parameters (de Niet et al., 2007). Accelerometery has also been used for estimation of limb inertial forces (Blank et al., 2001).

An internet based wearable motion tracker system that is designed for users with stroke to use at home has been recently reported (Zhang et al., 2008). This system is primarily designed for telerehabilitation, and requires several inertial sensors positioned near the wrist, and a belt-worn processor unit.

Other modalities have been applied to SMT, including video tracking with anatomical markers (Metcalf et al., 2008) and a 3D optoelectronic system (Caimmi et al., 2008). Sensorized gloves, such as the *Rutgers Master* II and others have been developed to encourage specific finger exercises and have demonstrated efficacy (Bouzit et al., 2002; Merians et al., 2006). A drawback of these technologies, such as wearable goniometers, markers and gloves, is the difficulty of donning and inconvenience in wearing by many persons with motor impairments.

Beyond ordinary computer games, virtual reality environments provide more realistic biofeedback and encouragement and may improve the prospects of physical exercise. Imagery has been used as biofeedback, whereby users practice watching a corrected image of their affected arm moving normally, done by projecting a mirror image of their sound arm (Stevens, 2005). While there are few devices that specifically provide users with feedback to help them regain fine motor control of the hand, there is much evidence that the paralyzed arm can be improved through repetitive training of isolated movements. One of the first demonstrations of this was with 27 hemiparetic patients who improved hand performance after several days of training with repetitive hand and finger flexions (Butefisch et al., 1995; Carey et al., 2002). Subjects who underwent 20 sessions of finger tracking exercises not only improved their function, but experienced plastic reorganization within the motor cortex. Subsequent studies have supported the benefit of repetitive training of the paretic hand (van der Lee et al., 2001).

EMG feedback of hand muscles is also efficacious, as shown by a recent study that randomly assigned stroke patients to either real or placebo EMG feedback, and applied it 5 times per week for 20 days (Armagan et al., 2003). Results showed that wrist range of motion and EMG potentials significantly improved in the test group. The efficacy of EMG biofeedback for stroke rehabilitation has been questioned in reviews of literature prior to 1992 (Glanz et al., 1995); recent reviews, however, and many controlled studies cited above have proven its efficacy (Ernst, 2003).

Vectorial maps (Fig. 1.5) can depict motor performance throughout the entire range of motion of a single joint, i.e. as a function of joint angle, not time. the method quantifies accelerative transients within a movement by summing the errors between segments of trajectory and progressively finer straight-lines. This iterative procedure presents a map of spontaneous accelerative transients (SATs) across the angular workspace, quantifying regional dyscoordination as color shades. The method employs a pseudo-wavelet paradigm to detect regions of stable velocity and depicts spontaneous accelerations as bright bands against a black background, as shown in Fig. 1.5. This transformation into the angular domain eliminates residual error associated with the repeated differentiation of discrete-time data, and obviates systematic bias of time-domain smoothness metrics, such as jerk, due to prolonged *stall* behaviors (time spent at low angular velocities) typical of spastic movements.

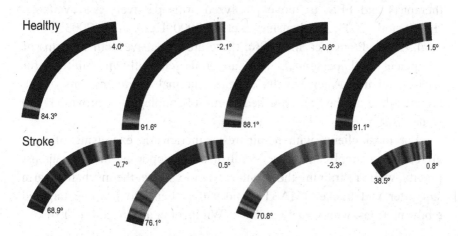

Figure 1.5. Sample traces from unimpaired subjects (*Top*) and chronic stroke patients (Bottom). The bright bands at the plot extrema reflect motion initiation and cessation. For stroke subjects, intermediary activity produces spontaneous accelerations of equal or greater magnitude to that of motion onset and cessation.

It can be seen from Fig. 1.5 that control subjects tend to produce doubly-peaked profiles, with thin bands only at the onset and cessation of activity (i.e. at plot extrema). This pattern is expected, since for normal motion, the greatest acceleration and hence the greatest error would be expected to occur at the reversals from flexion to extension. In contrast, stroke patients' movements exhibit large transient accelerations at intermediary angles.

SAT maps match well to ridges in the angular position trace (Fig. 1.5), and yield scalar metrics that resolve a significant performance deficit in a patient cohort with greater fidelity than time-domain metrics;

this discriminative power can be attributed to the transformation from temporal to angular domain, which eliminates bias associated with stall behaviors. The vectorial maps identify particular angular regions of impairment, and are useful biofeedback signals (Wininger et al., 2008).

1.2.6 *Repetitive task practice for the UL*

While methods and robotic devices, including manual assist from therapists and FES, to move paralyzed arms passively are available, (Eskes et al., 2003; Reinkensmeyer et al., 2000; Hesse et al., 2003; Volpe et al., 2004; Prange et al., 2006), these are expensive both in terms of equipment and personnel, and are thus currently prohibitive for widespread use. Alternatively, at least minimal active motions of the affected limb can be accomplished by most hemiplegics, if provided with some assistance.

For most clients with hemiparesis, therapeutic exercising of their affected arm simply can be accomplished by supporting the arm against gravity, while restraining the shoulder. For example, the mechanical arm supporter and tracker (MAST) guides the clients to practice targeted elbow motions, with visual feedback (Wininger et al., 2008; Fig. 1.6).

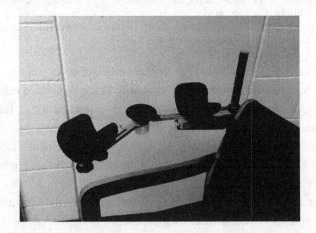

Figure 1.6. The Mechanical Arm Supporter and Tracker (MAST).

The MAST supports the arm, and stabilizes the shoulder, while the elbow flexions and extensions are recorded goniometrically. The user watches a display of his efforts in various formats. An engaging and useful targeting task is based on the Kinematic Speed- Accuracy (KSAT) task, using a Fitt's- type speed-accuracy tradeoff paradigm (Kim et al., 2007).

The subject interacts with a display as shown in Fig. 1.7, hitting alternating targets with his hand position as rapidly as possible. The two targets change randomly in size and spacing, and can be arranged so that they scan the right and left hemi-spaces, in order to map the subject's visual attention spaces. Performance is measured in terms of the speed and consistency of movements, using the slope of Fitts' log-linear plot.

A dynamic SAT test can be similarly applied to training grip force. A Grip force dynamometer was custom fabricated to ensure full radial contact between the five metacarpal bones and the sensors, measuring the true cylindrical grip force. Similarly to the standard Fitts' test, the user must hit alternating targets, that represent low and high grip force, as quickly as possible. The index of difficulty (ID) for a movement is proportional to the ratio of the spacing of the targets to their width. Movement times, MT, are acquired for all ID levels, and the average MTID across index of difficulty was fitted by a regression line, m, represented as:

$$MT = a + b \cdot \log_2 ID \qquad (1.1)$$

The slope of the regression line, b, measures grip proficiency in terms of the targeting frequency as a function of ID.

Typical grip force waveforms from a stroke subject are shown in Fig. 1.8, spanning all 5 ID levels of a single DSAT test. Each peak and valley corresponds to achievement of the grip force target (represented by red bands). Waveforms indicate that the subject reached the alternating force targets quickly, usually with some overshoot, but tended to release force more slowly.

Figure 1.7. Kinematic speed-accuracy tradeoff (KSAT) test. The tank display is shown at right. The subject is asked to hit each bar by reaching the appropriate elbow angle. Spacing between the bars is altered to change the difficulty level.

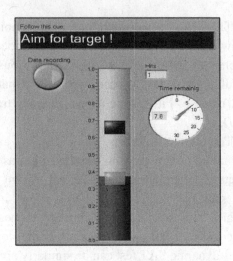

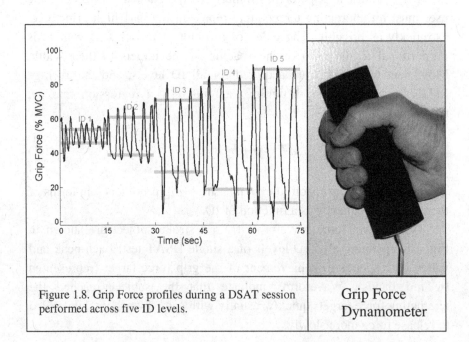

Figure 1.8. Grip Force profiles during a DSAT session performed across five ID levels.

Grip Force Dynamometer

Fitts' plots for a subject (Chedoke-McMaster score > 6) before and after 6 weeks of dynamic grip training are shown in Fig. 1.9. Correlations are high (R2=0.98), and there is a reduction in slope and movement times after training. Thus preliminary evidence indicates that hemiplegic subjects can readily accomplish Fitt's type SAT tests and potentially regain some arm and hand control.

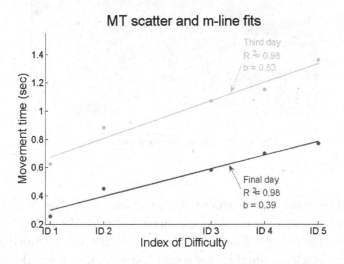

Figure 1.9. Scatter plots of average movement time (MT) against index of difficulty (ID) for a single subject. Note the R2 values of correlation are 0.98 for both the early test (Third day) and the late test (Final day). Both slope and intercept improved.

1.2.7 *Registering weak muscle activity*

Surface muscle pressure (SMP) is a highly sensitive and convenient register of muscle activity of the extrinsic muscles of the hand (Wininger et al., 2008). SMP sensor sleeves contain an array of force-sensitive resistors, that are applied to the limb surfaces, as shown for the arm in (Fig. 1.10). Such recording is useful for biofeedback, whereby the signals represent dynamic images of muscular activity, whose patterns can be learned by an adaptive processor, and associated with specific muscles (Craelius et al., 2002; Kuttiva et al., 2005).

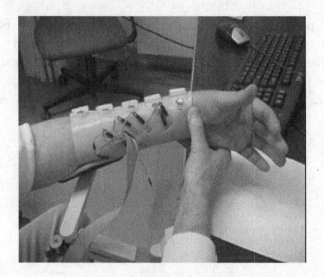

Figure 1.10. Surface muscle pressure sleeve.

SMP sleeves readily records finger motions, as seen in Fig. 1.11, wherein the subject was asked to extend and relax the index finger on both the affected and unaffected hand. Note that the rhythmic pattern from the muscles controlling the sound finger is clear, while the forearm muscles of the affected arm contracted strongly and relaxed slowly during the attempted motion. The sleeves can register and differentiate distinct motions of the digits, wrist, elbow, and shoulder.

Registration of forearm muscular activity by SMP sleeves can accurately predict relative grip force, as shown in Fig. 1.12 (Wininger et al., 2008). Here the subject grasped and released the dynamometer 3 times rhythmically while wearing the sensor sleeve.

In addition to movement individuation, the SMP method accurately represents neural coding of volitions. We have shown that simple algorithms applied to the signals from the UL, such as linear filters, can reliably distinguish finger motions and at least 5 different types of grasp (Curcie et al., 2001; Phillips, 2005; Yungher et al., 2006). These algorithms are useful as biofeedback cues in training specific gestures.

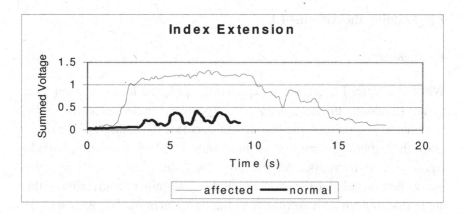

Figure 1.11. SMP Records from the forearm during attempted rhythmic extensions of the finger of the unaffected hand (lower) and affected hand (upper trace).

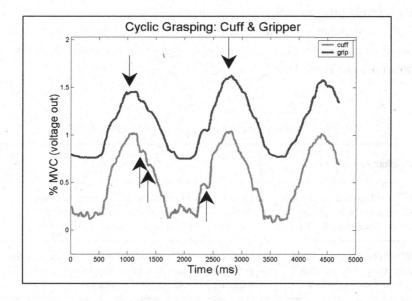

Figure 1.12. Comparison of SMP output with grasp force. Note the concordance of the overall signals as well as the small oscillations *(arrows)*.

1.3 Training the Affected LL

1.3.1 *General*

While the entire LL generally experiences profound loss of sensory and motor function in hemiplegia, the primary impediment to basic ambulation is drop foot, the inability to dorsiflex the ankle sufficiently to clear the ground during leg swing. Drop foot can manifest as ankle equinus or equinovarus. Ankle equinus is a deficiency experienced by many cerebral palsy patients, in which there is limited dorsiflexion of the ankle due to decreased flexibility in the gastrocnemius or soleus muscle groups. Most stroke patients experience equinovarus disorder, which is a weakness in both the ankle dorsiflexion and the ankle eversion muscles, as well as increased ankle stiffness. To compensate for decreased dorsiflexion, the subtalar and midtarsal joints may be overused resulting in a severely pronated foot (Thompson et al., 2004).

A somewhat oversimplified list of the problems commonly encountered by the LL after paralysis, and their potential solutions is shown below (Table 1.3):

Table 1.3 – Problems after LL Paralysis and Potential Solutions.

Problem	
Impaired gait due to damage to areas of the brain that controlled the ankle muscles.	Exploit CNS plasticity with repetitive task practice (RTP) in a rich sensorimotor environment. Possible use of inter-hemispheric learning transfer (IHLT).
Weak dorsiflexion and/or eversion combined with antagonistic hypertonia	Strength training and stretching in both planes with gravity-assist, possibly in conjuction with tone-reducing pharmacological treatments.
Spasticity	Stretching, weight bearing, and exercise to reset muscles.

Most hemiparetics cannot fruitfully execute RTP with their affected leg due to severe control deficiency, and therefore they do not generally participate in such physical therapies. Therapeutic options are further limited since the affected ankle is generally immobilized in an orthosis in order to restore a semblance of gait. Technology for If the affected limb could be improved by sustained exercises of the contralateral limb, this could ameliorate the complications caused its disuse and maximize the effectiveness of rehabilitation. In particular, restoring even a limited degree of ankle control could restore un-assisted gait and/or postural balance to many clients. The present results thus provide clear evidence for the potential benefit to the affected limb afforded by contralateral limb training, and studies are underway to test its efficacy

The standard treatment for drop foot is assisting weak muscles with the use of an ankle foot orthosis (AFO) to clear the foot from the ground during the swing phase of gait (Gok et al., 2003). Rehabilitative approaches to drop foot include muscle strengthening exercises, robotic gait trainers (Bharadwaj et al., 2005), functional electrical stimulation (Bogataj et al., 1997), biofeedback protocols (Basmajian et al., 1975) and treatment of the plantarflexor muscles with botulinum toxin (Reiter et al., 1998; Bayram et al., 2006).

1.3.2 *Assistive technology for the lower limb*

1.3.2.1 *Powered AFOs*

Mechanically powered AFOs are being developed to assist ankle dorsiflexion and knee extension (Durfee et al., 2005), however their external power requirements have limited their acceptance. An example of such a device is shown in Fig. 1.13, the Robowalker from Yobotics.

1.3.2.2 *FES of the LL*

Functional electrical stimulation (FES) of the ankle dorsiflexors can relieve drop foot and improve walking ability. Two commercial products, Bioness® and WalkAid, are ankle-foot orthoses instrumented with a battery-powered FES system for stimulating the Peroneal nerve.

The FES is triggered to stimulate the nerve near the time of late stance during walking, enabling the toe to clear the ground. The triggering event is sensed by either a tilt sensor, or ground force sensor in the heel.

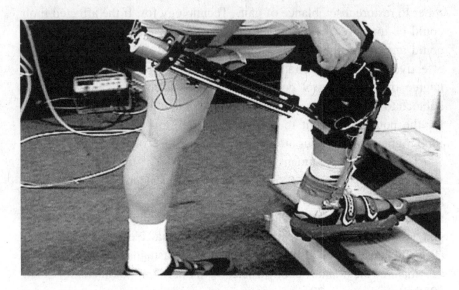

Figure 1.13. Robowalker by Yobotics.

1.3.3 *Contralateral training of the ankle*

While central motor control of the limbs is primarily contralateral, there is increasing evidence that specific types of learned motor actions can transfer across the hemispheres. Inter-limb transfer (ILT) of acquired motor skills, i.e., the ability of a limb to perform a task learned by the opposite limb, has been demonstrated for many activities such as drawing, writing, mirror tracing, ball catching, and pointing (Cook, 1933). Most ILT research focuses on the upper limbs and shows ILT to be either symmetric (bi-directional) or asymmetric, depending on the task studied. Learning of simple tasks, such as grasping, lifting small objects, or anticipatory timing, transfers across hemispheres symmetrically. ILT of more complex learned movements, such as reaching in the presence of visuo-motor (VM) rotations is generally asymmetric and correspondingly more complex. In these studies, the two major determinants of reaching effectiveness, initial trajectory and final hand position, are selectively learned and transferred by opposite hemispheres. Specifically, initial trajectory information transfers from the non-dominant (L) arm to the dominant (R) arm but not vice-versa, and the opposite occurs for final position information. These results have suggested that this type of asymmetric ILT reflects hemispheric specialization, wherein the dominant hemisphere specializes in movement trajectory information while the non-dominant hemisphere specializes in final position. According to this theory, both hemispheres receive similar information on visual rotation but specialized controllers in each hemisphere use it differently.

This study of ILT has important implications for functional rehabilitation of clients with hemiparesis due to stroke, CP or other central injury. Most hemiparetics cannot fruitfully exercise their affected leg due to severe control deficiency, and therefore do not generally participate in directed physical therapies. Therapeutic options are further limited since the affected ankle is generally immobilized in an orthosis in order to restore a semblance of gait. If the affected limb could be improved by sustained exercises of the contralateral limb, this could ameliorate the complications caused its disuse and maximize the effectiveness of rehabilitation. In particular, restoring even a limited degree of ankle control could restore un-assisted gait and/or postural balance to many clients.

Recent studies have shown that a single session of ankle training by the left ankle in healthy adults can significantly improve the right ankle (Morris et al., 2008). Subjects were divided into 2 groups, RL, that received right ankle training first, and LR, that received left ankle training first. After training to hit the targets by movement of the foot, a visuo-motor rotation was introduced that required learning. The paradigm is illustrated in Fig. 1.14 for group LR. The arrows depict the ideal movement vectors to the targets, for the left neutral and VMR conditions.

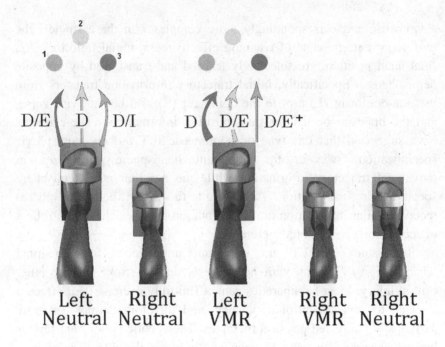

Figure 1.14. Experimental protocol for group LR. The task sequence and ideal direction of movements toward targets for a member of group LR are illustrated. Targets and trajectories to them (1,2,3 from left to right) are coded as shades from light to dark. The left foot (Left Neutral) initially trains to hit each target 24 times, using (ideally) dorsiflexion and inversion (D/I) for target 1, dorsiflexion only (D) for target 2, and dorsiflexion and eversion (D/E) for target 3. The right foot (Right Neutral) then performs the same task, however movements from targets 1 and 3 are reversed (arrows omitted). For Left VM rotation (30° ccw), movements must be shifted cw, as shown. For right VM rotation, the movements are also shifted cw (arrows omitted). For the neutral (catch) trial, the ccw rotation is nulled (arrows omitted).

At the start of each trial, subjects positioned the cursor inside of a start circle located in the center of the screen and held it for 0.3 seconds, using the foot attached to the platform. After receiving an audio and visual "go" cue, the subjects were given 800 ms to move the cursor to one of three targets that appeared at random. Targets were located around the base at radial distances of 250 pixels from its center, which represented approximately 5° of ankle rotation, as depicted in Fig. 1.15.

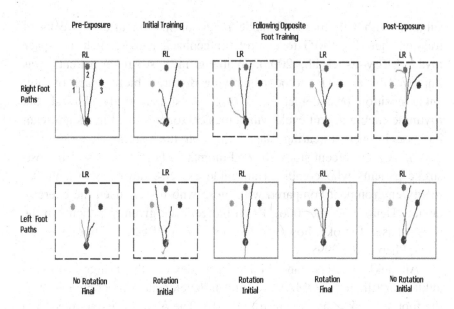

Figure 1.15. Sample Movement Trajectories of representative subjects. Trajectories from a subject in Group RL are in solid boxes, and trajectories from a subject in Group LR are in dashed boxes. Trajectories are shaded in accord with the target. The first column shows the last cycle of movements of each foot during the baseline condition. The second column shows the first cycle of movements during the initial training session. The third and fourth columns show the first and last cycle of movements following opposite foot training.

These results thus provide clear evidence for the potential benefit to the affected limb afforded by contralateral limb training, and studies are underway to test its efficacy.

1.3.4 *Biofeedback for the LL*

Many studies have shown that biofeedback sometimes using EMG or in combination with visual and auditory modalities, can improve ankle function in hemiplegia due to stroke or cerebral palsy (CP) (Skrotzky et al., 1978; Cozean et al., 1988; Mandel et al., 1990; Colborne et al., 1994). An early study showed that stroke patients gained conscious control of dorsiflexion after 5 weeks of biofeedback training, enabling unaided walking (Basmajian et al., 1975). More recently, four adult test subjects with CP improved ankle range of motion after 4 weeks of training their leg EMG to control biofeedback games, such as 'space invader' (Lyons et al., 2003). Walking in post-stroke patients was improved by an RTP protocol involving rhythmic biofeedback of their ankle position (Mandel et al., 1990). A similar study showed that rhythmic cueing of gait cycle with a musical tone resulted in a significant increase in weight-bearing stance time on the paretic side (Mauritz, 2002). A more recent study showed dramatically improved gait in post-stroke patients who combined an ankle exercise device with a virtual reality environment compared with those who merely used the exercise device (Deutsch et al., 2006). EMG biofeedback given to patients in the acute phase of stroke, however, has not proven effective (Bradley et al., 1998; Shepherd, 1999).

An ankle exercise and biofeedback device, the Range-of-motion ankle rehabilitator (ROMAR), has been developed to encourage RTP of the foot and ankle, as shown in Fig. 1.16. The platform is mounted on a bi-axial goniometer, which provides accurate   registration of ankle motion (Morris et al., 2007). The platform goniometer is calibrated to $\pm 1°$ and samples data at 1000 Hz. The interactive programs provide tracking games for the user to practice dorsiflexion and plantar flexion, inversion and eversion, and a combination of all four movements. Before each game or protocol the system is calibrated to fit the users' maximum range by having the user perform the necessary maximum movements. Once the game has started the user can decide to use either continuous movement or sustained contraction (in which the user must sustain a maximum inversion, eversion, plantar flexion or dorsiflexion) to play the games. The user can also increase or decrease the speed or shorten or lengthen the playing time.

During exercise, ankle muscle activity can be registered conveniently with a SMP bracelet on the calf. Figure 1.17 shows simultaneous ROMAR and SMP recordings of a foot rhythmically dorsi-flexing and plantar-flexing, with corresponding traces indicating angular motion (top) and muscle activity (bottom). Since the two traces correspond, either one can serve as a biofeedback signal.

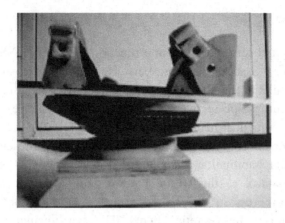

Figure 1.16. Range-of-motion ankle rehabilitator (ROMAR).

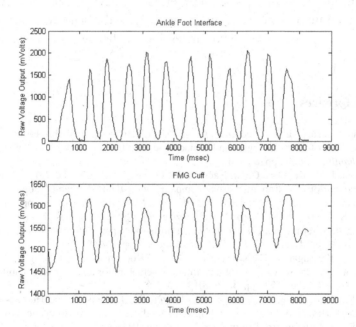

Figure 1.17. Simultaneous recording of plantar flexions and dorsiflexions using both the ROMAR and the SMO cuff placed over the calf muscle.

1.4 Summary

While significant restoration of limb function following CNS injuries is an uphill battle at best for most persons, many bionic strategies are becoming available to help the process. There are a plethora of tools to encourage neuroplastic recovery through intense, guided exercises, and there are also practical neuroprosthetic devices for stimulating muscles that are no longer connected to the brain. Herein we presented several new tools for rehabilitation, including, (1) new paradigms for restoring fine motor control to the UL; (2) new, more accurate methods for quantifying progress in UL motor control; (3) methods to improve ankle function in hemiparetic clients. The fundamental principle of neurorehabilitation is based on devices that assist and/or encourage the client to perform repetitive task practices over lengthy periods of time with the affected limb. The most effective devices are those which support the limb, either actively or passively, and engage the client in an interesting set of tasks, with increasing challenge, and rewards for success.

1.5 References

Armagan, O., Tascioglu, F. and Oner, C. (2003). Electromyographic biofeedback in the treatment of the hemiplegic hand: a placebo-controlled study. *Amer. J. Phys. Med. & Rehabilitation*, 82, pp. 856-61.

Basmajian, J. V., Kukulka, C. G., Narayan, M. G., and Takebe, K. (1975). Biofeedback treatment of foot-drop after stroke compared with standard rehabilitation technique: effects on voluntary control and strength. *Arch. Phys. Med. Rehabil.* 56, pp. 231-236.

Bayram, S., Sivrioglu, K., Karli, N., and Ozcan, O. (2006). Low-dose botulinum toxin with short-term electrical stimulation in poststroke spastic drop foot: a preliminary study. *Amer. J. Phys. Med. & Rehabilitation*, 85, pp. 75-81.

Bharadwaj, K., Sugar, T. G., Koeneman, J. B., and Koeneman, E. J. (2005). Design of a robotic gait trainer using spring over muscle actuators for ankle stroke rehabilitation. *J. Biomech. Eng.*, 127, pp. 1009-1013.

Blank, R., Breitenbach, A., Nitschke, M., Heizer, W., Letzgus, S. and Hermsdorfer, J. (2001). Human development of grip force modulation relating to cyclic movement-induced inertial loads. *Exp. Brain Res.*, 138, pp. 193-199.

Bogataj, U., Gros, N., Kljajic, M., and Acimovic-Janezic, R. (1997). Enhanced rehabilitation of gait after stroke: a case report of a therapeutic approach using multichannel functional electrical stimulation. *IEEE Trans. Rehabil. Eng.*, 5, pp. 221-232.

Bouzit, M., Burdea, G., Popescu, G. and Boian, R. (2002). The Rutgers Master II - New design force-feedback glove. *IEEE-ASME Trans. Mechatronics*, 7, pp. 256-263.

Bradley, L., Hart, B. B., Mandana, S., Flowers, K., Riches, M., and Sanderson, P. (1998). Electromyographic biofeedback for gait training after stroke. *Clinical Rehabilitation*, 12, pp. 11-22.

Butefisch, C., Hummelsheim, H., Denzler, P. and Mauritz, K. H. (1995). Repetitive training of isolated movements improves the outcome of motor rehabilitation of the centrally paretic hand. *J. Neurol. Sci.*, 130, pp. 59-68.

Caimmi, M., Carda, S., Giovanzana, C., Maini, E. S., Sabatini, A. M., Smania, N. and Molteni, F. (2008). Using kinematic analysis to evaluate constraint-induced movement therapy in chronic stroke patients. *Neurorehabitation and Neural Repair*, 22, pp. 31-39.

Carey JR, K. T., Lewis SM, Auerbach EJ, Dorsey L, Rundquist P, Ugurbil, K. (2002). Analysis of fMRI and finger tracking training in subjects with chronic stroke. *Brain*, 125, pp. 773-788.

Colborne, G. R., Wright, F. V. and Naumann, S. (1994). Feedback of triceps surae EMG in gait of children with cerebral palsy: a controlled study. *Arch. Phys. Med. Rehabil.*, 75, pp. 40-45.

Cook, T. W. (1933). Studies in cross education: I. Mirror tracing the star-shaped maze, *J. Exp. Psychol.*, pp. 144-160.

Cozean, C. D., Pease, W. S. and Hubbell, S. L. (1988). Biofeedback and functional electric stimulation in stroke rehabilitation. *Arch. Phys. Med. Rehabil.*, 69, pp. 401-405.

Craelius, W. (2002). The bionic man: restoring mobility. *Science*, 295, pp. 1018-1021.

Curcie, D. J., Flint, J. A., and Craelius, W. (2001). Biomimetic finger control by filtering of distributed forelimb pressures. *IEEE Trans. Neural. Syst. Rehabil. Eng.*, 9, 69-75.

de Niet, M., Bussmann, J. B., Ribbers, G. M. and Stam, H. J. (2007). The stroke upper-limb activity monitor: Its sensitivity to measure hemiplegic upper-limb activity during daily life. *Arch. Phys. Med. and Rehabilitation*, 88, pp. 1121-1126.

Deutsch, J. E., Mirelman, A., Patritti, B. and Bonato, P. (2006). Increased ankle moments and forces during walking as a result of lower-extremity virtual reality traning of persons post-stroke. *Joint ACRM-ASNR Annual Conference*, Boston, MA.

Duncan, P., Studenski, S., Richards, L., Gollub, S., Lai, S. M., Reker, D., Perera, S., Yates, J., Koch, V., Rigler, S., and Johnson, D. (2003). Randomized clinical trial of therapeutic exercise in subacute stroke. *Stroke*, 34, pp. 2173-2180.

Durfee, W. K. and Rivard, A. (2005). Design and simulation of a pneumatic, stored-energy, hybrid orthosis for gait restoration. *J. Biomechanical Engin.-Trans. of the ASME*, 127, pp. 1014-1019.

Edgerton, V. R., de Leon, R. D., Harkema, S. J., Hodgson, J. A., London, N., Reinkensmeyer, D. J., Roy, R. N., Talmadge, R. J., Tillakaratne, N. J., Timoszyk, W. and Tobin, A. (2001). Retraining the injured spinal cord. *J. Physiology-London*, 533, pp. 15-22.

Ernst, E., 2003. Systematic reviews of biofeedback. *Physikalische Medizin Rehabilitationsmedizin Kurortmedizin*, 13, pp. 321-324.

Eskes, G. A., Butler, B., McDonald, A., Harrison, E. R., and Phillips, S. J. (2003). Limb activation effects in hemispatial neglect. *Archives of Physical Medicine and Rehabilitation*, 84, pp. 323-328.

Fasoli, S. E., Krebs, H. I., Stein, J., Frontera, W. R. and Hogan, N. (2003). Effects of robotic therapy on motor impairment and recovery in chronic stroke. *Arch. Phys. Med. and Rehabilitation*, 84, pp. 477-482.

Fasoli, S. E., Krebs, H. I., Hughes, R., Stein, J. and Hogan, N. (2005). *Functionally-Based Rehabilitation: Benefit or Buzzword? Proceedings of the 2005 IEEE 9th International Conference on Rehabilitation Robotics*, Chicago.

Feys, H., De Weerdt, W., Verbeke, G., Steck, G. C., Capiau, C., Kiekens, C., Dejaeger, E., Van Hoydonck, G., Vermeersch, G. and Cras, P. (2004). Early and repetitive stimulation of the arm can substantially improve the long-term outcome after stroke: a 5-year follow-up study of a randomized trial. *Stroke*, 35, pp. 924-929.

Flint J. A., Phillips S. L., and Craelius, W. (2003). Myo-Kinetic Interface For A Virtual Limb. *2nd International Workshop on Virtual Rehabilitation*.

Glanz, M., Klawansky, S., Stason, W., Berkey, C., Shah, N., Phan, H. and Chalmers, T. C. (1995). Biofeedback Therapy in Poststroke Rehabilitation - a Metaanalysis of the Randomized Controlled Trials. *Arch. Phys. Med. and Rehab.*, 76, pp. 508-515.

Goffredo, M., Bernabucci, I., Schmid, M. and Conforto, S. (2008). A neural tracking and motor control approach to improve rehabilitation of upper limb movements. *J. NeuroEngineering and Rehabilitation*, 5: 5.

Gok, H., Kucukdeveci, A., Altinkaynak, H., Yavuzer, G. and Ergin, S. (2003). Effects of ankle-foot orthoses on hemiparetic gait. *Clin. Rehabil.*, 17, pp. 137-139.

Green, L. B. (2007). Assessment of habitual physical activity and paretic arm mobility among stroke survivors by accelometry. *Topics in Stroke Rehab.*, 14, pp. 9-21.

Hesse, S., Schulte-Tigges, G., Konrad, M., Bardeleben, A. and Werner, C. (2003). Robot-assisted arm trainer for the passive and active practice of bilateral forearm and wrist movements in hemiparetic subjects. *Arch. Physical Medicine and Rehabilitation*, 84, pp. 915-920.

Hogan, N., Krebs, H. I., Rohrer, B., Palazzolo, J. J., Dipietro, L., Fasoli, S. E., Stein, J., Hughes, R., Frontera, W. R., Lynch, D. and Volpe, B. T. (2006). Motions or muscles? Some behavioral factors underlying robotic assistance of motor recovery. *J. Rehabil. Res. Dev.*, 43, pp. 605-618.

Hung, G. K. (2003). Effect of putting grip on eye and head movements during the golf putting stroke. *ScientificWorld Journal*, 3, pp. 122-137.

Kim, N. H. and Craelius, W. (2007). Quantification of Motor Ability in Kinematic Speed vs. Accuracy Trade-off Test from Hemiparetic Populations. *Northeast American Society of Biomechanics Meeting*, College Park, MD.

Kottke, F. J., Pauley, D. L. and Ptak, R. A. (1966). The rationale for prolonged stretching for correction of shortening of connective tissue. *Arch. Phys. Med. Rehabil.* 47, pp. 345-352.

Krebs, H. I., Palazzolo, J. J., Dipietro, L., Volpe, B. T. and Hogan, N. (2003). Rehabilitation robotics: Performance-based progressive robot-assisted therapy. *Autonomous Robots*, 15, pp. 7-20.

Kuttiva, M., Burdea, G., Flint, J., and Craelius, W. (2005). Manipulation Practice for Upper-Limb Amputees Using Virtual Reality. *Presence*, 14, pp. 175-182.

Lam, P., Hebert, D., Boger, J., Lacheray, H., Gardner, D., Apkarian, J., and Mihailidis, A. (2008). A haptic-robotic platform for upper-limb reaching stroke therapy: Preliminary design and evaluation results. *J. NeuroEngin. Rehab.*, 5: 15.

Lum, P. S., Burgar, C. G., Shor, P. C., Majmundar, M. and Van der Loos, M. (2002). Robot-assisted movement training compared with conventional therapy techniques for the rehabilitation of upper-limb motor function after stroke. *Arch. Physical Medicine and Rehabilitation*, 83, pp. 952-959.

Lum P. S., Taub, E., Schwandt, D., Postman, M., Hardin, P., and Uswatte G. (2004). Automated constraint-induced therapy extension (AutoCITE) for movement defects after stroke. *J. Rehabilitation Research and Development*, 41, pp. 249-258.

Lyons, G. M., Sharma, P., Baker, M., O'Malley, S. and Shanahan, A. (2003). A computer game-based EMG biofeedback system for muscle rehabilitation. *Engineering in Medicine and Biology Society, Proc.25th Annual Internat. Conf. of the IEEE.*

Mandel, A. R., Nymark, J. R., Balmer, S. J., Grinnell, D. M. and O'Riain, M. D. (1990). Electromyographic versus rhythmic positional biofeedback in computerized gait retraining with stroke patients. *Arch. Phys. Med. Rehabil.*, 71, pp. 649-654.

Mauritz, K. H. (2002). Gait training in hemiplegia. *Eur. J. Neurol.*, 9 Suppl, 1, pp. 23-29; discussion 53-61.

Merians, A. S., Poizner, H., Boian, R., Burdea, G. and Adamovich, S. (2006). Sensorimotor training in a virtual reality environment: Does it improve functional recovery poststroke? *Neurorehabilitation. and Neural Repair*, 20, pp. 252-267.

Metcalf, C. D., Notley, S. V., Chappell, P. H., Burridge, J. H. and Yule, V. T. (2008). Validation and application of a computational model for wrist and hand movements using surface markers. *IEEE Trans. Biomed. Engin.*, 55, pp. 1199-1210.

Micera, S., Carrozza, M. C., Beccai, L., Vecchi, F. and Dario, P. (2006). Hybrid bionic systems for the replacement of hand function. *Proc. IEEE*, 94, pp. 1752-1762.

Morris, T., Escaldi, S., Glass, C. N., N.A. and Craelius, W. (2007). Quantifying ankle motion using the ankle-foot interface (AFI). ISPO: *The International Society of Prosthetics and Orthotics Annual Meeting,* Vancouver, British Columbia.

Morris, T., Newby, N. A., Wininger, M. and Craelius, W. (2008). Inter-limb Transfer of Learned Ankle Movements. *Exp. Brain Res.* 192, pp. 33-42.

Ouellette, M. M., LeBrasseur, N. K., Bean, J. F., Phillips, E., Stein, J., Frontera, W. R., and Fielding, R. A. (2004). High-intensity resistance training improves muscle strength, self-reported function, and disability in long-term stroke survivors. *Stroke*, 35, pp. 1404-1409.

Page, S. and Levine, P. (2003). Forced use after TBI: promoting plasticity and function through practice. *Brain Injury*, 17, pp. 675-684.

Page, S. J., Levine, P., and Leonard, A. C. (2005). Modified constraint-induced therapy in acute stroke: A randomized controlled pilot study. *Neurorehab. and Neural Repair,* 19, pp. 27-32.

Pang, M. Y., Harris, J. E., and Eng, J. J. (2006). A community-based upper-extremity group exercise program improves motor function and performance of functional activities in chronic stroke: A randomized controlled trial. *Archives of Physical Medicine and Rehabilitation*, 87, pp. 1-9.

Phillips, S., and Craelius W. (2005). Residual kinetic imaging as a control source for a multi-finger prosthesis. *Robotica*, 23, pp. 277-282.

Platz, T. (2003). Evidence-based arm rehabilitation - a systematic review of the literature. *Nervenarzt*, 74, pp. 841-849.

Platz, T., Winter, T., Muller, N., Pinkowski, C., Eickhof, C. and Mauritz, K. H. (2001). Arm ability training for stroke and traumatic brain injury patients with mild arm paresis: A single-blind, randomized, controlled trial. *Arch. Phys. Med. and Rehabilitation*, 82, pp. 961-968.

Popovic DB, P. M., Sinkjaer T. (2002). Neurorehabilitation of upper extremities in humans with sensory-motor impairment. *Neuromodulation*, 5, pp. 54-67.

Prange, G. B., Jannink, M. J. A., Groothuis-Oudshoorn, C. G. M., Hermens, H. J., and Ijzerman, M. J. (2006). Systematic review of the effect of robot-aided therapy on recovery of the hemiparetic arm after stroke. *J. Rehabilitation Research and Development*, 43, pp. 171-183.

Reinkensmeyer, D. J., Emken, J. L. and Cramer, S. C. (2004). Robotics, motor learning, and neurologic recovery. *Annual Review of Biomedical Engineering*, 6, pp. 497-525.

Reinkensmeyer, D.J., Kahn, L.E., Averbuch, M., McKenna-Cole, A, Schmit, B.D., Rymer, W.Z. (2000). Understanding and treating arm movement impairment after chronic brain injury: Progress with the ARM guide. *J. Rehabilitation Res. and Development*, 37, pp. 653-662.

Reinkensmeyer, D. J., Pang, C. T., Nessler, J. A. and Painter, C. C. (2002). Web-based telerehabilitation for the upper extremity after stroke. *IEEE Trans. Neural Systems and Rehabilitation Engin.*, 10, pp. 102-108.

Reinkensmeyer, D.J., Takahashi, C.D., Timoszyk, W.K., Reinkensmeyer, A.N., Kahn, L.E. (2000). Design of robot assistance for arm movement therapy following stroke. *Advanced Robotics*, 14, pp. 625-637.

Reiter, F., Danni, M., Lagalla, G., Ceravolo, G. and Provinciali, L. (1998). Low-dose botulinum toxin with ankle taping for the treatment of spastic equinovarus foot after stroke. *Arch. Phys. Med. Rehabil.*, 79, pp. 532-535.

Riener, R., Lunenburger, L., Jezernik, S., Anderschitz, M., Colombo, G. and Dietz, V. (2005). Patient-cooperative strategies for robot-aided treadmill training: First experimental results. *IEEE Trans. Neural Sys.Rehab. Engin.*, 13, pp. 380-394.

Salter, A. C. D., Bagg, S. D., Creasy, J. L., Romano, C., Romano, D., Richmond, F. J. R. and Loeb, G. E. (2004). First clinical experience with BION implants for therapeutic electrical stimulation. *Neuromodulation*, 7, pp. 38-47.

Scheidt, R.A., Reinkensmeyer, D.J., Conditt, M.A., Rymer, W.Z., Mussa-Ivaldi, F.A. (2000). Persistence of motor adaptation during constrained, multi-joint, arm movements. *J. Neurophysiology*, 84, pp. 853-862.

Shepherd, R. (1999). Electromyographic biofeedback following stroke slightly increases ankle dorsiflexion strength but not ankle range - Commentary. *Australian J. Physiotherapy*, 45, pp. 47-47.

Skrotzky, K., Gallenstein, J. S. and Osternig, L. R. (1978). Effects of electromyographic feedback training on motor control in spastic cerebral palsy. *Phys. Ther.*, 58, pp. 547-552.

Stevens, J. A. (2005). Interference effects demonstrate distinct roles for visual and motor imagery during the mental representation of human action, *Cognition*, 95, 329-350.

Thomson, C. E., Campbell, R. H., Wood, A. R., and Rendall, C. C. (2004). Chapter 5: Adult foot disorders. *Neale's Disorders of the Foot: Diagnosis and Management*. Elesevier Limited, pp. 123-125.

Turton, A. & Pomeroy, V. (2002). When should upper limb function be trained after stroke? Evidence for and against early intervention, *Neurorehab.*, 17, pp. 215-224.

van der Lee, J. H., Snels, I. A., Beckerman, H., Lankhorst, G. J., Wagenaar, R. C. and Bouter, L. M. (2001). Exercise therapy for arm function in stroke patients: a systematic review of randomized controlled trials. *Clin. Rehab.*, 15, pp. 20-31.

Volpe, B. T., Ferraro, M., Lynch, D., Christos, P., Krol, J., Trudell, C., Krebs, H. I., and Hogan, N. (2004). Robotics and other devices in the treatment of patients recovering from stroke. *Curr. Atheroscler. Rep.*, 6, pp. 314-319.

Volpe, B.T., Krebs, H.I., and Hogan N. (2001). Is robot-aided sensorimotor training in stroke rehabilitation a realistic option? *Curr. Opin. Neurol.*, 14, pp. 745-752.

Wininger, M., Kim, N., and Craelius, W. (2008). Pressure Signature of the Forearm as a Predictor of Grip Force. *J. Rehab. Res. and Development*, 45, pp. 883-892.

Wininger, M., Kim, N. H. and Craelius, W. (2008). Spontaneous accelerations in single joint motions. *J. Biomechanics*, 42, pp. 29-34.

Winstein, C. J., Rose, D. K., Tan, S. M., Lewthwaite, R., Chui, H. C. and Azen, S. P. (2004). A randomized controlled comparison of upper-extremity rehabilitation strategies in acute stroke: A pilot study of immediate and long-term outcomes. *Arch. Phys. Med. and Rehabilitation*, 85, pp. 620-628.

Woldag, H., Waldmann, G., Heuschkel, G. and Hummelsheim, H. (2003). Is the repetitive training of complex hand and arm movements beneficial for motor recovery in stroke patients? *Clin. Rehabilitation*, 17, pp. 723-730.

Wolf, S. L. (2007). Revisiting constraint-induced movement therapy: Are we too is all nonuse "learned"? and other quandaries. *Physical Therapy*, 87, pp. 1212-1223.

Yasukawa A, M.B. and DJ, G.-A. (2003). Efficacy for maintenance of elbow range of motion of two types of orthotic devices: a case series. *J. of Prosthetics and Orthotics*, 15, pp. 72-77.

Yungher, D. A., and Craelius, W. (2006). Discriminating 5 Grasps Using Force Myography of the Forearm. *BMES Annual Fall Meeting*, Chicago, IL.

Zhang, S. M., Hu, H. S. and Zhou, H. Y. (2008). An interactive Internet-based system for tracking upper limb motion in home-based rehabilitation. *Med. & Biological Engin. & Computing*, 46, pp. 241-249.

1.6 Review Questions

Q1.1　Compare and contrast non-invasive and invasive methods for re-animating paralyzed limb musculature.

Q1.2　Compare and contrast neurorehabilitation strategies based on passive and active approaches.

Q.1.3　State the meaning of Fitt's law and how it applies to functional measurement of human performance. Give an example.

Q1.4　State the two major sources of ankle stiffness in central paralysis.

Q1.5　State two measures of motion smoothness.

Q1.6　What is meant by compliance in a robot?

II

EYE

Chapter 2

Vision Correction Surgery: Refractive Surgery and Intraocular Lens Implants

Daniel J. Hu, M.D.[1] and Peter A. Rapoza, M.D.[2]

[1] New England Eye Center
Department of Ophthalmology, Tufts Medical Center
Tufts University School of Medicine
800 Washington Street, Box 450, Boston, MA 02111
PH: 617-636-1128; FX: 617-636-4866; EM: DHu@tuftsmedicalcenter.org

[2] Ophthalmic Consultants of Boston
Department of Ophthalmology, Tufts Medical Center
and Department of Ophthalmology, Harvard Medical School
50 Staniford Street, Boston, MA 02114
PH: 617-314-2684; FX: 617-723-7028; EM: parapoza@eyeboston.com

2.1 Introduction

Vision correction surgery has been practiced for 3,000 years. In its earliest form, surgery focused on the treatment of the eye in a pathologic state: that of cataract or opacification of the eye's crystalline lens. As early as 800 BC, surgeons in India performed a procedure known as couching. The surgeon sat facing the patient while an assistant kept the head still. A needle was introduced through the sclera behind the iris towards the lens. The opacified lens was then pushed posteriorly to displace it out of the visual axis. A surgical success was the restoration of the patient's ability to again see shapes and figures and possibly ambulate independently. Couching was performed into the Middle Ages.

The procedure was fraught with complications including a high rate of infection and inflammation often leading to total loss of the eye. It was therefore only used in eyes with no useful vision due to the presence of a dense cataract.

Significant progress was made during the 17th and 18th centuries, when surgeons improved on the technique by not simply pushing the cataract out of the visual axis, but by removing it from the eye. This brought forth the era of intracapsular and extracapsular cataract extraction. Intracapsular cataract extraction removes the lens in its entirety while extracapsular cataract extraction leaves a portion of the lens capsule intact. By the early 20th century, the expectations for vision after cataract extraction had evolved from perception of motion and shapes to corrected visual acuity of 20/30 or better. Corrected vision however was dependent on the use of thick magnifying aphakic spectacles, which posed a difficult adjustment for patients. In the mid-20th century, cataract surgery took its next leap forward. First came the advent of the intraocular lens implant, introduced by Sir Harold Ridley, M.D. Then Dr. Charles Kelman developed phacoemulsification, which used ultrasound to emulsify the cataract and allowed aspiration of the cataract fragments through small incisions. Phacoemulsification significantly decreased the risks of severe intraoperative and post-operative complications. This technique, along with the use of intraocular lens implantation for visual rehabilitation, became the standard for cataract surgery in the developed world. With this great technological advance in the surgical approach to cataract removal and the advances in intraocular lens design, the expectation of patients and surgeons for perfect visual outcomes continues to grow.

No longer is vision correction surgery limited to the removal of cataracts causing profound levels of visual loss, but also to those with far lesser degrees of treatable visual disability. In today's environment, refractive surgery has come to replace the use of spectacles and contact lenses even in young healthy eyes. Gone are the days where spectacle correction following cataract surgery is adequate. Patients increasingly expect spectacle independence for all tasks following surgery. How can we achieve this "holy grail" of vision correction surgery for today's patients? Current high patient expectations warrant even greater caution on the part of the surgeon to be certain that the patient is a good candidate for a specific surgical technique or prosthesis, and that the patient's expectations are on par with the usual expected surgical outcome.

2.2 Background

2.2.1 *Basic optics of the eye*

The refractive power of the eye is determined essentially by three variables: the power of the cornea, the power of the lens and the length of the eye. If these variables are appropriately balanced, this emmetropic eye is able to focus a ray of light from infinity directly onto the retina. This allows for any image in front of the eye to infinity to be projected in focus on the retina. If these three variables are not appropriately balanced, then the eye is left with ametropia. When the image is focused in front of the retina, this is called myopia. This can result from imbalance in the above variables where the refracting power of the cornea or lens is too strong for the length of the eye. If the image is focused behind the retina, this is called hyperopia. In hyperopia the refractive power of the cornea or lens is too weak for the length of the eye. An additional category of refractive error, astigmatism, is caused by a toric cornea, and crystalline lens that can add to the overall refractive error of the eye.

Accommodation is the eye's ability to change its refractive power by changing the shape of the crystalline lens. This is necessary for the eye to maintain focus as objects are viewed closer to the eye. Presbyopia is an acquired loss of the ability to see at near with onset in the emmetropic eye during the fifth decade of life.

2.2.2 *Refractive procedures*

Refractive procedures seek to reduce the need for spectacle or contact lens correction of ametropia by eliminating the imbalance between the refractive power of the cornea and lens, and the length of the eye. Adjusting the ratio of these variables with a change in the corneal shape/refractive power can alter the refractive power of the eye. Refractive imbalance can also be managed at the lenticular plane.

The cornea accounts for approximately 2/3 of the eye's refractive power at the air-tear interface of the cornea. As such, the cornea is a perfect target for refractive surgery. Corneal refractive surgery is performed via procedures that add to, subtract from, relax or shrink the corneal tissue. Procedures performed on the cornea are not intraocular procedures so they generally pose less significant risks than lenticular procedures that are intraocular in nature. Procedures altering the length of the eye have been described, but they are no longer in use.

2.3 Corneal Surgical Techniques

2.3.1 *Incisional refractive surgical techniques*

The surgical correction of refractive errors dates back to incisional techniques applied a century ago. The initial surgical procedure was that of creating partial thickness corneal incisions to reduce astigmatism by flattening the steep meridian of the cornea. During World War II, Japanese ophthalmologists, attempted to correct nearsightedness in troops by creating radial incisions in the inner layers of the cornea to flatten that tissue. While reduction in myopia was achieved, the surgical technique caused significant collateral damage to the treated eyes, which ultimately resulted in adverse outcomes including irregular astigmatism, cataracts and corneal edema.

Modern incisional corneal surgery, also termed radial keratotomy (RK) and astigmatic keratotomy (AK), was pioneered in the 1970s by the Russian ophthalmologist Fyodorov. The commonly accepted tale is that a patient sustained corneal trauma from a shattered spectacle lens resulting in radial incisions inscribed through the external layers of the cornea. These radial incisions created a change in the refractive error of the eye by flattening the cornea. The application of externally created radial incisions to reduce myopia, sometimes coupled with arcuate or tangential incisions to reduce astigmatism, provided a technique for reducing these refractive errors in a systematic way with a reasonable risk-to-benefit ratio. Two approaches were developed which were often termed the "Russian" or the "American" techniques. Both techniques required the reproducible measurement of the corneal thickness at one or more points utilizing ultrasonography. A diamond blade with a guard that only allowed the exposed portion of the blade to penetrate into the corneal tissue to a prescribed depth was moved across the cornea to incise the tissue. A variable effect of corneal flattening resulted depending upon the primary factors of the length and depth of the incisions. In the Russian technique an "uphill" incision was inscribed in which the diamond knife would enter the cornea at the limbus (junction of the clear cornea and white sclera), then be advanced towards the apex of the cornea. The American technique used a "downhill" incision in which the diamond knife entered the cornea towards the apex and was drawn peripherally towards, but not crossing the limbus.

Surgery was usually carried out in a minor operating room utilizing an oral medication for sedation and topical eye drops for anesthetic. The surgery required a patient who was cooperative and a surgeon comfortable with operating upon an eye that had the ability to move during the procedure.

Eyes with variable amounts of nearsightedness ranging from one towards seven diopters and astigmatism from one to three diopters were deemed appropriate candidates for incisional refractive surgery. The surgical approach to each eye was determined primarily by the patients' age and severity of refractive error. Other factors including gender and measures of corneal curvature and rigidity were variably included in the algorithms. In general, higher refractive errors could be corrected in older than in younger patients. Surgical planning required consulting tables or computer programs to provide a surgical plan specifying the number of incisions suggested and length of the incision referable to the corneal apex. Other tables and programs detailed the number and length of tangential or curvilinear incisions for correction of astigmatism.

In the US, most refractive surgeons initially practiced the "downhill" technique, but later incorporated a "combination approach" in which a second "uphill" stroke with the same diamond blade that was specifically shaped to allow uphill cutting at the base of the incision. This blade allowed the deeper cutting associated with the Russian technique and its ability to correct higher degrees of myopia than the American system while not risking entry too far into the center of the cornea. In practice, the incisions were created by first marking the center of the pupil, then indenting the cornea with a metal ring affixed to a handle that was placed concentric with the centering mark. Commonly, the smallest optical zone used was down to 3.0 mm in diameter. Smaller optical zones were associated with increased glare and "starbursts", especially noted during night driving. The surgeon would select what he/she felt was the optimal combination of optical zone and number of incisions. Usually, surgeons employed a minimum of three to a maximum of eight radial incisions to correct myopia and up to two arcuate or tangential (to the radial) incisions to correct astigmatism (Fig. 2.1). If the treatment goal was not reached with the first surgical attempt, an enhancement or retreatment could be performed during which the incisions were deepened and lengthened to increase the myopic and/or astigmatic correction.

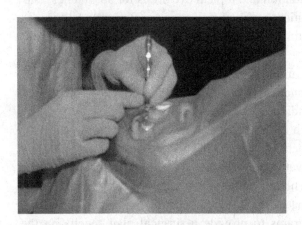

Figure 2.1. Surgeon performing radial keratotomy using a diamond blade.

The results of incisional keratorefractive surgery varied with the exact system performed and the surgeon. There was a large degree of "art" to the science of radial and astigmatic keratotomy. Two well-accepted multicenter controlled clinical trials of "combined" incisional keratotomy techniques representing the zenith of incisional surgery were published using the Genesis technique and the Casebeer system (Verity et al., 1995; Werblin and Stafford, 1996). The Genesis technique achieved 20/40 or better uncorrected visual acuity in 97% of eyes at one year while the Casebeer system achieved 20/40 or better visual acuity in 96% of eyes at three years follow-up.

Not all ophthalmic surgeons were capable of performing such complex surgery on an eye with the capability to move during the procedures. Incisions were sometimes not well inscribed resulting in less than expected results. More severe complications including cutting across the corneal apex, perforating the cornea, or even worse incising the iris and even the lens causing a cataract were described in the most extreme cases. In addition, there remained significant questions regarding the long-term safety and efficacy of the procedures especially in light of reports of significant ocular damage from trauma and the tendency towards developing overcorrections and even frank hyperopia or far-sightedness over time. Researchers turned to alternative techniques to achieve a reduction in refractive error.

2.3.2 *Intacs: intracorneal segments*

An alternative approach to incisional keratotomy was to implant plastic segments, either arcs or rings, into the peripheral stroma of the cornea to correct low to moderate degrees of myopia in eyes with little to no significant astigmatism. As with radial keratotomy, patients received oral sedation and topical anesthetic. A suction ring held the eye reasonably still while an arcuate blade entered the stroma and was manually rotated to create tunnels for the placement of the plastic segments. A single suture closed the slit like entry site. The most popular implant is called "Intacs". It had a brief bubble of popularity for the treatment of myopia as it was viewed as a safe and reversible alternative to radial keratotomy for lower degrees of nearsightedness with 20/40 or better uncorrected visual acuity in 95% of eyes at three months (Schanzlin et al., 1997). The advent of a new means of applying the excimer laser for refractive vision correction eclipsed the use of intracorneal segment technology for myopia.

Intacs are still utilized as refractive surgical implants, but usually only for the treatment of irregular astigmatism for corneal ectasia related to naturally occurring ecstatic conditions such as of keratoconus or pellucid marginal degeneration or keratoectasia induced by previous excimer laser ·treatments to correct myopia (Fig. 2.2). Ablation of excessive amounts of tissue or eyes that have sub-clinical ectasia can result in the outcome of excessive weakening of the residual tissue and bulging of the cornea simulating keratoconus. For these conditions, Intacs provide an excellent alternative to corneal transplantation with the placement of Intacs associated with significantly less risk and cost than penetrating or lamellar corneal transplantation techniques. Five year follow-up of Intacs for keratoconus demonstrated that 59% of eyes had uncorrected visual acuity of 20/50 or greater (Kymionis et al. 2006). The use of the femtosecond laser to create implantation tunnels has increased the popularity of Intacs for the treatment of ectasias.

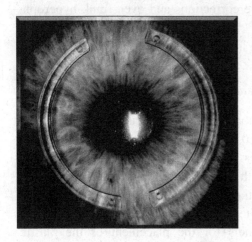

Figure 2.2. Eye with Intacs.

2.3.3 *Excimer laser vision correction*

The excimer laser, an industrial tool utilized to etch computer chips, was initially used in refractive surgery to apply computer and laser technology to cut radial incisions that were equally spaced of a standard length and depth. Because the excimer laser removes tissue rather than simply cutting it, this application failed as the resulting incisions were subject to variable healing. The excimer laser continued to receive further attention as a means for performing laser vision correction. Myopia, the most common form of non-presbyopic refractive error was the initial disorder studied. The original work focused upon using large spots or broad beams of laser light to ablate corneal tissue flattening the anterior curvature of the cornea to refocus light rays upon the retina.

In order to apply the excimer laser at the appropriate layer of the cornea, the constantly renewing corneal epithelium had to be removed. A variety of techniques were developed including the application of blunted or sharp epithelial scrapers, rotating brushes, application of dilute ethanol and even utilizing the excimer laser itself in what is termed "laser scrape". Removal of the epithelium was the most work intensive portion of photorefractive keratectomy and had the highest potential for inducing iatrogenic damage to the cornea. The Amoils brush removed the epithelium by rotating soft bristles. It was a reasonably safe technique, but the time required to remove all of the epithelium in the zone requiring treatment was variable and patients sometimes found the torsional movements and vibrations disconcerting.

Alcohol was found to be an effective means of removing epithelium. It was initially applied to a surgical sponge and kept in contact with the epithelium. The sponge was then removed and the eye copiously irrigated. Alcohol would commonly spread onto the conjunctiva inducing a chemical conjunctivitis and undoubtedly contributing to the pain that was an unfortunate hallmark of early PRK surgery. Later techniques utilized placement of radial keratotomy optical zone markers indented into the superficial cornea to hold a small quantity of dilute alcohol against the targeted area of the epithelium requiring removal. The alcohol was next aspirated using a dry surgical sponge and the remaining film of alcohol diluted via copious irrigation of balanced salt solution into the optical zone marker, then over the entire surface of the eye. This technique limited any exposure of the conjunctiva to alcohol successfully, as long as the optical zone stayed in contact throughout the 30-second exposure time.

The application of excimer lasers for vision correction surgery (Fig. 2.3) was carefully initiated on cadaver and animal eyes, then advanced onto human "blind eyes" scheduled for removal or having limited visual potential due to other diseases prior to the application of the technology on healthy eyes. Initial reports noted achieving 20/40 or better visual acuity in 82% of eyes at the 3-month post-operative exam (Salz et al. 1993).

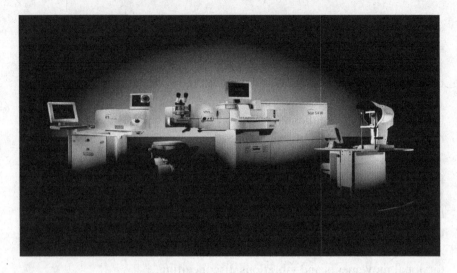

Figure 2.3. Laser vision correction suite including IntraLASE Femtosecond laser, VISX Star S4 excimer laser and VISX Wave Front Analyzyer.

With the initial safety and efficacy of the excimer laser in myopia successfully demonstrated, each laser manufacturer conducted more extensive clinical trials, and submitted data for approval to the Food and Drug Administration. Several manufacturers obtained approval for their excimer lasers initially for myopia, then later for hyperopia and eventually astigmatism. The surgical results were quite remarkable and took vision correction from the artistry of the individual surgeon to results that were more easily reproduced by numerous individuals using the same equipment and techniques. However, some significant problems kept the technique out of the mainstream.

Two important issues limited a wider acceptance of early PRK. The first was post-operative pain. The second was a tendency for superficial scarring or haze to develop in excimer laser treated eyes, particularly with higher attempted corrections. In modern PRK the use of topical nonsteroidal anti-inflammatory agents (NSAIDS) pre- and post-operatively has made surface ablation a procedure that now causes only mild irritation for the majority of patients. Most refractive surgeons now apply the antimetabolite Mitomycin C 0.02% to the ablated corneal stroma for 12 to 15 seconds. This practice has resulted in a significant reduction of corneal haze and scarring (Thornton et al., 2008).

During the early years of PRK, surgeons often separated the treatment of the two eyes by weeks or months. This was done due to the pain and temporarily decreased vision associated with the surgery. This fact made it difficult to successfully have the eyes working together especially in patients with higher degrees of myopia or hyperopia who were unable to wear a contact lens in the unoperated eye. The use of spectacles for eyes with significant differences in refractive error usually results in double vision based on unequal image size in each eye. An additional feature of PRK treatments was the tendency to obtain significant overcorrections, greater in the treatment of hyperopia than myopia. These factors lead to an alternative approach to laser vision correction.

2.3.4 *Laser-assisted in-situ keratomileusis (LASIK)*

A different approach to vision correction surgery termed keratomileusis utilized a mechanical device called a microkeratome to excise the anterior cornea from the subject's eye (Barraquer, 1949). Initially, the removed tissue was subjected to deep-freezing then mounted on a surgical lathe, which would remove a specified amount of the corneal stroma from the inner surface. Later, in the technique termed automated lamellar keratoplasty (ALK), the microkeratome was used to make a second cut from the subject's eye to remove a specified amount of tissue to flatten the cornea and treat the myopia. In both cases, the excised anterior corneal "cap" was replaced and either sutured into a stable position or simply placed on the corneal tissue bed and allowed to heal. While ALK was successful in treating a wide range of myopic eyes, the instrumentation was difficult to use and the results not very reproducible.

During the late 1980s, several independent researchers combined the use of keratomileusis and the excimer laser to develop what was termed LASIK, or Laser-Assisted in situ Keratomileusis (Ruiz and Rowsey, 1988; Pallikaris, 1990). The technique initially involved using the mechanical microkeratome to create a cap of corneal tissue for removal, then treating the remaining cornea with the excimer laser and replacing the cap into position (Fig. 2.4). LASIK evolved into performing an incomplete microkeratome cut leaving a hinge of tissue intact so that the corneal "flap" could be lifted, the remaining corneal tissue reshaped by the excimer laser, then the flap lowered into its exact prior position.

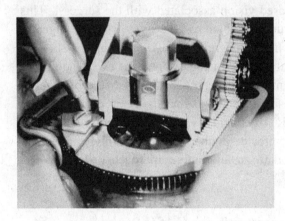

Figure 2.4. Mechanical microkeratome.

LASIK allowed for both of a patient's eyes to be treated during the same surgical session because the few hours of discomfort associated with LASIK was significantly less than the days of discomfort associated with PRK as performed in its early period of adoption. In addition, visual recovery was rapid with satisfactory vision being present within a few hours of LASIK surgery versus several days to weeks for PRK. While LASIK treatments might result in overcorrections, these were in general minimal compared to those seen with PRK, especially for hyperopes.

LASIK required surgeons to learn new skills including that of using potentially damaging instruments on an eye receiving only topical anesthetic. Iatrogenic complications included producing "free caps" versus "flaps" which could potentially be lost from the surgical field or displaced from the postoperative eye; incomplete incisions not exposing enough corneal bed for excimer laser treatment and poorly made flaps incorporating "buttonholes" or inadvertently produced incisions in the visual axis. In addition, the interface of the flap was a newly created "potential space" which could harbor infection or inflammation. For months to years, physical trauma to the eye could potentially wrinkle the flap or in extreme cases result in a severed hinge and actual loss of the flap by avulsion. Nevertheless, the advance of LASIK over PRK, at least as practiced in the late 1980s and early 1990s, advanced laser vision correction into the public eye.

LASIK, utilizing one of several mechanical microkeratomes in conjunction with one of several FDA approved excimer lasers, became the industry standard for laser vision correction between the mid 1990s and the early 2000s. Each microkeratome and laser had various advantages and disadvantages touted by their manufacturers, proponents and detractors. In capable hands, the combined technologies were readily applied initially to myopes and later hyperopes. During the earlier years of use of the excimer laser for vision correction surgery, astigmatic corrections could not be performed with the laser. If a patient with astigmatism was to undergo excimer laser treatment, the myopia or hyperopia would be treated first and then the patient could undergo astigmatic keratotomy for any remaining astigmatism. Most surgeons would wait two or more months for initial healing to occur so that a stable refraction was obtained and the flap was less likely to move while placing the arcuate or tangential incisions. Eventually, each of the major manufacturers received FDA approval for astigmatism as a stand-alone disorder or myopia and hyperopia with astigmatism.

2.3.5 *Advanced surface ablation*

While LASIK was accepted by most of the ophthalmic community as the preferred technique for laser vision correction in most eyes, there were patients that were not well suited for the technique. Patients could be poor LASIK candidates due to vocational requirements, avocational pursuits, higher refractive corrections with relatively thinner corneas or preexisting ocular surface diseases such as dry eyes that were more easily exacerbated by LASIK. In addition, some surgeons felt that PRK provided a superior result to LASIK as the mechanically constructed flaps of LASIK could induce optical irregularities into the visual system or be traumatized during or following surgery resulting in visual compromise.

Advances in PRK kept the technique active at least for a minority of treated patients. The use of topical NSAIDS pre and postoperatively substantially reduced the amount of pain that post-PRK patients experienced. Surgeons began to use topical Mitomycin C, an antimetabolite used in ophthalmology to reduce scarring for glaucoma filtration surgery and in the removal of ptergyia (lesions growing across the cornea). Mitomycin C, especially when used with newer generation excimer lasers, was found to reduce the incidence of haze or scarring in PRK patients. The application of bandage soft contact lenses at the conclusion of surgery also reduced pain and allowed patients to have at least moderately good vision in their PRK treated eyes soon after the procedures were completed.

A novel technique attempting to combine the safety of PRK with the faster healing of LASIK was described: Laser Assisted Sub-epithelial Keratectomy (LASEK). This procedure was similar to PRK using ethanol to assist in loosening the epithelium, but preserved the loosened tissue rather than discarding it. Several variants existed with the primary difference being either creating an epithelial flap or opening a "fish mouth" in the epithelium, which would expose the anterior stroma for excimer laser ablation. In both cases, the epithelium was replaced and a bandage contact lens inserted to hold it in position while new epithelium grew in to cover the ablated corneal stroma. No significant differences have been described in comparing LASEK versus PRK regarding resulting uncorrected and best-corrected visual acuity or epithelial healing time. LASEK treated eyes were more painful, but showed less inflammation than PRK treated eyes (Ghirlando et al., 2007).

A potential disadvantage of using alcohol to loosen the epithelium is that the epithelial cells are usually killed by the alcohol exposure. An alternative technique, Epi-LASIK, was developed utilizing an epithelial separator. This instrument was essentially an unsharpened keratome blade that was used to lift the epithelium away from Bowman's membrane without exposing the epithelial cells to the potential for alcohol toxicity. While the technique did work to loosen epithelium, it was subsequently discovered that epithelial flaps created mechanically were often not viable. When investigators examined the healing patterns and speed of visual recovery in Epi-LASIK where epithelium was repositioned versus removed, the latter technique produced a more rapid visual recovery than actually keeping the cells intact (Kalyvianaki et al. 2008). LASEK and Epi-LASIK appear to offer no significant advantages to a properly performed alcohol assisted epithelial debridement for PRK, a low cost technique with no specialized equipment to maintain.

2.3.6 *Excimer laser ablation profiles*

Current innovations in excimer laser treatment involve improved laser treatment profiles that are specific for each patient. The new technology will better specify the amount and location of tissue that is ablated or removed to produce the intended visual improvement. Conventional ablation, performed since the outset of excimer laser vision correction surgery, involves careful measurement of an eye's refractive error. This is done using an interactive technique in which the examiner presents various lens choices to the patient to try to determine which combination of lens provides the best visual acuity. The technique is subjective and different examiners might have slightly different results for the same patient's eye. Nevertheless, clinical refraction has been the primary tool for determining the amount and location of tissue removal with the excimer laser.

Two alternative techniques for specifying ablation profiles are (1) wavefront-guided and (2) topography-guided ablations. Wavefront-guided ablation software is available from most of the major excimer laser manufacturers. In addition to the conventional measures of refractive error, some patients also have significant higher order aberrations that degrade image quality. In theory, higher order aberrations or irregularities in the visual system are measured by one of several proprietary systems that determine how light rays through the eye are altered by the ocular structures. The information gathered can be analyzed and small laser spots selectively placed to make the corneal surface more regular in shape and improve both visual acuity and visual quality. Wavefront treatments often improve other visual symptoms such as glare and "starbursts" which were common accompaniments of conventional laser vision correction. This type of treatment allows the surgeon to direct the laser treatment to the individual eye's specific irregularities creating a custom treatment that is truly unique to that patient. Wavefront-guided ablation profiles can be specified for myopia, hyperopia and astigmatism. Each laser system has a specific range of refractive error that can be treated with custom ablation software. At this time, wave front-guided ablations are only FDA approved for primary treatments and not for retreatments of eyes that have had prior laser vision correction surgery. Nevertheless, in clinical practice, many surgeons use custom ablation profiles if the wavefront determined refraction is similar to the clinical refraction. Custom ablation profiles have been determined to give more accurate results when compared to conventional treatments with the same laser system (Alpins and Stamatelatos, 2008). In addition, a lessened percentage of patients require retreatments to achieve their visual goals. The most commonly used excimer laser platform in the United States is the VISX Star S4. The FDA labeling of the VISX Star S4 for LASIK with wavefront guided ablations indicates uncorrected visual acuity results as follows:

Indication	$\geq$20/40	$\geq$20/20
Low-moderate myopia		
Spherical	100%	100%
With astigmatism	100%	97%
High myopia	100%	86%
Hyperopia		
Spherical	97%	66%
With astigmatism	93%	56%
Mixed astigmatism	97%	75%

Topography-guided ablations are not yet FDA approved. A topographic map of the cornea to create an ablation profile that makes the cornea more symmetrical in shape guides the excimer laser. This is particularly important in certain patients that might have undergone prior LASIK, LASEK or PRK and require additional treatment of an eye with a decentered ablation or irregular healing (Lin et al, 2008). In addition, the technique will probably be useful for the treatment of full thickness and anterior lamellar corneal transplants that have resulted in significant refractive error, especially in cases where there exists irregular astigmatism.

Additional systems have been developed for measuring and reorienting the excimer laser to torsional movements of the eye, which can occur when a patient is supine versus in an upright position (Ghosh et al., 2008). Iris recognition or registration not only directs the ablation to correct astigmatism at the appropriate axis, but also serves as a safety check to reduce the possibility of treating a patient with a custom treatment specified for another patient's eye.

2.3.7 *Femtosecond laser for LASIK*

While mechanical microkeratomes combined with advanced generation excimer lasers provided reasonably safe and effective surgical results, the persistent occurrence of cases of flap complications remained a visually threatening entity. Investigators looked at the potential role for intrastromal ablation where laser energy would be focused in the middle layers of the cornea to change its shape without the need for removing epithelium or creating a flap. Unfortunately, the technique failed to produce the hoped for results, but led to the use of femtosecond lasers that could be programmed to cut a planar flap safely with little chance of resulting in a flap complication (Nordan et al, 2003). The current generation of the IntraLASE femtosecond laser can now create a flap in under 20 seconds time. Use of the accompanying software allows the surgeon to determine flap diameter, thickness, hinge location and size, construction of a gas release pocket and alter the steepness of the flap incision. The surgeon can also use the software to accurately align the incision with the pupil to avoid decentered flaps and decrease the chance of decentered or incomplete excimer ablations (Fig. 2.5). Other manufacturers have designed competing femtosecond lasers each with their inherent advantages and disadvantages. Wavefront analysis has confirmed that the femtosecond laser induces less higher order aberrations than mechanical microkeratomes positioning the femtosecond laser as a safer and more effective means of creating a flap for LASIK (Medeiros et al., 2007). The femtosecond laser can also be utilized to create accurately placed and depth determined astigmatic keratotomies, channels for Intacs and incisions for penetrating keratoplasties (corneal transplantations).

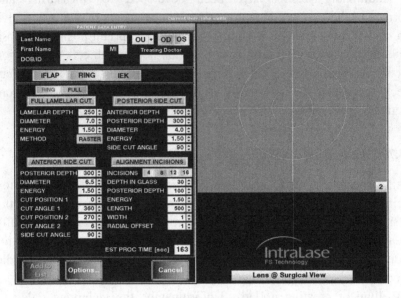

Figure 2.5. IntraLASE screen.

2.3.8 *Excimer laser retreatment of eyes with prior refractive surgery*

Laser vision correction is now commonly performed to enhance results from incisional refractive surgery or early generation lasers. PRK or surface ablation with the application of Mitomycin C is usually used to retreat patients that previously had incisional surgery, PRK, those that had LASIK over two years prior to the retreatment and LASIK patients who do not have an ample amount of residual corneal tissue remaining for additional excimer laser ablation below the flap (Alio et al., 2008).

2.3.9 *Excimer laser treatment of eyes with prior cataract surgery*

Either LASIK or PRK can be used to correct residual refractive error after implantation of monofocal, toric or presbyopic IOLs (Dvali et al.,

2009). This technique, sometimes called "bioptics" is especially important with the latter lenses where overall distance and near visual acuity and patient satisfaction are primarily determined by achieving an accurate distance correction. Patients that had prior laser vision correction, then cataract surgery, are those with the least tolerance for residual refractive error following their cataract extraction as they well remember their years of lack of reliance on spectacles or contact lenses.

2.4 Intraocular Refractive Surgery

One of the major functions of the crystalline lens of the eye is to refract light onto the fovea of the retina. Surgical treatments to augment or replace the crystalline lens with a manufactured optical prosthesis are alternative means of treatment in refractive surgery. The refractive power of the eye can be altered by placing an intraocular lens (IOL) in front of the crystalline lens or by replacing the crystalline lens itself. For patients with presbyopia, an age-acquired reduction of the ability to see at near, removal of the crystalline lens and replacement with a monofocal IOL can result in spectacle independence for distance visual tasks while maintaining a need for spectacles or contact lenses for near work. In younger patients, who have not developed presbyopia, removing the crystalline lens and replacing it with a monofocal IOL improves distance vision, but will reduce the ability to see at near. Lenticular surgery therefore can be approached in different fashions for patients of various ages with or without actual vision-limiting cataracts.

2.4.1 *Phakic intraocular lens implantation*

Phakic intraocular lens (pIOL) implantation has grown as a technique for refractive surgery in which an IOL is implanted in front of the crystalline lens to correct refractive error. These lenses are supported in the anterior chamber angle, iris-fixated, or placed in the posterior chamber.

The benefits of pIOL implantation include a potentially reversible procedure, maintenance of accommodation with the patient's own crystalline lens and generally excellent refractive results. Challenges in this type of procedure include the requirement for intraocular surgery and the risks inherent to it including: intraocular infection, surgically induced astigmatism, corneal decompensation due to surgically induced and ongoing endothelial cell loss, pupil ovalization, chronic inflammation, zonular damage, cataract formation, and pupillary block glaucoma. In addition, special measurements are required for IOL calculations and the long-term impact of pIOLs remains uncertain. Implantation of pIOLs remains an option for patients who are not candidates for corneal refractive surgery (Lovisolo et al., 2005).

2.4.1.1 *Angle-supported phakic IOLs*

Angle-supported lenses have been used in the treatment of high myopia for 20 years. The anterior chamber angle was first described as a fixation site for pIOLs in the 1950's. Due to complications including cataract formation and corneal decompensation following implantation of these IOLs, they were abandoned for use in phakic eyes. By the late 1980's, the angle fixated PMMA IOLs had been improved by increased haptic flexibility and alternative optic designs decreasing the occurrence of intraocular complications. The current generation of angle-supported IOLs consists of foldable lenses that can be introduced through small incisions. These lenses are made of acrylic optics with variable haptic designs and materials. Current lenses include the Vivarte/GBR lens (Zeiss-Meditec, Jena, Germany), I-CARE (Corneal, Pringy, France), Kelman Duet Implant (Tekia, Irvine, California), Acrysof ACP-IOL (Alcon, Ft. Worth, Texas), and the ThinPhAc (ThinOpt-X, Medford Lakes, New Jersey). Studies regarding these lenses have shown great

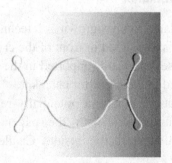

Figure 2.6. Acrysof Phakic Intraocular Lens.

initial promise. Unfortunately, complications developed over time and the Vivarte/GBR and I-CARE were removed from the market for the reason of excessive corneal endothelial cell loss. The Acrysof lens (Figure 2.6) has shown great stability, predictability, and endothelial cell counts post-operatively. While these lenses hold promise; none are approved for use in the US at this time (Espandar et al., 2008, Lovisolo et al., 2005).

2.4.1.2 *Iris-fixed phakic IOLs*

Iris-fixed pIOLs were developed as an alternative pIOL to reduce the occurrence of the problems that arose from the original generation of angle fixated IOLs. The 1950s saw several designs that were supported by the iris sphincter with anterior and posterior loops. These lenses led to progressive intraocular damage from inflammation including corneal and macular edema and their use was abandoned. Dr. Jan Worst then designed the "lobster-claw" lens, which was a single piece PMMA IOL. The haptics had a fine fissure meant to capture or enclevate a small knuckle of mid-peripheral iris that is virtually immobile with changes in pupil size. Use of a small portion of iris for fixation was thought to create less trauma thereby reducing damage to the iris so that the pupil could retain its constricting and dilating functions. The Artisan/Verisyse lens (AMO, Abbott Park, Illinois) is the current generation of this IOL platform (Fig. 2.7). It has essentially remained unchanged from its original design. The Verisyse is capable of correcting hyperopia, myopia, and astigmatism. These lenses are made of PMMA, and need to be implanted through a 5.5 to 6.5 mm incision. Post-operative astigmatism induced because of the large wound size is a concern in the

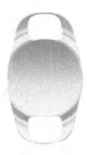

Figure 2.7. Verisyse lens.

use of these lenses as are pupil ovalization and endothelial cell loss. Recent advances in this technology include an injectable lens known as the Artiflex/Veriflex that is a polysiloxane foldable optic with PMMA haptics that can be injected through a 3.2 mm incision. Smaller incisions decrease the induction of wound related astigmatism. This lens has the longest track record of all the pIOLs with over 65,000 implanted in aphakic and phakic eyes (Lovisolo et al., 2005; Guell et al., 2008; Moshifar et al., 2007; Espandar et al., 2008).

2.4.1.3 *Posterior chamber phakic IOLs*

The use of posterior chamber IOLs intended for the replacement of cataractous crystalline lenses, into the anterior chamber of the phakic eye was investigated in the 1980's, but this lens position was subsequently abandoned due to complications including nighttime vision disturbance, light sensitivity, inflammation, pupil block glaucoma, cataract and corneal decompensation. In response to these significant complications related to anterior chamber IOLs, specific posterior chamber pIOLs designed to reside in the ciliary sulcus posterior to the iris and anterior to the crystalline lens were first developed in 1986. Current lenses include the Visian Implantable Collamer Lens (ICL), (Staar Surgical, Monrovia, California) and the Phakic Refractive Lens (PRL), (Ciba Vision/Medennium, Duluth, Georgia), and Sticklens (IOLTECH, LaRochelle, France). The Visian ICL (Fig. 2.8), the only posterior chamber pIOL currently FDA approved for use in the US, is made from Collamer that is composed of hydrophilic collagen. This lens is placed in the posterior chamber, in the ciliary sulcus, and vaults over the

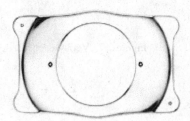

Figure 2.8. Visian ICL.

anterior surface of the crystalline lens. Results using the ICL have been promising with the ICL performing equal to or better than keratorefractive surgery (ICL in Treatment of Myopia Study Group, 2004). A toric ICL with similarly good results is on the way for patients who may not have been ideal candidates for ICL currently because of astigmatism (Sanders et al., 2007). The PRL is a one-piece silicone lens. It has been shown to be a predictable pIOL with stable postoperative refractions, however, there were reports of PRL subluxations (Donoso and Castillo, 2006). The Sticklens is made of hydrophilic soft acrylic with four closed loop haptics. Unlike the other posterior chamber pIOLs, vaulting over the crystalline lens is not necessary. The anterior radius of curvature varies, while the overall length, posterior shape, and curvature are fixed to match the anterior curvature of the crystalline lens. A smooth slippery surface optimizes the contact with the crystalline lens and posterior iris surfaces. Despite these new lens designs, concerns with the posterior chamber pIOL still include cataract, angle closure glaucoma, lens subluxation, zonular loss, and endothelial cell loss (Lovisolo et al., 2005; Espandar et al., 2008).

Phakic IOLs are proving to be a viable option for patients seeking spectacle independence. These lenses provide predictability equivalent to keratorefractive procedures and may provide better quality of vision with fewer surgically induced higher order aberrations especially in eyes with higher magnitudes of refractive errors (Malecaze et al., 2002). The use of pIOLs for the treatment of high ametropia continues to advance. These lenses are also being studied for the treatment of presbyopia with multifocal phakic IOLs (Baikoff et al., 2004). The risks of intraocular surgery must be balanced with the perceived benefit of spectacle independence in these patients. Challenges that remain in the development and advancement of these lenses include minimizing the constellation of post-operative complications that can arise from the implantation of these lenses, as well as biocompatibility of the lens material, optimal lens position and centration, optical performance, and lens sizing (Lovisolo et al., 2005; Espandar et al., 2008).

2.5 Treatment for Presbyopia

2.5.1 *Optics of accommodation and presbyopia*

The onset of presbyopia brings forth the loss of accommodation. Accommodation is the eye's ability to increase the refractive power of the crystalline lens to keep objects in focus as they approach the eye. In the unaccommodated state, the crystalline lens is relatively flat as a result of outward resting tension on the elastic zonular fibers. Accommodative stimulus causes contraction of the ciliary muscle, loosening tension on the zonules. This initiates a forward movement of the anterior lens surface, as well as an increase in lens curvature, increasing the refractive power of the eye (Glasser, 2006).

The exact mechanism by which accommodation is lost is incompletely understood. Accommodation begins to decline in the second decade of life with 2/3 of accommodative amplitude lost by age 35. By age 55, accommodation is completely lost. Conventionally, the loss of accommodation has been attributed to hardening of the crystalline lens. Hardening prevents the accommodative mechanism from increasing the curvature of the lens. It is unlikely that this is the only change that results in accommodative loss. Studies have shown that there is some loss of ciliary muscle as well as neuromuscular alterations associated with aging. MRI studies in humans have shown decreased ciliary body movement and decreased lens movement with age, but residual movement does indeed remain present. The decrease in ciliary movement does not correlate to the loss of accommodation. There seems to be enough residual ciliary body muscle as well as function left to provide enough movement of the lens to retain some accommodation. Loss of ciliary muscle action may be part of the change in aging that result in loss of accommodation. As the crystalline lens ages, the anterior and posterior lens surfaces become more curved as well as thicker due at least in part to the addition of layers of cells deposited in the lens cortex. These changes should make for a more powerful refractive lens, but a concurrent change in the refractive index of the lens is thought to prevent this change. These findings are likely to induce the hardening and loss of elasticity of the lens with age. The lens capsule also thickens with age and becomes more brittle. The change in lens size induces an anterior shift in the anterior zonular attachments. This could influence the force generated by the zonules, and may not allow for enough force to induce a change in the shape of the hardening lens capsule complex. The vitreous may play a role as well. A pressure gradient has been shown to be present in the eye during accommodation with vitreous forces pushing toward the anterior chamber. This movement or anterior force may have a role in supporting the lens thickening and rounding of the lens with accommodation. Lens changes with aging certainly play a major role in the loss of accommodation. However, there are other changes in the lens, capsule, ciliary body complex that play a role in the loss of accommodation. (Croft and Kaufman, 2006; Menapace et al., 2007) An understanding of presbyopia by the patient is critical as presbyopia may require the patient to remain dependent on spectacles for near work.

There are now available technologies that seek to diminish the effect of presbyopia by attempting to restore accommodation or by using a multifocal effect. The answer to achieving spectacle independence after cataract surgery lies in solving the problem of presbyopia, and loss of accommodation following implantation of an intraocular lens. Cataract surgery and implantation of a monofocal intraocular lens can result in pseudoaccomodation, but a return of true accommodation is not achieved (Menapace et al., 2007).

2.5.2 *The treatment of presbyopia*

Attempts to duplicate the accommodation of the youthful eye in presbyopic eyes come in several forms: monovision, conductive keratoplasty, lensectomy with implantation of monofocal, multifocal or accommodating IOLs and multifocal phakic IOL.

2.5.2.1 *Monovision*

Monovision can be created with the excimer laser via PRK or LASIK, CK, as well as by crystalline lens removal and the placement of an IOL. The goal of the treatment is to leave one eye (usually the dominant eye) for distance vision while creating or leaving residual myopia in the non-dominant eye in order to allow for near vision. While results are good, there remain issues that may arise from loss of stereopsis, loss of contrast sensitivity, depth of focus, and the difficulty of tolerating the difference in residual refractive error between the two eyes (Braun et al. 2008). Patient selection and a trial of monovision with either contact lenses or spectacles is essential in the success of this technique. Now that the FDA has approved the use of the excimer laser for monovision treatment of presbyopia, wavefront-guided treatments can also be performed.

2.5.2.2 *Conductive keratoplasty*

Conductive keratoplasty (Near Vision CK, Refractec, Irvine, California) is a technology that uses low level radio-frequency energy directed at predetermined spots of the cornea. The energy is delivered at a specified optical zone around the visual axis that creates shrinkage of the collagen fibrils and thus changes the refractive power of the cornea by steepening the area central to the ring of treatment. This technique has been shown to be predictable and relatively stable way of treating presbyopia, and hyperopia (Du et al., 2007) (Fig. 2.9).

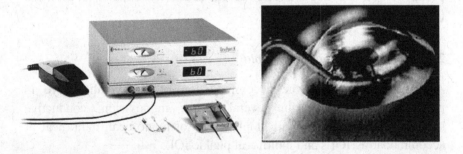

Figure 2.9. Conductive keratoplasty. Instrumentation (left), and eye procedure (right).

2.5.2.3 *Multifocal intraocular lenses*

Multifocal IOLs project multiple images into the eye. These lenses distribute light onto 2 or more foci. On the retina, these lenses produce superimposed images of observed objects. One image will be in sharp focus, and the other will be blurred by the set defocus aberration. These lenses can allow for spectacle independence for distance and near, but often at the expense of image degradation, decreased contrast sensitivity, and disturbing optical phenomena (Menapace et al., 2007). These are true for both the diffractive (Alcon ReStor, AMO Tecnis multifocal) and refractive optics (AMO Array and ReZoom) used in multifocal IOLs. Currently available lenses exist in both diffractive and refractive optics, for placement in the capsular bag and ciliary sulcus. (Figs. 2.10a-d) They have even been adapted for use in the anterior chamber for use as a multifocal phakic IOL (Baikoff et al., 2004).

a   b

c   d

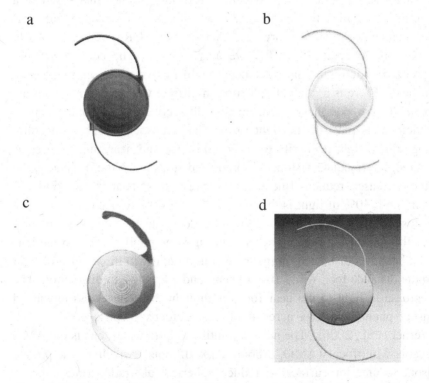

Figure 2.10. Multifocal IOLs: a. ARRAY, b. Rezoom, c. ReStor, d. Tecnis multifocal.

Refractive optics of the first multifocal IOL approved by the FDA, the AMO ARRAY, and its next generation counterpart, AMO ReZoom (AMO, Abbott Park, Illinois), have concentric refractive zones with each zone alternating for distance or near vision. The ARRAY is a distance dominant, silicone IOL with the center of the optic set for distance. Each of the 4 other zones are a mix of distance and near with 50% of light directed to the distance focus, 13% to intermediate, and 37% to near. The ReZoom is a hydrophobic acrylic lens, with zones 1, 3, and 5 being distance dominant, zones 2 and 4 near dominant, and aspheric transitions between each zone. The distribution of light with this refractive IOL is dependent on the size of the pupil. With a 2-mm pupil, 83% of light is driven to distance focus and the remaining 17% to intermediate focus. With a 5-mm pupil, 60% of light is directed to distance focus, 30% to near focus, and the remaining 10% to the intermediate focus.

Diffractive optics have concentric diffractive zones that result in a continuum of light that is directed at 2 primary foci, distance and near, independent of pupil aperture. The Acrysof ReSTOR (Alcon, Ft. Worth, Texas) is an apodized, diffractive acrylic IOL. The central 3.6 mm apodized optic region has 12 concentric diffractive zones on the anterior surface. There is a gradual reduction in diffractive step heights from the center to the periphery. The largest diffractive step is at the center, which sends most of the light to the near focus. These 12 concentric rings direct light primarily to 2 foci, distance and near, and to a lesser degree, intermediate vision. As apodized steps reach the periphery, the step decreases, reducing the amount of light to the near focus. With a 2 mm pupil, 40% of light is distributed to near, 40% to distance, and 20% is lost to diffraction. This allows for adequate reading vision with a small pupil during reading tasks. During large pupil situations, the lens then becomes distance dominant. A 5 mm pupil will direct 84% of light to the distance foci, while 10% to near, and 6% is lost in diffraction. The decrease in light to the near focus is thought to produce less unwanted visual phenomenon as a result of near defocus (Pepose et al., 2007; Werner et al., 2006). The newest multifocal intraocular lens is the AMO Tecnis Multifocal (AMO, Abbott Park, Illinois), which has a prolate aspheric anterior surface to reduce spherical aberration and improve contrast sensitivity. It also has a fully pupil-independent diffractive posterior surface. The diffractive surface consists of 32 concentric rings on the posterior surface of the lens. These rings allow for the IOL to produce a near focus (Cillino et al., 2008).

Attempts have been made to minimize unwanted visual phenomenon associated with multifocal IOLs. Studies comparing the optical trade offs between multifocal and monofocal IOLs did not reveal any surprising information. Uncorrected distance visual acuity was good in both groups. Multifocal IOLs had better uncorrected near vision, and those patients had greater spectacle independence. Glare and halos were present in the multifocal patients. Study of contrast sensitivity by Montes-Mico et al. (2004) showed that multifocals performed more poorly in mesopic conditions at both distance and near, as well as photopic conditions at near. Further study by Montes-Mico and Alio (2003) indicated patients' ability to adjust and adapt to the blur caused by multifocal IOLs. After 3 months post-op, patients demonstrated varying degrees of neuroadaptation and there were no significant differences in contrast sensitivity in all lighting conditions between multifocal and monofocal IOLs (Bellucci, 2005). Continued improvements in IOL technology will seek to further improve existing multifocal IOLs to minimize the optical effects that currently limit these lenses.

2.5.2.4 *Accommodating intraocular lenses*

Accommodating IOLs are designed to restore the accommodation lost with or removal of the crystalline lens by implanting an IOL that replicates accommodation. Some patients with traditional monofocal IOLs are happy with their uncorrected near visual acuity. Ciliary muscle contraction allows for anterior bowing of the lens optic, which is thought to increase the dioptric power of the eye. Movement of conventional IOLs has been reported with near stimulus as well as pharmacologic stimulation. This is the basis for the development of the current generation of accommodating IOLs (Dick and Dell, 2006; Menapace et al., 2007; Doane et al., 2007).

2.5.2.5 *Single optic accommodating intraocular lenses*

There are several iterations of single optic accommodating IOLs. The first accommodating IOL on the market was the Morcher BioComFold ring-haptic IOL (Stuttgart, Germany). It is a one-piece IOL made of hydrophilic acrylic. It has a 5.8 mm optic with a total lens diameter of 10.2 mm. The lens has 3 haptics, angled anteriorly, with a perforated transition zone attached to a discontinuous ring at the end of the haptics. The mechanism of action is thought to be due to compression of the haptics by the contracting ciliary muscle resulting in anterior displacement of the lens optic and posterior movement of the IOL with ciliary muscle relaxation. Another single optic accommodating IOL is the HumanOptics 1CU (Erlangen, Germany) which sits in the capsular bag. It is an acrylic single optic IOL with 4 hinged plate haptics that allow for anterior displacement of the lens optic. The proposed mechanism of accommodation is presumed to be related to relaxation of the zonular fibers leading to relaxation of the capsular bag. The contraction of the ciliary muscle turns the haptics anteriorly. This results in forward movement of the IOL optic.

The Crystalens (Bausch and Lomb, Aliso Viejo, California) is the only commercially available accommodating lens in the US at this time. It has a biconvex optic made of Biosil, a 3rd generation silicone, with a modified plate haptic that is hinged adjacent to the optic (Figure 2.11). The haptics have small looped polyimide feet, which fixate firmly in the capsular bag. The mechanism of action is thought to be related to an increase in vitreous pressure resulting from a change in ciliary body position with accommodative effort. This increase in vitreous pressure moves the lens optic anteriorly increasing its plus power. The FDA clinical trial for the Crystalens showed excellent uncorrected distance visual acuity, as well as good uncorrected intermediate and near visual acuity. Spectacles could further increase the quality of near visual acuity. However, studies using pharmacologic or optical stimulus to facilitate movement of the lens optic show opposing views on whether there is true accommodation of the Crystalens. It is possible that any near vision is still gained through pseudoaccommodation (Dick and Dell, 2006). As we look to the future, a more consistent driving force must be found to push the lens optic forward. In addition capsular fibrosis as well as posterior capsule opacification must be well controlled to prevent immobilization of the IOL and the resting IOL position should be positioned as posteriorly as possible, to allow for maximal anterior optic shift for near tasks. Other single optic lenses in various stages of development that function based on the anterior displacement of the optic during accommodative effort include the Kellan Tetraflex KH-3500 (Lenstec, St. Petersberg, Florida), Opal IOL, (Bausch and Lomb, Rochester, New York) C-Well IOL (Acuity Ltd, OrYehuda, Israel), and the Tek-Clear IOL (Tekia, Irvine, California)(Harman et al, 2008; Menapace et al., 2007; Doane et al, 2007).

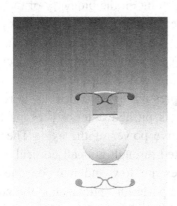

Figure 2.11. Crystalens.

2.6 Next Generation Intraocular Lenses

Newer designs attempt to improve the safety and efficacy of the next generation of lenses including spring-driven single-optic, dual-optic, magnet-driven and "lens-refilling" IOLs.

2.6.1 *Dual optic intraocular lenses*

Dual optic designs are currently in development, including the Sarfarazi Elliptical Accommodating IOL(Bausch and Lomb, Rochester, New York) and Visiogen Synchrony accommodating IOL (Irvine, California).

The mechanism of accommodation is slightly different between these 2 designs. The Sarfarazi IOL is designed to mimic the crystalline lens' change in antero-posterior dimension with accommodation and therefore change in optical power. It employs two-silicone lens optics connected by three haptics that serve both to center the IOL in the capsular bag as well as to produce the spring-like resistance that separates the two-lens optics. Studies have shown accommodation of up to 4 diopters. Near vision is achieved by the 2 lens optics moving closer together during accommodation (Sarfarazi, 2006). The Synchrony IOL has a posterior optic that is essentially stationary, and accommodation and near vision occurs as the anterior lens optic moves forward. The posterior minus-powered optic, which is varied depending on the biometry of the eye for lens implantation, is meant to be fixed posteriorly. The anterior optic has a fixed power of +32 D that is designed to move forward with accommodation. This IOL system is meant to completely occupy the capsular bag with the haptics resting in the capsular fornix. As the haptics are circumferentially compressed or extended as a result of zonular tension, the anterior optic is pushed anteriorly or posteriorly increasing or decreasing the refractive power of the eye. The lens is made of silicone, and can be injected through a small corneal incision. Posterior capsule opacification rates are low and may be due to the spring driven design that presses the posterior optic against the posterior capsule. Of concern is the possibility of intralenticular opacification. Preliminary results with this lens showed promising accommodative range of approximately 3 diopters in a small cohort of patients (McLoed et al., 2007; Ossma et al., 2007; Menapace et al., 2007).

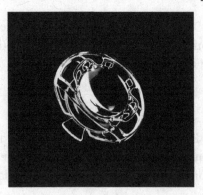

Figure 2.12. Synchrony dual optic accommodating IOL.

2.6.2 *Deformable accommodating intraocular lenses*

Other accommodating lenses in development include the Quest Vision FlexOptic deformable accommodating IOL (Austin, Texas), the FluidVision lens (PowerVision, Belmont, California), and the NuLens (HerzLiya Pituach, Israel). The FlexOptic IOL is a silicone lens shaped like a ball situated anteriorly in the capsular bag. The hollow, globe-shaped IOL is reshaped by the accommodative forces of the eye, increasing the radius of curvature of the lens optic. The FluidVision lens is designed to accommodate via a series of deformable cells attached to the anterior and posterior surface of the lens with channels for fluid flow. As the ciliary muscle contracts, this forces fluid to the lens, causing it to thicken, and increasing the power of the lens (Doane et al., 2007). The NuLens uses an anterior lens optic that presses through a diaphragm during accommodation decreasing the radius of curvature while increasing the power of the lens. This system is modeled after the lens of waterfowl, which demands a high accommodative range. The crystalline lens in these birds is forced through the rigid iris, creating a bulge, increasing the refractive power of the lens. For the human eye, the ciliary processes and capsule have been deemed a functional unit termed the capsular diaphragm. This unit is capable of active positional changes related to the contraction-relaxation status of the ciliary muscles and forms the back part of the compressible compartment for this lens. A rigid plate is placed in the ciliary sulcus, with an aperture in the center. The space between the sulcus plate, and the capsular diaphragm is filled with the flexible material. When pressure is applied by the capsular diaphragm according to the contraction-relaxation status of the ciliary muscles, the flexible material will bulge through the central aperture, increasing the lens power. The lens uses the brain's natural control of accommodation for choosing the lens power that gives the optimal image of the object. In monkey models, this lens system has shown up to 40 diopters of accommodation. This lens may allow people to harness the diminished accommodative effects of the aging eye (Ben-nun, 2006).

2.6.3 *Lens-filling accommodating intraocular lenses*

Presbyopia is thought to be in part due to hardening of the crystalline lens related to aging. As such, the concept of replacing the hardened crystalline lens with an implanted soft lens material might restore accommodation. Kessler described this in 1964. After removing the crystalline lens through a small incision at the pars plana, he used an injectable silicone to fill the capsular bag. He reported that capsules of treated eyes remained clear out to 2 years after implanting these silicone lenses. Additional studies of capsular filling techniques showed some accommodation with the replacement of the crystalline lens with their injectable lens. Posterior capsule opacification remained a problem with these methods.

Norby developed an injectable IOL, a tercopolymer, that cures into a network when exposed to the normal temperature of the eye. This lens is injected via a dual-chamber syringe containing the catalyst and the polymer. This injectable IOL was shown to have 3-5 diopters of pharmacologically induced accommodation. Fifty percent of the primates tested maintained the same accommodative amplitude at 1 year. There was only minimal capsular opacification in the lens periphery.

The SmartIOL (Medennium, Irvine, California) is a capsular filling design currently being studied, in which an acrylic material transforms to a preset dioptric power when placed in the eye, and completely fills the capsular bag. It is thought that this soft, gel-like material will behave more like the crystalline lens of youth. While lens capsule filling techniques show promise, many problems remain, including achieving emmetropia in the relaxed state, adequate accommodative response with zonular relaxation, adequate optical clarity, image quality, prolonged functionality, and posterior capsular opacification (Norby et al., 2006).

2.6.4 *Adjustable intraocular lenses*

Adjustable lens implants are an important next step in crystalline lens replacement. Following lensectomy with IOL implantation, the eye can exhibit mild degrees of either myopia or hyperopia reducing uncorrected visual acuity. This is particularly true in patients that have had previous keratorefractive surgery where IOL selection is much less predictable. Accuracy of IOL selection and residual post-operative refractive error has improved dramatically with improved biometry techniques. As the demands for excellent uncorrected post-operative vision increase, surgeons will seek to be within 0.25 diopters of the desired post-operative correction. While new techniques have lessened the occurrence of large refractive surprises, small ones are still commonly encountered. Currently, in cases where significant refractive error remains, restoration of good uncorrected visual acuity can be obtained via IOL exchange, "piggybacking" a second IOL alongside the initial one implanted and keratorefractive surgery. Adjustable lens implants may allow for the correction of residual refractive error at the lens plane without significant surgical risks as well as the potential for the correction of higher order corneal aberrations.

2.6.4.1 *Lens adjustable intraocular lenses*

Lenses currently under investigation include the Werblin lens, which has a 3-component lens system. Removing or exchanging a combination of 2 of the 3 components adjusts post-operative refractive error. The disadvantage of this system is the need for further intraocular surgery. Other systems include an adjustable PMMA lens optic that requires intraocular adjustment by turning the lens optic, thus adjusting the lens location within the eye (Matthews et al., 2003). An alternative design by Eggleston et al is a lens whose position is adjusted using external magnets (Matthews et al., 2003).

2.6.4.2 *Light adjustable intraocular lenses*

The light adjustable lens of Calhoun Vision (Pasadena, California) works on the principle of adjusting the refractive power of the lens in situ without any additional intraocular surgery. The IOL optic is composed of partially polymerized macromers with a bonded photosensitizer. When the lens is exposed to the appropriate wavelength of light, the photosensitizer will cause reorganization and polymerization of the IOL macromer to a degree that is proportional to the amount of light used.

This changes the refractive power of the IOL with great precision. Up to 6.0 diopters of refractive adjustments have been made with this design. Human clinical trials have shown this system to achieve refractive results following adjustment to within 0.25 diopters of the desired refractive change. However, hurdles still exist in the development of this technology. One hurdle was the development of a precise light delivery system. The Zeiss Digital Light Delivery Device has proven to be incredibly precise as well as offering a wide array of light patterns that can be delivered. The issue of UV exposure to the eye has been resolved by adding a UV filter to the posterior aspect of the lens optic. Corneal surface abnormalities blocking the introduction of light have also been resolved with this system by using a contact lens to introduce the light. The Calhoun lens is currently able to treat only spherical refractive error. Cylindrical and wavefront treatments are currently being studied. The IOL plane is ideal for this type of correction because it is not subject to the forces of healing that may influence correction performed at the corneal plane. The current generation of this lens is locked after the desired refractive effect has been achieved so that no further light adjustment can be carried out following the locking procedure. Locking is required as ambient light, especially intense sunlight, could theoretically readjust the refractive power of the lens. In the future, the hope is that the lens will always remain adjustable, but not be subjected to possible change by environmental light sources. This would allow for multiple adjustments through life if the refractive parameters of the eye altered over time. Another potential application of this technology is in the treatment of presbyopia. Multifocal rings can be induced or "imprinted" into this lens as well. The benefit would be that if the patient was unable to tolerate symptoms related to the multifocal lens, that function could be reversed. This light adjustable technology could also potentially be combined with capsular filling techniques that would allow for the return of accommodation, as well as correction of residual refractive error and higher order aberrations on the lens implant. This is a promising technology that could help surgeons achieve the "holy grail" of vision correction possibly on its own, or in combination with some of the other technologies discussed.

While intraocular implants that are currently available or under development have generated great excitement for their potential for enhancing vision correction, intraocular complications from surgery or ongoing ocular damage from the lenses residing in the eye might negate the intended value of these lenses. The exceedingly common outcome of cataract extraction, capsular opacification, could render much of the refractive advances of new IOLs moot. One idea for minimizing posterior capsule opacification is the "Perfect Capsule" approach, which uses sterile water to destroy residual lens epithelial cells and impair capsular opacification (Agarwal et al., 2003). An alternative technique of impairing capsular opacification is the use of polymers in the IOL to prevent residual lens epithelial proliferation via an exothermic reaction or cross-linking to the capsule. Limiting this common post-operative event is paramount to the long-term effectiveness of the new generation of intraocular lenses (Olsen et al., 2006; Schwartz et al., 2003; Werner et al., 2006).

2.7 Summary

Vision correction surgery has progressed dramatically during the past two decades. Ocular surgery, once performed primarily on older individuals with disease states, is now commonplace on individuals of all ages expecting excellent post-operative visual acuity at all ranges of vision including far, intermediate and near. The paradigm has shifted from excellent best spectacle corrected post-operative vision to excellent uncorrected post-operative vision minimizing the need for any glasses or contact lens. These demands have resulted in the treatment of healthy eyes of all ages with keratorefractive surgery and implantation of phakic IOLs as well as lensectomy for spectacle independence of presbyopic patients without significant cataracts. While the technology for treating ametropia and presbyopia have advanced, no ideal treatment is yet available. Various techniques, alone or in combination, can be offered to address the visual needs over a patient's lifespan. Critically important is the full discussion of the risks and benefits now and in the future for patients undergoing vision correction surgery of any type. The limits of technology and possible unwanted visual effects must be explored. New treatments continue to be developed with the goal of complete independence from optical aids of spectacles and contact lenses while minimizing risks to the eye and reducing unwelcome visual phenomenon. This is an exciting time in vision correction surgery and the future appears to be even more promising.

2.8 References

Agarwal, A., Agarwal, S., Agarwal, A., et al. (2003). Sealed Capsule Irrigation Device. *J. Cataract Refract. Surg.,* 29, pp. 2274-2276.

Alio, J. L., Elkady, B., Ortiz, D., et al. (2008). Clinical outcomes of intraocular optical quality of a diffractive multifocal intraocular lens with asymmetrical light distribution. *J. Cataract Refract. Surg.,* 34, pp. 942-948.

Alio, J. L., Pinero, D. P., and Puche, A. B. P. (2008). Corneal wavefront-guided photorefractive keratectomy in patients with irregular corneas after corneal refractive surgery. *J. Cataract Refract. Surg.* 34, pp. 1727-1735.

Alpins, N., and Stamatelatos, G. (2008). Clinical outcomes of laser in situ keratomileusis using combined topography and refractive wavefront treatments for myopic astigmatism. *J. Cataract. Refract. Surg.,* 34, pp. 1250-1259.

Baikoff, G., Matach, G., Fontaine, A., et al. (2004). Correction of presbyopia with refractive multifocal phakic intraocular lenses. *J. Cataract Refract. Surg.,* 30, pp. 1454-1460.

Barraquer J.I. (1949), Oueratoplastia refractive. *Estudios Inform. Oftal. Inst. Barraquer,* 10, pp. 2-21.

Bellucci, R. (2005). Multifocal intraocular lenses. *Curr. Opin. Ophthal.,* 16, pp. 33-37.

Ben-nun J. (2006). The NuLens Accommodating Intraocular Lens. *Ophthalmology Clinics of North America.* 19, pp. 129-134

Braun, E. H. P., Lee, J., and Steinert, R. F. (2008). Monovision in LASIK. *Ophthlamology,* 115, pp. 1196-1202.

Cillino, S., Casuccio, A., Di Pace, F., et al. (2008). One-year outcomes with New-Generation Multifocal Intraocular Lenses. *Ophthalmology,* 115, pp. 1508-1516.

Croft, M. A., and Kaufman, P. L. (2006). Accommodation and presbyopia: The ciliary neuromuscular view. *Ophthalmology Clinics of North America,* 19, pp. 13-24.

Dick, H. B., and Dell, S. (2006). Singgle Optic Accommodative Intraocular Lenses. *Ophthalmology Clinics of North America.* 19, pp. 107-124.

Doane, J. F., and Jackson, R. T. (2007). Accommodative intraocular lenses: considerations on use, function and design. *Curr. Opin. Ophthal.,* 18, pp. 318-324.

Donoso, R and Castillo, P. (2006). Correction of high myopia with the PRL phakic intraocular lens. *J Cataract Refract Surg.* 32, pp. 1296-300.

Du, T. T., Fan, V. C., and Asbell, P. A. (2007). Conductive keratoplasty. *Current Opinion in Ophthalmology.* 18, pp. 334-337.

Dvali, M. L., Tsinsadze, N. A., and Sirbiladze, B. V. (2009). Bioptics with LASIK flap first for the treatment of high ametropia. *J. Refract. Surg.*, 25, pp. S160-S162.

Espandar, L., Meyer, J. J., and Moshirfar, M. (2008). Phakic intraocular lenses. *Current Opinion in Ophthalmology.* 19, pp. 349-356.

Ghirlando, A., Gambat, C., and Midena, E. (2007). LASEK and photorefractive keratecotomy for myopia: clinical and confocal microscopy comparison. *J. Refract. Surg.*, 23, pp. 694-702.

Ghosh, S., Couper, T. A., Lamoureaux, E., Jhanji, V., Taylor, H. R., and Vajpayere, R. B. (2008). Evaluation of iris recognition system for wavefront-guided laser in situ keratomiluesis for myopic astigmatism. *J. Cataract Refract. Surg.*, 34, pp. 215-221.

Glasser, A. (2006). Accommodation: Mechanism and Measurement. *Ophthalmology Clinics of North America,* 19, pp. 1-12.

Guell, J. L., Morral, M., Gris, O., et al. (2008). Five-year follow-up of 399 phakic Artisan-Verisyse implantation for myopia, hyperopia, and/or astigmatism. *Ophthalmology,* 115, pp. 1002-1012.

Harman, F.E., Maling, S., Kampougeris, G., Langan, L, Khan, I, Lee, N, Bloom, P.A. (2008) Comparing the 1CU accommodative, multifocal, and monofocal intraocular lenses: a randomized trial. *Ophthalmology* 115, pp. 993-1001.

ICL in Treatment of Myopia Study Group. (2004). United States Food and Drug Administration clinical trial of the Implantable Collamer Lens (ICL) for moderate to high myopia. *Ophthalmology.* 111, pp. 1683-1692.

Kalyvianaki, M. I., Kymionis, G. D., Kounis, G. A., Panagopoulou, S. I., Grentzelos, M. A., and Pallikaris, I. G. (2008). Comparison of Epi-LASIK and off-flap Epi-LASIK for the treatment of low and moderate myopia. *Ophthalmology,*115, pp. 2174-2180.

Kymionis, G. D., Siganos, C. S., Tsiklis, N. S., Anastasakis, A., Yoo, S. H., Pallikaris, A. I., Astyrakakis, N., and Pallikaris, I. G.. (2007). Long-term follow-up of Intacs in Keratoconus. *Am. J. Ophthalmol.*, 143, pp. 236-244.

Lin, D. T. C., Holland, S. P., Rocha, K. M., and Krueger, R. R (2008). Method for optimizing topography-guided ablation of highly aberrated eyes with the Allegretto Wave excimer laser. *J. Refract. Surg.*, 24, pp. S439-S445.

Lovisolo, C. F., and Reinstein, D. Z. (2005). Phakic Intraocular Lenses. *Survey of Ophthalmology.* 50(6), pp. 549-587

Malecaze, F.J., Hulin, H, Bierer, P, et al. (2002) A randomized paired eye comparison of two techniques for treating moderately high myopia: LASIK and artisan phakic lens.*Ophthalmology* 109, pp. 1622-1630.

Matthews, M. W., Eggleston, H. C., and Hilmas, G. E. (2003). Development of a repeatedly adjustable intraocular lens. *J. Cataract Refract. Surg.*, 29, pp. 2204-2210.

Matthews, M. W., Eggleston, H. C., Pekarek, S. D., et al. (2003). Magnetically adjustable intraocular lens. *J. Cataract Refract. Surg.,* 29, pp. 2211-2216.

McLoed, S. D., Vargas, L. G., Portney, V., et al. (2007). Synchrony dual optic accommodating intraocular lens, Part 1: Optical and Biomechanical Principles and design considerations. *J. Cataract Refract. Surg.*, 33, pp. 37-46.

Medeiros, F. W., Stapleton, W. M., Hammel, J, Krueger R. R., Netto, M. V., and Wilson, S.E. (2007). Wavefront analysis comparison of LASIK outcomes with the femtosecond laser and mechanical keratomes. *J. Refract. Surg.*, 23, pp. 880-887.

Menapace, R., Findl, O., Kriechbaum, K., et al. (2007). Accommodating intraocular lenses: a critical review of present and future concepts. *Graefe's Archive for Clinical and Experimental Ophthalmology*. 245, pp. 473-489.

Montes-Mico, R., and Alio, J. L. (2003). Distance and near contrast sensivity function after multifocal intraocular lens implantation. *J. Cat. Refract. Surg.*, 29, pp. 703-711.

Montes-Mico, R., Espana, E., Bueno, I., et al. (2004). Visual performance with Multifocal Intraocular Lenses. *Ophthalmology*. 111, pp. 85-96.

Moshirfar, M., Holz, H. A., and Davis, D. K. (2007). Two-year follow-up of the Artisan/Verisyse iris-supported phakic intraocular lens for the correction of high myopia. *J. Cataract Refract. Surg.*, 33, pp. 1392-1397.

Norby S., Koopmans, S., and Terwee, T. (2006). Artificial crystalline lens. *Ophthalmology Clinics of North America*. 19, pp. 143-146.

Nordan, L. T., Slade, S. G., Baker, R. N., Suarez, C., Juhasz, T., and Kurtz, R. (2003). Femtosecond laser flap creation for laser in situ keratomileusis: six month follow-up of initial US clinical series. *J. Refract. Surg.*, 19, pp. 8-14.

Olsen R., Mamalis, N., and Gaugen, B. (2006). A light Adjustable Lens with Injectable Optics. *Ophthalmology Clinics of North America*. 19, pp. 135-142.

Ossma, I. L., Galvis, A., Vargas, L. G., et al. (2007). Synchrony dual optic accommodating intraocular lens, Part 2: Pilot clinical evaluation. *J. Cataract Refract. Surg.*, 33, pp. 47-52.

Pallikaris, I. G., Papatzanaki, M. E., Stathi, E. Z., Frenschock, O., and Georgiades, A. (1990). Laser in situ keratomileusis. *Laser Surg. Med.,* 10, pp. 463-468.

Pepose, J. S., Qazi, M. A., and Davies, J., et al. (2007). Visual performance of patients with bilateral vs combination Crystalens, ReZoom, and ReSTOR Intraocular Lens Implants. *American Journal of Ophthalmology*. 144, pp. 347-357.

Ruiz, L. A., and Rowsey, J. (1988). In situ keratomileusis. *Invest. Ophthalmol. Vis. Sci.*, 29(suppl.), pg. 392.

Salz, J. J., Maguen, E., Nesburn, A. B., Warren, C., Macy, J. I., Hofbauer, J. D., Papaioannou, T., and Belin, M. (1993). A two-year experience with excimer photorefractive keratectomy for myopia. *Ophthalmology,* 100, pp. 873-882.

Sanders, D. R., Schneider, D., Martin, R., et al. (2007). Toric Implantable Collamer Lens for moderate to high myopic astigmatism. Ophthalmology, 114, pp. 54-61.

Sarfarazi, F. M. (2006). Dual Optic Accommodative Intraocular Lens. *Ophthalmology Clinics of North America.* 19, pp. 125-128.

Schanzlin, D. J., Asbell, P. A., Burris,T. E., and Durrie, D. S. (1997). The intrastromal corneal ring segments; phase II results for the correction of myopia. *Ophthalmology*, 104, pp. 1067-1078.

Schwartz, D. M. (2003). Light-Adjustable Lens. *Transactions of the American Ophthalmological Society.* 101, pp. 411-430.

Thornton, M. D., Xu, .M,., and Krueger, R. R. (2008). Comparison of standard (0.02%) and low dose (0.002%) mitomycin C in the prevention of corneal haze following surface ablation for myopia. *J. Refract. Surg.*, 24, pp. S68-S76.

Verity, S. M., Talamo, J. T., Chayet, A., Wolf, T. C., Rapoza, P. A., Schanzlin, D. J., Lane S., Kenyon, K., and Assil, K. K. (1995). The combined Genesis) technique of radial keratotomy. A prospective, multicenter study. Refractive Keratoplasty Group. *Ophthalmology*, 102, pp. 1908-1917.

Werblin, T. P., and Stafford, G. M. (1996). Three year results of refractive keratectomy using the Casebeer system. *J. Cataract Refract. Surg.*, 22, pp. 1023-1029.

Werner, L., Olsen, R. J., and Mamalis, N. (2006). New technology IOL optics. *Ophthalmology Clinics of North America*. 19, pp. 469-483.

Werner, L., Yeh, O., Haymore, J., et al. (2007). Corneal endothelial safety with the irradiation system for light-adjustable intraocular lenses. *J. Cataract. Refract. Surg.*, 33, pp. 873-878.

2.9 Review Questions

Q2.1 What factors are primarily responsible for determining the refractive power of the eye?

A. cornea

B. crystalline lens

C. axial length of the eye

D. all of the above

E. none of the above

Q2.2 What ophthalmic laser is utilized to perform laser vision correction for both photorefractive keratectomy (PRK) and Laser Assisted in situ Keratomileusis?

A. excimer laser

B. YAG laser

C. argon laser

D. CO_2 laser

E. femtosecond laser

Q2.3 To date, laser vision correction is least successful in which of the following conditions?

A. myopia

B. hyperopia

C. astigmatism

D. presbyopia

E. pseudophakia

Q2.4 Wavefront guided ablations are not FDA approved for the treatment of which condition?

A. myopia

B. hyperopia

C. astigmatism

D. pseudophakia

E. eyes needing laser enhancements following initial laser vision correction surgery

Q2.5 Accommodation is usually completely lost by age

A. 25 years

B. 35 years

C. 45 years

D. 55 years

E. 65 years

Q2.6 Presbyopia is caused by

A. loss of ciliary muscle function

B. hardening of the crystalline lens

C. changes in the lens capsule

D. all of the above

E. none of the above

Q2.7 The least invasive treatment for presbyopia is

A. conductive keratoplasty

B. phakic intraocular lens

C. eye lengthening

D. lensectomy with intraocular lens implant

E. penetrating keratoplasty

Q2.8 A weakness of multifocal IOL when compared with accommodating IOL is

A. disruptive optical phenomena

B. poor uncorrected near vision

C. decrease contrast sensitivity

D. A and C

E. none of the above

Chapter 3

Applications of Advanced Technologies to Retinal Prosthesis

Dean Scribner[1] and Lee Johnson[2]

[1] Northrop Grumman, 5113 Leesburg Pike, Falls Church VA 22041
PH: 703-845-8311; FX: 20703-575-3527; EM: dean.scribner@ngc.com

[2] Optical Sciences Division, Naval Research Laboratory; 4555 Overlook Ave.
SW, Washington, DC 20012; EM: lee.johnson@nrl.navy.mil

3.1 Introduction

The aging process tends to degrade the human visual system. Even in those fortunate few individuals with "perfect vision", most will require some corrective devices (spectacles) during middle age. A more serious problem is the formation of cataracts, which is a clouding of the lens in the eye thus degrading visual acuity. Although cataracts can form early in life, they are generally considered to be part of the aging process. Cataracts are very common in older people. By age 80, more than half of all Americans have cataract problems, but surgetical treatment consisting of artificial lens implants has been highly successful in recent decades (Friedman, 2002).

But other afflictions can be more catastrophic, bringing with them major loss of vision. The leading causes of blindness in the developed world are Retinitis Pigmentosa (RP) and Age-Related Macular Degeneration (AMD). Both of these two serious eye diseases also progress with aging. Neither have treatment options at this time that can reverse the effects of the disease – although recently there has been some success with gene therapy drugs that give some encouragement to AMD patients in terms of stopping the progression of the disease provided it is detected early.

Biomedical engineers are currently developing retinal prosthesis implants that could provide a form of artificial vision to severely blind individuals (Zrenner, 2002). The purpose of this chapter is to provide an overview of the concept of retinal prosthesis and discuss advanced technologies that promise to not only make this possible, but to also provide a very high degree of visual acuity to blind patients. There is no firm consensus at this time as to what a final retinal prosthesis system will be – in fact different types of blindness and different levels of visual impairment may dictate different system architectures. Thus the discussion here will remain fairly broad and general. However, because RP and AMD are the leading causes of blindness in the developing world, effecting approximately 30 million people, most of the discussion here will emphasize prosthetics for these two diseases.

Retinitis Pigmentosa (RP) is the name given to a group of hereditary eye disorders, all of which involve the eye's retina, the light-sensitive nerve layer that lines the back of the eye This disease causes a gradual, yet progressive, loss or reduction in visual ability. RP is caused by a variety of different inherited retinal defects - all of which affect the ability of the retina to sense light. The retinal defect may be found in the rod cells (a type of retinal cell found outside of the central portion of the retina that help to transmit dim light and allow for peripheral vision), the cone cells (a type of retinal cell found inside the center of the retina that help to transmit the color and detail of images), and in the connection between the cells that compose the retina.

In the progression of symptoms RP generally precedes <u>tunnel vision</u> by years or even decades. Many people with RP do not become legally <u>blind</u> until their 40s or 50s and retain some sight all their life while others go completely blind from RP, in some cases as early as childhood. Unfortunately, there is currently no specific treatment for RP, however, there are some treatments that may slow the progression of the cell degeneration such as nutritional supplements, neurotropic factors, antioxidants, and reduced light exposure.

AMD is a degenerative condition of the central <u>retina</u>. It is the most common cause of vision loss in the developed world in those 50 years of age or older. Its prevalence increases with age. AMD is generally caused by hardening of the arteries that nourish the retina. This deprives the sensitive retinal tissue of oxygen and nutrients that it needs to function and thrive; as a result, central vision deteriorates, but peripheral vision remains relatively unchanged. AMD varies widely in levels of severity. In the worst cases, it causes a complete loss of central vision, making reading or driving impossible while for others it may only cause slight distortion. AMD is classified as either the wet from or dry form.

Wet AMD occurs when abnormal blood vessels behind the retina start to grow under the macula (see Fig. 3.1). These new blood vessels tend to be very fragile and often leak blood and fluid. The blood and fluid raise the macula from its normal place at the back of the eye. Damage to the macula occurs rapidly. With wet AMD, the loss of central vision can occur quickly. Wet AMD is also known as advanced AMD and about 10% of patients who suffer from macular degeneration have wet AMD. However, if only advanced AMD is considered, about two-thirds of patients have the wet form. Wet AMD can be treated with laser surgery, photodynamic therapy and injections into the eye. However, none of these treatments completely cures wet AMD and the disease often progresses despite treatment.

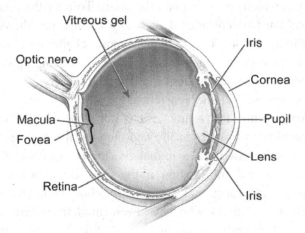

Figure 3.1. Eye diagram showing the macula and fovea (National Eye Institute).

More than 50 million people worldwide are estimated to have irreversible blindness as a result of AMD, making it the most common cause of blindness for those over 60. It's estimated that 30 percent of the population will have some form of AMD by the time they reach the age of seventy-five. Currently, 15 million seniors in the United States suffer from some form of AMD, with 1.6-1.75 million experiencing the active blood vessel growth and blood vessel leakage associated with wet AMD. There are approximately 200,000 new cases of wet AMD each year and this number is expected to increase significantly as the baby boomer generation ages and overall life expectancy increases. Owing to the rapid aging of the US population, this number will increase to almost three million by 2020 and over six million people by 2030.

It should be noted that in both RP and AMD the progression of the diseases is over a time period of several decades and that any successful retinal prosthesis system needs to understand the pathophysiology of the diseases and their long term progression. This understanding will also need to consider how electrical stimulation will affect the tissue (Rizzo et al., 2001).

The third leading cause of blindness worldwide is optic nerve damage from glaucoma (Hetling and Baig-Silva, 2004) that can render the retina ineffective. In these cases, retinal prosthesis is obviously not an option because of the severe loss of all retinal function or the loss of connectivity between the retina and the brain. To treat these conditions, other options must be considered such as a cortical prosthesis (Hetling and Baig-Silva, 2004). This is much more challenging for several reasons, not the least of which is the lack of understanding of complex brain structure and the difficulties of intracranial surgery.

Another important issue for retinal prosthesis is the state of the patients visual cortex. For example, it is not clear whether individuals who became blind very early in life and then spent many years without full vision will benefit from a retinal prosthesis. The visual cortex is desensitized to visual information if the eyes are deprived of visual stimuli during a critical period during early childhood. This process is called amblyopia. Patients who have been blind from early childhood may have lost their ability to process visual stimuli in the visual centers of their cortex and therefore may not benefit from any type of visual prothesis.

A strategy for successfully treating the large population of AMD and RP patients is based on the premise that even in advanced stages of these diseases, the inner retinal layers remain viable for long periods of time. By stimulating these remaining functional retinal layers, it may be feasible to restore visual perception. Thus the goal of biomedical researchers is to design and fabricate safe and effective devices that create a neural-electronic interface between an electrode array and the retinal surface. A fully engineered system would also need to provide input imagery and electrical power to operate the array.

Based on this belief, a number of research groups have proposed retinal prostheses devices that can electrically stimulate these intact cell layers and create visual perception in blind patients. Experiments with human subjects in the 1990's indicated that retinal prosthesis might be feasible (Humayun et al., 1996). During the past decade, a number of groups have been developing retinal prosthesis devices with a few dozen electrodes, where the individual electrodes have diameters of >100 microns and even greater center-to-center spacing. Subsequent chronic tests in blind human subjects have demonstrated that these devices were able to generate the perception of light and the detection of simple large shapes (Chow et al., 2004; Yanai et al., 2007; Rizzo et al., 2003; Gekeler et al., 2007).

Recent results with isolated animal retina (rat guinea pig, and non-human primate) indicate that high resolution stimulation of the retina is possible (Sekirnjak et al., 2008). Although these successes have generated much optimism, the technological path to a high resolution device with a wide field-of-view remains unclear at this time. There are a number of approaches that have been proposed which involve different device structures to achieve an electrode-neuron interface and different system architectures to transport image data and power to the device. There are also many challenges ahead in terms of forming a reliable and safe neural-electronic interface with retinal tissue.

Section 3.2 gives the basic concepts of retinal prosthesis based on electrical stimulation; Section 3.3 discusses device structures for creating an electrical interface with the curved surface of the retina; Section 3.4

describes different system architectures for retinal prosthesis, mainly addressing the issues of inputting image data and providing electrical power to the stimulating array; Section 3.5 gives an overview of advanced technologies that will provide pathways to high resolution systems.

3.2 Basic Concepts of Retinal Prothesis

The basic operation of a retinal prosthesis device is straightforward in theory. Localized electrical stimulation of neurons elicits a neural response by creating an electric field outside a retinal neuron thus activating voltage sensitive ion channels causing the cell to fire. Visual images can be produced in the brain by patterned electrical stimulation of retinal cells - in place of an optical image that otherwise would stimulation the photoreceptor cells - so as to provide a one-to-one mapping to areas in the visual cortex. A layer of retinal cells, such as the ganglion layer, can be electrically stimulated by an electrode array that inputs electrical impulses as shown in Fig. 3.2. Placing the device against the inner-most surface of the retina is known as epiretinal prosthesis. The axons of the stimulated ganglion cells then transmit the image through the optic nerve to other areas of the brain, specifically the lateral geniculate nucleus and visual cortex to create the perception of an image.

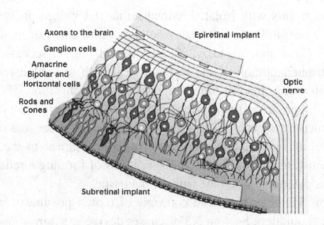

Figure 3.2. Two modes of retinal implantation (Rattay and Resatz, 2004).

Studies performed at Johns Hopkins Wilmer Eye Institute in the 1990's, demonstrated that epiretinal stimulation of ganglion cells can create visual precepts in blind patients (Humayun et al., 1996). The first set of experiments were acute tests in which the retina of blind subjects was stimulated by a single electrode and the patients reported the correct relative location and time dependency of the stimulation pulse. A second study showed that when multiple electrodes were positioned against the retina, the human subjects could perceive the crude patterns (Humayun et al., 1999). Subretinal stimulation, in the area of the rods and cones, is also a possible mode to stimulate the retina as shown in Fig. 3.2. There are a number of reasons, both mechanical and neurological to consider both modes of stimulation, as briefly summarized below:

3.2.1 *Epiretinal implantation*

Epiretinal implantation has the advantage of leaving the retina intact by placing the implant in the vitreous cavity, a naturally existing and fluid-filled space. However, implantation requires a vitrectomy and placement of a stimulation array against the retina. Studies at John Hopkins University Hospital have demonstrated that this array position is biocompatible (Majji et al., 1999). Preliminary versions of this technique involve mounting a miniature video camera (e.g., charge-coupled device - CCD) on a pair of glasses. The video signal and power of the output will be processed by a data processor, and the information is transmitted to intraocular electronics by electromagnetic coupling with an external metal coil to an intraocular coil (Heetderks, 1988; Troyk and Schwan, 1992). The power and data transmitted is converted to electrical stimulation pulses by other intraocular electronics that then control the distribution of current to the epiretinal electrode array. Section IV of this chapter discusses more details regarding system aspects of retina prosthesis.

3.2.2 Subretinal implantation

Subretinal implantation of a retinal prosthesis is being developed by Zrenner (Guenther et al., 1999; Zrenner et al., 1999), Chow (Peachey and Chow, 1999; and Chow et al., 2004), and Rizzo. This approach essentially replaces the diseased photoreceptors with a microelectronic stimulator device. However, the implantation requires special surgical procedures such as detaching the retina or invasive surgery through the sclera. Furthermore, the location of the device may be disruptive to the health of the retina (Zrenner et al., 1999). The histology of the retina after chronic device implantation showed declining of inner nuclear and ganglion cell layer densities (Peyman et al., 1998).The nourishment of the outer retinal layers of the retina comes from the choroid. For this reason, Zrenner's group implemented nutrition openings in each unit of their device.

To summarize, an epiretinal device is positioned in front of the retina, whereas a subretinal placement refers to placing the device behind or underneath the retina. Besides the difference in physical location there are a number of contrasting advantages and disadvantages for both placement options. Subretinal electrodes preferentially stimulate horizontal, bipolar and amacrine cells which utilize remaining retinal processing. Epiretinal placement preferentially stimulates ganglion cells, providing direct connection to higher visual structures. Subretinal surgeries can be complicated and require novel procedures. The surgical procedure for epiretinal placement uses standard techniques such as vitrectomy, lensectomy and retinal tacks. Light is imaged by the subretinal device through the retina eliminating the need for an external camera and allowing for natural control of the visual field. However, while the retina is clear in cases of RP, it can be clouded from drusen with advanced AMD and may reduce light reaching the subretinal implant. For most epiretinal devices, the scene is imaged with an external camera. Thus the epiretinal design avoids possible problems with drusen. Only chronic stimulation with an epiretinal device has been proven to work in patient testing. Chronic subretinal stimulation, while promising, still requires research in humans to achieve perception of light patterns.

3.2.3 *Other major considerations*

Regardless of the positioning of the electrode array, the development of an implantable retinal prosthesis system for chronic use is a complex undertaking. Ultimately any commercial device must meet stringent biocompatibility requirements and have a lifetime of several decades. However, recent technological advances in retinal surgery, microelectronics, and materials science have encouraged biomedical researchers that retinal prosthesis is feasible. The success of cochlear implant systems for the deaf has also been an encouragement in terms of forming biocompatible neural-electronic interfaces that are safe and effective (Makhdoum et al., 2007). Currently, most prototype designs for retinal prosthesis are attempting to provide only the rudimentary vision or a very limited field-of-view. A major limitation of these designs is that the underlying technologies are not scalable to higher resolution, that is, electrode arrays with thousands of elements.

One of the biggest issues for retinal prosthesis design is that of biocompatibility and safety. Whether or not retinal tissue will reject a prosthetic device can only be determined empirically. Therefore, that question can not rigorously be address here, but we will comment as appropriate. Biocompatibility has two aspects: first, the device cannot cause damage to the retina: and second, the intraocular environment cannot corrode or damage the device.

Aside from biocompatibility there are many other basic considerations for developing a high-resolution retinal prosthesis device. First, the electrode array must have a spherical shape to conform to the spherical surface of the retina such that the individual electrodes are in very close proximity to the neurons they are to stimulate. (Hetling, 2004) If the electrodes are not in close proximity, the electrical current outputs will diffuse, essentially blurring the image and losing effective resolution. Second, the electrical stimulation pulse shapes, amplitudes, and repetition rates should be capable of covering the full dynamic range of the retinal neurons (Weiland et al., 2005) and yet have minimum power dissipation so as not to exceed the level of safe electrical stimulation currents (both for neurons and electrodes). In general, for functional electrical stimulation of neural tissue, a biphasic pulse of current is required (Weiland et al., 2005). By varying the current amplitude, from pixel-to-pixel, image contrast can be achieved. Third, direct electrical stimulation of the ganglion cells precludes certain image processing functions that normally would have occurred in earlier layers of the retina – although these processing functions are not known in detail, it is well known that they exist. Therefore, image pre-processing operations may need to be performed on the image before stimulation of the retina. Fourth, a means of delivering electrical signals and power to the device needs to be engineered, designed, and verified. Fifth, because a normal retina processes images layer-by-layer starting with the photoreceptors, it is assumed that a prosthesis device should similarly excite retinal cells in a simultaneous manner (as opposed to a sequential raster scan like that used in video displays).

In an effort to define the minimum acceptable resolution for useful vision, several psychophysical experiments have been performed. In seminal work in 1965 Brindley suggested that 600 electrodes or points of stimulation would be sufficient for reading ordinary print (10 letters per presentation and 120 presentations per minute) (Brindley, 1965). More recent studies confirmed these estimated numbers (Cha et al., 1992; Dagnelie et al., 2006). Therefore, even with a low-resolution retinal prosthesis system, the brain might be able to extract a useful amount of information. Nevertheless, it is expected that the better the resolution of the system, and the better the associated preprocessing, the more the brain will be able to perceive. For minimal reading skills and visual–manual coordination, a device should have more than 600 resolution elements (pixels) with approximately a 10 x 7 degree field-of-view. But with all human viewing systems, more resolution is always better and will always be a primary consideration in developing a retinal prosthesis system.

Probably the most practical path to developing commercial retinal prosthesis systems would be to first start by developing systems for RP patients who have near total vision loss. This is in contrast to AMD patients, most of whom typically retain good peripheral vision and approximately 20/400 "central vision". Therefore a future retinal prosthesis system aimed at AMD patients would have to provide a significant improvement over 20/400 vision and not degrade the patient intact peripheral vision. One factor to consider when working with RP patients with severe vision loss is the fact that over many years of blindness, any remaining retinal neurons that still function tend to "remodel" (Marc et al., 2003).

It should be noted that "non-electrical" stimulation of the retina has been proposed using micro-fluidic delivery of neurotransmitters to retinal neurons (Peterman, Mehenti et al., 2003; Peterman, Bloom et al., 2003). This avoids all the problems of electrical stimulation and offers the possibility of selectively activating different types of ganglion cells, but it raises many other problems not the least of which is a renewable supply of neurotransmitters.

Another area of interest is tissue engineering which is now being studied as a potential alternative to tissue or organ transplantation. With this technology, artificially generated tissue can be used to replace lost or failed organs. This tissue can be employed as a biological substitute or alternatively with *ex vivo* perfusion. The tissue-engineered products may be fully functional at the time of treatment (e.g., liver assist devices, encapsulated islets), or have potential to integrate and form the expected functional tissue upon implantation (e.g., chondrocytes embedded in a matrix carrier). In some cases, biomaterials are modified to enhance migration and attachment of the specific cell populations, which repair or replace the damaged tissue. This is considered a very promising area for the development of simple cornea and lens tissue and could possibly be a source of retinal tissue at some point in the future (Ito et al., 2005; Winter et al., 2008; Kubota et al., 2006). At this time, most of this work involves stem cell projects.

Finally it should be noted that there are new treatments for AMD that involve injection therapies for wet AMD offered by Lucentis and Visudyne (there are no current effective therapies for RP). Lucentis is given as an injection into the eye typically starting with four monthly injections, followed by a regiment of once every three months. These injections primarily attempt to stop the progression of the disease by blocking the growth of the abnormal blood vessels that are characteristic of wet AMD. Approximately 40% on the patients receiving Lucentis measure some improvement in vision, while the remainder reported that their sight stayed the same, but got no worse. The treatment is new, so long term efficacy is unknown, but the gains in vision have been sustained through two years of testing with monthly Lucentis treatments. However, Genentech, the manufacturer of Lucentis, recently warned doctors that Lucentis may increase the risk of stroke in some patients (Chyu and Shah, 2007). It is noteworthy that the current annual cost of Lucentis is over $2,000 per injection.

3.3 Interfacing Electrical Devices to the Retina

One of the biggest challenges for creating a high resolution retinal prosthesis is the design and fabrication of a device with high density electrodes in very close proximity to retinal neurons. The device must conform precisely to the curved surface of the retina and of course be biocompatible. A basic tenet of neural prosthetics is to intervene in the central nervous system at a point that is closest to the damaged or diseased area. Direct electrical stimulation of the retinal cells in lieu of optical activation of the photoreceptors takes advantage of the spatially organized neural structure of the retina. As mentioned above, both epiretinal and subretinal placement of a stimulating array have been studied.

Epiretinal placement requires electrodes positioned very close to the ganglion cells, but the input images may require more preprocessing before stimulation to make up for that lost from the bypassed bipolar, horizontal and amacrine cells. However, in the severest form of AMD, the retina becomes more opaque. This opaqueness could make it difficult for subretinal devices with electronic imaging arrays located behind the retina to collect sufficient light to form an image. Furthermore, the surgical approach is different for epiretinal verses subretinal implantation. The epiretinal approach requires a vitrectomy and intraocular surgery. A vitrectomy is a standard procedure for a retinal surgeon. Subretinal placement may also be performed with intraocular surgery, but can also be accomplished by penetrating the sclera from outside the eye.

Aside from device positioning, many specific physiological questions and concerns arise when interfacing an electronic device to neural tissue. A number of these questions are addressed individually below:

3.3.1 *What is the minimum electrical current for neuron activation?*

The signaling mechanisms between neurons have been intensely studied for over 50 years. Neurons are connected in dense networks via dentrides and axons which transmit information through electrochemical interactions. If the sum of all the signals transmitted through dentrites to a neuron reaches a threshold level, then the neuron fires and an output is sent through the cell axon to the dentrides of other neurons. The actual firing of a neuron is described by the Hodgkin-Huxley model of neuronal stimulation; an action potential involves the following sequence of events: a depolarization of the membrane causes Na+ channels to open rapidly resulting in an inward Na+ current (because of a higher concentration of this ion *outside* the cell membrane). This current causes further depolarization, thereby opening more Na+ channels and results in increased inward current; the regenerative process causes the action potential.

For the case of retinal prosthesis, a neuron is artificially caused to fire by applying electrical stimulation which elicits a neural response by "turning on" the voltage sensitive ion channels, bypassing the chemically gated channels in the stimulated cell. To achieve stimulation, electric fields can be applied in different sequences. The first is cathodic threshold activation. This is the minimum stimulus amplitude and duration required to initiate an action potential. Once the membrane reaches a certain potential, a trigger mechanism is released and an action potential results (all-or-nothing mechanism). Other methods to stimulate neurons are anodic pulses and biphasic pulses. There are well-defined relationships between the threshold charge and pulse duration (West and Wolstencroft, 1983). Charge and threshold have different minimum requirements during neuronal stimulation. A minimum charge is required for shorter pulse duration in contrast to threshold current, which is minimized at long pulse duration. Experiments were performed at Johns Hopkins University to define threshold currents for retinal electrical stimulation. One study assessed the effect of changing parameters of the stimulating electrode and the stimulus pulse by recording electrically elicited action potential responses from retinal ganglion cells in isolated rabbit retina. The study demonstrated successful stimulations with currents as low as $0.14 - 0.29$ µA (Grumet et al., 2000)

A second type of experiment compared the electrical stimulation threshold in normal mouse retina versus different aged retinal degenerate (rd) mouse retina (Suzuki et al., 2004). Retinal ganglion cell recordings were obtained from anesthetized 8- and 16-week old rd mice, and 8-week old normal mice in response to a constant current electrical stimulus delivered via a platinum wire electrode on the retinal surface. The excitation thresholds were significantly higher in the 16-week old rd mouse (0.075 µC for 0.08 msec square pulse) versus the 8-week old rd (0.048 µC for 0.08 msec square pulse) ($P < 0.05$) and versus normal mouse rd (0.055 µC for 0.08 msec square pulse) ($P < 0.05$). In all groups, short-duration pulses were more efficient than longer pulses (lower total charge) ($P < 0.05$).

In human experiments at Johns Hopkins University Hospital, typical thresholds observed for retinal stimulation of RP patients was 500 µA with a 2 msec half-pulse stimulus duration (1 µC/phase) using electrode sizes from 50 µm to 200 µm diameter disks that were very near, but not touching the retina (Humayun et al., 1996). The quantity *charge-per-phase* is defined as the integral of the stimulus current over one half-cycle of the stimulus duration. In summary, the measurements that have been made to date serve as useful guides for threshold levels needed to stimulate retinal neurons, however, a quantitative relationship between minimum currents, electrode size, proximity, and pulse shape is still incomplete.

In spite of the encouraging progress discussed above, there remain several critical questions regarding the stimulation of neurons in any future retinal prosthesis device. Three important questions are discussed below.

3.3.2 *What is the maximum current that can be used and what electrode materials support these current levels?*

Among the early studies that have addressed this issue are the histopathological studies of long-term stimulation by Pudenz et al. (Pudenz, Bullara, Jacques, and Hambrecht, 1975; Pudenz, Bullara, and Talalla, 1975; Pudenz, Bullara, Dru et al., 1975). Lilly (1961) demonstrated the relative safety of biphasic, charge-balanced waveforms compared to monophasic waveforms.

McCreery et. al. (1990) showed that the threshold of tissue damage from electrical stimulation is dependent on current amplitude and pulse frequency, but more importantly, on charge density and charge per phase (McCreery et al., 1990). Charge density is defined as *charge-per-phase* divided by the electrochemically active electrode surface area. Since total charge density is responsible for the damage of tissue and electrodes, there is a theoretical limit to how small the electrodes can be (Brown et al., 1977; Tehovnik, 1996). Most of the studies that were done to determine these limits were performed with superficial cortical electrodes (McCreery et al., 1990), or intracortical microstimulation (Bullara et al., 1983). Chronic *in vivo* retinal stimulation tests still need to be performed to define tissue damage thresholds.

Even though the "noble" metals (platinum, iridium, rhodium, gold, and palladium) corrode to some degree when used as stimulating electrodes (Cogan et al., 2004; McHardy et al., 1980; Laing et al., 1967) - platinum and its alloys with iridium are the types most widely used. Using simple waveforms, conservative charge density limits for chronic stimulation with platinum electrodes are 100 $\mu C/cm^2$ and 1 $\mu C/phase$ (Rose and Robblee, 1990; Robblee and Rose, 1990). Platinum-iridium alloys are mechanically stronger then platinum alone.

Iridium oxide electrodes belong to a new category termed "valence change oxides." Iridium oxide layers can be formed by electrochemical activation of iridium metal, by thermal decomposition of an iridium salt on a metal substrate, or by reactive sputtering from an iridium target. Activated iridium is exceptionally resistant to corrosion. It appears to be a very promising electrode material. Most neural prostheses use platinum electrodes, the exception being the BION microstimulator (Advanced

Bionics, Sylmar, California), which uses iridium oxide. For activated iridium oxide electrodes, the limit is 1 mC/cm^2 and 16 nC/phase (Robblee and Rose, 1990). Other materials may have potential in comparison to iridium oxide. A paper reported a titanium nitride, thin-film electrode demonstrated charge injection limits higher than both platinum and iridium oxide (Janders et al., 1996). A subsequent study suggested the limit was $0.78mC/cm^2$ (Weiland et al., 2002). Still, titanium nitride may be worth further study.

3.3.3 *What are the optimum conditions for stimulating retinal neurons and what is the desired response?*

One of the conditions for safe electrical stimulation of neural tissue is a reversible faradaic process. These reactions involve electron transfer across the electrode-tissue interface. Some chemicals are either oxidized or reduced during these reactions. These chemicals remain bound to the electrode surface and do not mix with the surrounding solution. It is also necessary to know the chemical reversibility of electrode materials and stimulation protocols. Chemical reversibility requires that all processes occurring at an electrode due to an electrical pulse, including H_2 and O_2 evolution, will be chemically reversed by a pulse of opposite polarity.

Over time, any net DC current can lead to charge accumulation and irreversible electrolyte reactions. A biphasic current waveform consisting of two consecutive pulses of equal charge but opposite polarity generally avoids these problems. A simple monophasic waveform is similarly unacceptable. Studies with both isolated rabbit retina and mice retina (normal and *rd*) showed that the electrophysiological response has the lowest threshold when using a cathodic wave first. These studies also showed that response threshold was lower when using square-wave electrical stimulus (Suzuki et al., 2004; Jensen and Rizzo, 2006).

3.3.4 *What attachment methods should be used for minimizing any possible damage to neural tissue?*

Because any future implantable device could be positioned against neural tissue for very long periods of time, potentially decades, a number of biocompatibility issues need to be addressed. The biocompatibility between an implanted medical device and the host tissue is as important as its mechanical durability and functional characteristics. This includes the effects of the implant on the host and vice versa. Effects of the implant on the tissue include inflammation, sensitivity reactions, infections, and carcinogenicity. Effects of the tissue on the implant are corrosion and other types of degradation. Sources of toxic substances are antioxidants, catalysts, and contaminants from fabrication equipment.

Microfabricated electrodes were initially conceived in the early 1970s (Wise et al., 1970). In subsequent years, the dimensions of these electrodes have been decreased, using concurrent advances in the microelectronics industry. Today, micromachined silicon electrodes with conducting lines of 2 μm are standard (Hetke et al., 1994; Blanche et al., 2005). Methods for depositing thin-film metal electrodes have been established. Chronic implantation and *in vivo* testing have demonstrated the ability of silicon devices to maintain electrical characteristics during long-term implantation (Weiland and Anderson, 2000)

Stabilizing the electrode array on the surface of the retina is an especially formidable problem. The biocompatibility and the feasibility of surgically implanting an electrode array onto the retinal surface has been examined Johns Hopkins University Hospital. In one experiment, a 5 × 5 electrode array (25 disc-shaped platinum electrodes in a silicone matrix) was implanted on to the retinal surface using retinal tacks in each of four mixed-breed sighted dogs for a maximum period of time of one year. No retinal detachment, infection, or uncontrolled intraocular bleeding occurred in any of the animals. Retinal tacks and the retinal array remained firmly affixed to the retina throughout the follow-up period. It was concluded that implantation of an electrode array on the epiretinal side is surgically feasible, with little if any significant damage to the underlying retina, and that platinum and silicone arrays as well as the metal tacks are biocompatible in the eye (Majji et al., 1999).

Another method for attaching electrode arrays is by biocompatible adhesives. Nine commercially available compounds were examined for their suitability as intraocular adhesives: commercial fibrin sealant, autologous fibrin, Cell-Tak®, three photocurable glues, and three different polyethylene glycol hydrogels. One type of hydrogel (SS-PEG,

Shearwater Polymers, Inc.) proved to be nontoxic to the retina (Margalit et al., 2000). Hydrogels proved superior for intraocular use in terms of consistency, adhesiveness, stability, impermeability, and safety.

3.4 System Architecture for Retinal Prothesis

As of 2008, a number of research centers and commercial biomedical companies are developing prototype systems for use in clinical trials with the intent to develop an eventual commercial product. These efforts included both epiretinal and subretinal devices and represent a diverse set of system architectures. At present there are at least four small companies conducting clinical trial with retinal implants and other research groups working on various biomedical engineering aspects of the problem. All of the systems used in clinical trials are low resolution - none of these groups have revealed their future plans for obtaining higher resolution and a wider field-of-view. The four companies that have been actively developing retinal implants are summarized below:

3.4.1 *Second sight*

Second Sight (Sylmar, California) was founded in 1998 by entrepreneurs Al Mann, Sam Williams and others to create an epiretinal prosthesis to provide sight to patients blinded from outer retinal degenerations, particularly RP (see Fig. 3.3). Their device consists of a tiny camera and transmitter mounted in eyeglasses, an implanted receiver, and a 60 electrode-studded array that is secured to the retina in an epiretinal position with a retinal tack. A wireless microprocessor and battery pack worn on the belt powers the ARGUS device. Second Sight recently received FDA approval to begin clinical trials. Second Sight is probably the most well-funded and well-positioned company in terms of having a large, experienced team in place with continuous, long-term funding and enjoys first mover status. Second Sight is closely aligned with the Doheny Eye Institute at the University of Southern California where they perform clinical testing. Although their devices are low resolution that is typical of early prototypes, Second Site has been successful at demonstrating basic feasibility with human test subjects. The Argus II version of their device has 60 electrodes and is in clinical trials internationally.

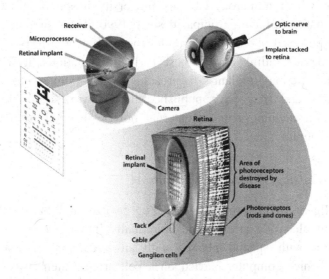

Figure 3.3. Retinal prosthesis system under development by Second Sight LLC (Mlhanasankar, pp. 2631-2632).

3.4.2 *Optobionics*

Optobionics (Naperville, Illinois) has developed the subretinal Artificial Silicon Retina™ (ASR) microchip to stimulate damaged retinal cells, allowing them to send visual signals to the brain. The ASR microchip is 2 mm in diameter and contains approximately 5,000 microscopic photovoltaic cells called "microphotodiodes," The ASR microchip is powered solely by incident light and does not require the use of external wires or batteries. In clinical trials that began in June 2000, Optobionics implanted its microchip into the subretinal space of ten patients with RP, to study its safety and feasibility in treating retinal vision loss. However, the company states no evoked lights spots with the ASR microchip. The company was in bankruptcy in 2007.

3.4.3 *Retinal implants*

Retina Implant (Reutligen, Germany) is a medical technology start-up company founded in 2003 that is building upon the results of a research project in which numerous German university hospitals and German research institutes have participated since 1996. Their subretinal 1,500 electrode powered photodiode array has been implanted in two patients with the device failing during these early implantations. It should be noted that Retina Implant's approach is very similar to that of Optobionics and they have published design work describing their approach for adding gain via external power obtained from electro-magnetic coupling.

3.4.4 *IMI Intelligent Medical Implants AC*

IMI Intelligent Medical Implants AG (Zug, Switzerland) has developed a 49-element electrode array to be epiretinally implanted in the eye in conjunction with special glasses with an integrated camera and a "learning" microcomputer carried on a belt around their waist. Visual information received by the glasses is converted into electrical pulses by the microcomputer and the pulses are then used to stimulate the patient's ganglion cell layer. Of the 20 patients suffering from RP who participated in a study, 19 reported that their visual perception had been triggered by electrical stimulations from IIP's retina implant (Gekeler et al., 2007).

In the future it is expected that retinal prosthesis systems will strive for higher resolution and fully integrated, compact designs that will allow patients to lead more natural lives. To achieve this goal, supporting advanced technologies will need to be developed in the future (these will be discussed in Section V). The design of a fully integrated retinal prosthesis system must consider the overall system architecture that includes not only the actual stimulation of retinal neurons (as described in Section III above), but also a means of delivering image data and power. It may also be the case that some image processing must be performed on the input image before the retina is stimulated. These three points are addressed below:

3.4.5 *How is the image acquired; for example, an external cameral versus and intraocular imaging array?*

An external camera has the advantage of simplicity over functionality. That is, conventional off-the-shelf miniature cameras can acquire imagery and process it before transmitting it to a retinal stimulator array. The disadvantage of this approach is that it decouples the view direction from the natural ocular motion of the eye – in essence, the patient must perform all visual tracking by head motion only. It also requires transmission of image data, which for a high resolution system will require higher carrier frequencies due to the increased bandwidth. Direct connections through the eye wall are probably not desirable for chronic implants.

A more elegant design than an external camera is to use the natural lens of the eye to image light onto a microelectronic imaging array positioned against the retina. A major advantage of this approach is that the patient uses his natural ocular motor system to control his viewing direction. For an epi-retinal device, one means of accomplishing this is to use a backside-illuminated imaging array as shown in Fig. 3.4 (Scribner et al., 2007).

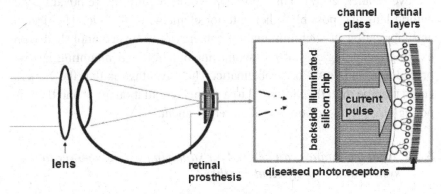

Figure 3.4. System concept for a backside illuminated retinal prosthesis.

A backside imaging array (Culurciello and Andreou, 2004; Fish et al., 2007; Bebek et al., 2004) is typically fabricated using a *silicon-on-insulator* (SOI) structure. The SOI technique creates transistors on a thin top silicon layer that is electically insulated from the substrate which is either an insulator itself or possesses a thin insulating layer of silicon dioxide. There are basically two choices for backside illuminated SOI arrays. One method of forming this insulating layer is the Separation by Implantation of Oxygen (SIMOX) technique, which implants oxygen into a silicon wafer under intense heat. A second is to deposit silicon on an insulating substrate, typically sapphire. SOI structures have recently gone through a period of rapid development and large-scale production. This is primarily because the SOI structure can greatly reduce any capacitance between the silicon circuitry and the substrate, thus increasing the transistor switching speed and permitting large increases in communication band width. This high speed capability has become extremely important for use in the high frequency circuits of cell phones and for satisfying the high bandwidth requirements of HDTV. High frequency capabilities are not necessary for retinal prosthesis, however, the intense commercialization of SOI has made it a viable and affordable technology.

An alternative to using an external camera or an imaging array positioned near the retina is to mount a miniature camera at the front of the eye (Hauer, 2007). This approach would require the removal of the natural lens and possibly other anterior elements of the eye. The design and fabrication of such a miniature camera could be accomplished with existing technologies, but the actual implantation and mounting has no precedence and could be problematic. The advantage is that the camera could then be directly hardwired to a retinal stimulation array and there is no high frequency RF transmission requirement.

3.4.6 *What techniques can be used for supplying wireless power to the system and how efficient are they?*

Supplying power to a retinal prosthesis is a major challenge because the requirements are quite demanding in terms of high power and limited space. In general biomedical implants such as cardiac pacemakers have traditionally used non-rechareable batteries that last 7-10 years (Gerrish et al., 2005).

The level of power required by a retinal prosthesis system makes a large storage battery awkward because of the limited intraocular space available. As a comparison, cardiac pacemakers are typically rated around 2.0 *A-hrs* (operating at slightly more than 2 volts) and have a volume of less than 8 cm^3 (ironically about the same volume as the intraocular region of an adult eye). A high resolution retinal prosthesis most likely will require constant power in the range of 1-10 *mW*. This implies that a retinal prosthesis device using a *Li*-ion battery the size of the human eye would be depleted in roughly 1-6 months. As alternatives, there are other techniques for supplying power from an external source to an implanted prosthesis. These include electromagnetic inductive coupling, photovoltaic optical conversion, and thermoelectric devices that exploit temperature differences (Weiland et al., 2005). Of these possible options, electromagnetic inductive coupling appears to be the most practical (Margalit et al., 2002).

3.4.7 *What image processing is necessary before stimulating the retina and how can it be accomplished?*

The basic operating within a diseased retina in logical spatial patterns that will create image perception in the visual cortex. The point of any neural prosthetic intervention should be as close as possible to the diseased neurons. For the case of an epiretinal prosthesis that is designed to stimulate the ganglion cells, there is an absence of image processing that would normally have occurred in the earlier retinal layers. The loss of natural retinal image processing poses two fundamental problems in terms of developing a retinal prosthesis system, namely determining what image processing was lost and how can it be replaced. Regarding the former, research in the neuroscience community is still incomplete as to how the retina processes visual images. Another important aspect of this question is the degree to which the visual pathways at the higher levels will naturally adapt to artificial stimulation and learn to process that information. On the other hand, if preprocessing of the input image is required, then what algorithms are needed and where can the supporting electronic image processing be done.

The development of successful image processing methods for a retinal prosthesis system should logically begin with a complete understanding of the visual system. This would include the visual pathways, of which there are several that functionally branch apart in the retina and propagate through the lateral geniculate nucleus and then to the visual cortex. To fully understand these pathways, one must learn the hierarchy of image processing functions performed as information proceeds from the photoreceptors through the retina and into the higher processing levels of the brain.

Unfortunately, a complete understanding of the visual pathways and their image processing functions does not exist at this time. Nevertheless, many interesting research results can be used collectively to construct a general representation of information flow and processing in the human visual system. Because the retina is at the beginning of the visual system and very accessible, it has been extensively studied and some models of retinal processing have been conjectured (Field and Chichilnisky, 2007; Kolb, 1994; Jacobs and Werblin, 1998).

The retina is a highly complex biological system that has been extensively studied over the past century. Nevertheless, there are still many unknowns regarding the anatomy, pharmacology, and flow of information. The field has attracted many renowned biologists, and a full description of this topic is beyond the scope of this paper. Image information is converted from photons into neural signals by the photoreceptors (either rods or three types of cones). The image information flows through the retina in a synchronous, parallel manner through as many as 10 types of bipolar cells and finally to the ganglion cells, of which there may be 20 to 25 types. The signals from the ganglion cell bodies flow through their output axons, which converge to form the optic nerve that channels the signals on to higher processing levels in the brain.

The image information goes through a number of transformations before leaving the retina. Some of this processing is spatial in nature and is performed predominantly by the intermediate cell layers containing the horizontal cells and the amacrine cells (see Fig. 3.2). Mathematically, one of the processing functions performed by these lateral layers of cells can generally be represented as a spatial convolution. Another form of processing that occurs is temporal in nature. Specifically, as information flows directly from layer to layer, the individual cells perform adaptive processing functions. For example, the photoreceptors adapt their response to the ambient light levels, and the bipolar cells may perform temporal filtering. Ganglion cells receive input processed by the previous layers and generate coded pulses that are transmitted through the optic nerve to the higher visual processing centers.

Depending upon where along the pathway a retinal prosthesis system stimulates neural cells, neuroscientists hope to develop image processing algorithms that can be applied to the incoming image. For example, assume an array stimulates ganglion cells, than it may not be desirable to stimulate these cells with the raw image. Instead, the stimulating image should be like that processed and transmitted by the photoreceptors and earlier layers in the retinal processing pathway. Regardless of our knowledge of the visual system, it will not be easy to develop artificial stimulation for the blind that completely replicates those natural processes that occur in healthy, functioning, retina. It needs to be clear from the outset that our ability to understand this processing and substitute for it in blind subjects will be quite limited. However, as has been the case with cochlear prosthesis devices, even a less than optimal stimulation capability can be successful since the human brain is highly adaptable.

3.5 Advanced Technologies for High Resolution Devices

A retinal prosthesis device presents a unique design challenge: how to electrically stimulation neurons on the curved retinal surface? More specifically, the challenge is to fabricate a highly dense electrode arrays on a spherical surface. The exact proximity of the electrodes to the retina is important because increased distance requires increased stimulation charge and reduces visual acuity due to charge dispersion. Even flexible substrates, such as polyamide, which can flex naturally into a cylindrical shape do not readily transform into a spherical shape. From an advanced electronics perspective, it would be highly advantageous to use standard silicon microelectronics as an interface to neural tissue. The problem becomes clear: how to bridge the gap between a flat silicon chip and a curved retina. This section discusses advanced technologies that provide unique geometries, structures, and materials for future retinal prosthesis systems.

One basic requirement for a stimulator array is to provide a conformal fit against an adult human retina that has a nominal radius of curvature of approximately 12 *mm*. If the fit is not conformal, then two problems immediately arise, increased electrode current is needed to activate neurons, and there will be a loss of visual acuity proportional to the dispersion of the electrical current across the retina. The neuron stimulation threshold in terms of current density is dependent on distance because the current, moving from an electrode toward the retinal surface, will disperse with something like an inverse squared law. The resolution is lost because the same electrical current dispersion will cause a blurring effect.

A comparison of two early studies of human retinal stimulation shows that reduced distance between the electrode and the retina may reduce thresholds. In one study a gold weight fixation method was used with arrays of electrodes of 100μm or 400μm diameters (Rizzo et al., 2003). They found that the majority of the reported thresholds were lower than in a study using a handheld electrode more distant from the retina (Humayun et al., 1996), 0.28–2.8 mC/cm2 vs. 0.16–80 mC/cm2 respectively. Even within the study by Rizzo et al., they found lower thresholds in general for a smaller, weighted 100 micron diameter electrode versus a 250 micron hand held electrode, 50μA versus 500μA. A seemingly contrary position is taken in a recent paper by Mahadevappa et al. (2005), which suggests that the distance from the retina is not a factor in thresholds in practice until the distance is greater than 500 μm. Analysis by Palanker et al. (2005) indicates that this would likely be the case for a larger 400 μm electrode studied by Mahadevappa et al. (2005). However, 400μm electrodes will not result in high resolution retinal prostheses. The smaller electrodes required for a high resolution retinal prosthesis will require close contact.

3.5.1 *Flexible electrode designs*

Many of the research groups developing retinal prostheses use metal electrode disks embedded in polyamide, parylene-C, polydimethylsiloxane or similar materials as electrode arrays. The designs of most devices using flexible materials are placed directly against the retina. The limitation of this design is that a dedicated lead is required to connect each electrode back to the control electronics. This will reduce the density of the electrodes because of space limitations and routing complications. Most systems using flexible electrode arrays are currently configured with less than 100 electrodes. In fact, the four groups described in Section IV above have used flexible substrates with fewer than 30 electrodes per array. Using the latest technology DRC Metrigraphics Inc. specifies 5 microns as the smallest lead width and spacing between electrical leads to achieve a reliable cable. Therefore, each line requires 10 microns which implies that the limit for a 3mm wide polyamide cable would be 300 lines. This is far fewer than the thousands required for reading and face recognition. Layering signal lines is possible, but could create capacitive coupling problems and reduce polyamide array flexibility.

Polyamide and other flexible electrodes are formed using standardized methods as shown in Fig. 3.5 (Stieglitz et al., 2004). The first step is to spin a layer of polyamide (or similar material) onto a solid substrate such as a silicon wafer and cure it in an oven. In some facilities, large pre-fabricated sheets of polyamide are used instead. The thickness of the base layer can vary but 5 to 15 μm is typical. The next step is to deposit a layer of metal, typically sputtered gold, to act as the interconnections. Lift-off technology is used to pattern the interconnections and features in a photoresist and remove excess gold to reveal the desired pattern.

An additional metallization step to add patterned biocompatible electrode materials such as platinum or iridium may be performed if those metals have not been used as the base metal. A second layer of polyamide is spun to provide insulation of the metal features. In some cases before the second layer of polyamide is added, a layer of silicon nitride is used to improve impedance. Sputtered and wet etched aluminum can then be used as a mask to allow the selective reactive ion etching of the polyamide to reveal windows to the electrodes and other polyamide device features.

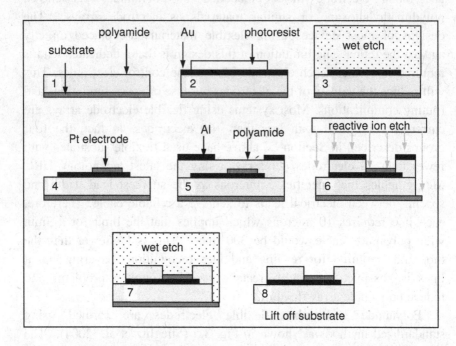

Figure 3.5. Steps to fabricate polyamide electrode arrays and cables. Polyamide is spun onto a substrate and gold and/or other metals are patterned on (1,2,3,4). After a second layer of polyamide is spun onto the device, aluminum is patterned as a mask to block the reactive ion etch of polyamide in selected areas (5,6). A thin wet etch removes the Al (7). Finally the device is lifted off the substrate (8).

The Tubingen, IIP and Boston VA groups all use variations of polyamide with metal traces leading to openings in the top layer polyamide to form the electrode sites (see Fig. 3.6). The Tubingen group has fabricated a device with 16 electrodes on polyamide (Gekeler and Zrenner, 2005). Their device is for subretinal implantation and the active area covers approximately 1mm x 1mm. The Boston VA group has a number of designs for both epiretinal and subretinal implantation - their subretinal array is similar to the Tubingen group. They have the ability to make their electrode array from either polyamide or parylene-C and have reported results of a device that has 25 electrodes in an 1mm x 1mm array (Yamauchi et al., 1992). The IMI group also uses a flat polyamide array with exposed electrodes to connect their electronics to the retina (Hornig et al., 2005). The device, as with the Tubingen and Boston VA groups has a portion of the polyamide which acts as a cable to transmit current laterally from the electronics before directing current into the retina. The IIP device is different in that they plan to create an epiretinal device.

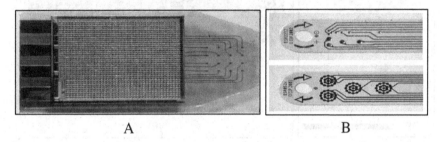

A   B

Figure 3.6. Three examples of polyamide arrays/cables used for prototype retinal prostheses. A) The Tubingen group device with array attached. B) Two test versions of the IIP device.

Two other unique electrode designs that are also being developed using MEMS fabrication methods to achieve close approximation to the retina as shown in Fig. 3.7. A design of the Boston VA group, in collaboration with the Cornell Nanofabrication Institute and MIT, involves a flexible epiretinal array which can unfold when inserted into the eye through a narrow incision. The design allows for a large area of retina (9mm diameter) to be covered by a device that could be implanted through a 3mm incision in the sclera (incisions in the sclera are typically limited to approximately 5mm). In addition, inflatable channels within the device would gently press the arms of the device and the electrodes against the retina to improve contact (Shire et al., 2001). The Stanford/Palanker group has a different approach. They hope to bring the retina closer to the electrodes by creating chambers in a multilayer polyamide membrane. Their experimental results from *in vitro* cultures and *in vivo* 9 day implantations show that the outer retinal cells will migrate into the recesses of the subretinal device (Palanker et al., 2005).

Their concept for a subretinal device would require lower current levels because of the close approximation of the electrodes and the cells. Some issues remain such as how well the cells will survive in the recesses.

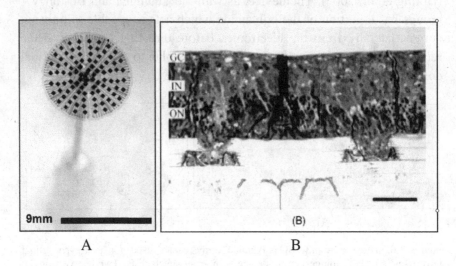

A   B

Figure 3.7. MEMS type flexible devices with 3 dimensional structure. (A) Boston VA group inflatable array with 100 electrodes supported by a cannula (image courtesy of D. Shire). (B) Stanford/Palankar recessed holes design showing migrated retina cells (scale bar is 50 μm).

Two other flexible designs use a silicon rubber, or PDMS (polydimethylsiloxane), to create retinal electrode arrays as shown in Fig. 3.8. Lawrence Livermore National Laboratory has a PDMS device which is very similar to the flat polyamide devices with gold traces described above (Güven et al., 2006). As with most polyamide designs, this structure allows for a cylindrical curvature but not a spherical curvature to fit the retina correctly. The thin PDMS can be distorted towards a spherical curvature but then the electrodes will not have regular contact with the retina due to folds. Another difference from the previous polyamide devices is the addition of a thicker PDMS "rib" which extends along the cable portion of the device for additional support.

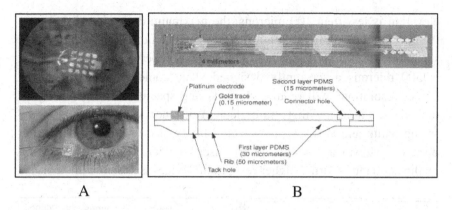

Figure 3.8. Two flexible PDMS (Polydimethylsiloxane) devices. (A) Doheny/Second Sight 16 electrode device is a thick PDMS array molded to have a curvature to fit the retina. (B) A polyamide like electrode array developed at the Lawrence Livermore National Laboratory.

Second Sight, Inc has a device made of silicon rubber which is currently under clinical testing by Doheny Eye Institute (Mahadevappa et al., 2005). This device has 16 electrodes, 500µm in diameter embedded in the silicon rubber and a continuous cable which contains the wire leads connecting to the current source. Unlike flat polyamide or PDMS devices the silicon is molded into a spherical geometry to fit the surface of the retina and make good contact to reduce thresholds. The difficulty in this design is how to scale up to hundreds or thousands of electrodes.

To meet the challenge of configuring a device with a spherical curvature that conforms to the retina, researchers at Sandia National Laboratory have a developed a unique MEMS structure (Ameri et al., 2005; Okandan et al., 2003a,b). Their design incorporates springs that act as electrode posts which "float" as shown in Fig. 3.9. The springs assembly is made from micromachined silicon which is implemented as a 5mm x 5mm array with 81 electrodes. They reported a few minor problems with inserting the device through the scleral incision. Related issues include positioning all the electrodes in contact with the retina and avoiding damage to the electrode posts. Some problems were resolved by developing an insertion sleeve. The obvious advantage of this device is that it can match the curvature of any retina if the difference in surface elevation is less than 100 microns, the maximum deflection distance of the springs. A high resolution device would require electrodes with a separation of 50 microns or less. The separation between their electrodes is 500 microns as currently designed. This could be problematic, as higher resolutions will require closer spring spacing. The geometry of their device indicates that the deflection distance is proportional to the spring width and closer spacing would likely lead to reduced deflection distance. However, as the device uses standard MEMS fabrication methods, manufacturing higher resolution devices is possible in theory.

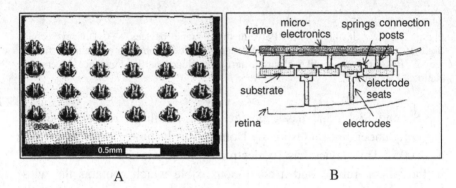

A   B

Figure 3.9. SEM image of the Sandia device (A) and a cross sectional diagram of the same (B). In the SEM picture, the white bar is 500 microns.

3.5.2 Rigid electrode designs

One of the earliest rigid designs is that of Optobionics, Inc. (see Fig. 3.10) (Chow et al., 2004). The prosthesis is a subretinal 25 μm thick silicon chip with 5000 photodiode electrodes. The device is flat and non-conforming to the shape of the retina. However, as the device is implanted subretinally some soft deformation of the retina may occur. The device is 2mm in diameter, which implies that geometrically there is a 30 μm distance from the edges of the device to the retina. This distance may be small enough that the increase in current and loss of resolution may be minimal. The Optobionics device suggests that smaller devices may be a way to approximate a conformal fit to the shape of the retina.

Of course, the field of view for such a small device is very limited; in this case, less than six degrees.

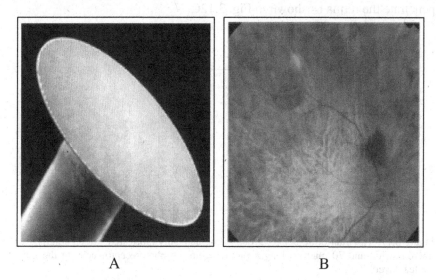

A   B

Figure 3.10. The Optobionics retinal prosthesis. The 2mm silicon disk (A) is placed behind the retina (B).

Two groups working at Stanford have produced rigid devices with protruding electrode columns. An interesting rigid design developed by the Stanford/Harris group (Wang et al., 2006) involves an array of carbon nanotube (CNT) columns. The columns are grown on a rigid silicon substrate. The CNT electrode array is designed to penetrate the retina to allow for close contacted between the retinal neurons and the electrodes. The carbon nanotube columns have some degree of flexibility, which should cause less damage as they penetrate the retina. The design makes some accommodation to the curvature of the retina in that electrodes at the edges of the device could penetrate slightly into the retina to allow center electrodes to get closer to the retina. The columns have been grown to heights of 100 µm, at a height:width aspect ratio of 4:1.

The Stanford/Palanker group has a concept for a pillared electrode array made on a lighographically fabricated silicon wafer (see Fig. 3.11) (Palanker et al., 2005). The device would be 3mm in diameter. They implanted a prototype device with 10 micron columns in a RCS rat for 15 days. Their experiment demonstrated the ability of the columns to penetrate the retina as shown in Fig. 3.12C.

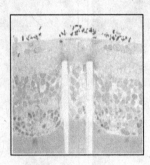

Figure 3.11. The Stanford/Palanker group lithographically fabricated silicon columns 10 microns wide and 70 microns long penetrate from the photoreceptor cells to the inner nuclear layer.

The Naval Research Laboratory has developed a microwire glass electrode array that has embedded electrodes with 5 μm diameters in a hexagonal configuration with 7.5 μm center-to-center spacing as shown in Fig. 3.12, (Johnson et al., 2002; Panigrahi et al., 2005; Scribner et al., 2007; Johnson et al., 2007). The electrode array was designed so that it could be hybridized to a silicon microelectronic integrated circuit with 3200 unit cells (or pixels). The test device is 6mm long and 3mm wide and designed to operate as an epiretinal device for use in acute experiments in an operating room environment. The microwire glass can be polished to a curved surface, thus obtaining a conformal fit against the retina. The microwire glass array acts as a bridge material spanning the gap between the flat silicon chip and the spherical shape of the retina. The microwires conduct the stimulus currents from the microelectronic device to the retina, while the glass matrix material electrically insulates each microwire from the others.

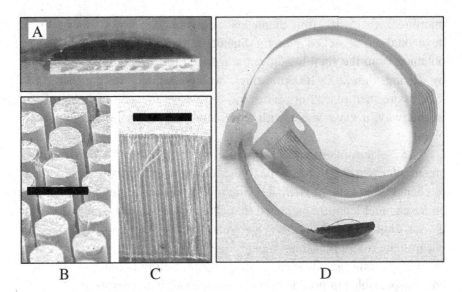

Figure 3.12. The NRL stimulation array developed for acute testing: A) The side view of a partially encapsulated device showing the curvature of the device surface; B) A high magnification SEM of the 5.5 µm microwires (bar is 10µm); C) A low magnification SEM of the side of the microwire glass - note a few microwires can be seen as bent away from the side wall as a result of the cleaving process (bar is 100µm); D) the completed retinal prosthesis - the surgical sponge on the polyamide cable is used to reduce leakage of saline during the acute implant procedure.

Microchannel glass electrodes arrays are fabricated using a starting material known as *microchannel plates* which are used extensively as compact electron multiplier tubes in particle and photon detection systems. An acetic acid-etchable glass rod, nominally one inch in diameter and four inches in length, is inserted into a non-acetic acid-etchable glass tube. This pairing of dissimilar glasses is *drawn* at an elevated temperature into a fiber of smaller diameter. Several thousand of these fibers are then cut and stacked in a hexagonal-close-packed arrangement, yielding a hexagonal-shaped bundle that is several inches in length. This bundle is subsequently drawn at an elevated temperature, fusing the individual composite fibers together while reducing the overall bundle diameter to that of a fiber. The process can be repeated several times until the desired dimensions are obtained. At this stage, the fibers are hexagonal-shaped and contain a fine structure of several thousand micron-sized (5–10 μm diameter) acid-etchable glass fibers in a hexagonal-close-packed pattern. Standard microchannel plate glass is obtained from the final bundle (now referred to as a boule) at this point by slicing thin 200–1000μm thick wafers, which are polished flat. Wafers are then placed in acetic acid to remove the acid-etchable glass. In this way, a glass wafer with extremely uniform, hollow channels is obtained.

Next, electroplating is performed to fill the channels with a metal to create microwires. With a typical aspect ratio of 200:1 (channel length to channel diameter) it is challenging to electroplate a metal through the entire channel length. One metal that electroplates easily is nickel, but it is not biocompatible as an electrode. However, it is possible to encapsulate the protruding nickel microwires with a layer of gold, platinum or other suitable electrode material. Solid platinum microwires are also possible but producibility issues are still being resolved.

Microwire glass electrodes used for eventual *in vivo* testing with the NRL stimulation array will have one side of the electrode curved to create a spherical surface to allow positioning of the high-density electrode array in extremely close approximation to the retinal tissue. The radius of curvature is nominally 12.7 mm to provide a conformal fit against the retina. The NRL device could be custom made with diamond turning or other polishing methods standard in the optics industry, to match any curvature of the patient's retina as measured by a profilometry device.

The polishing process will create slightly recessed microwires with respect to the curved microwire glass surface because the metal is softer than the glass. Therefore, further processing is necessary to create electrodes that protrude slightly above the curved surface. This can be accomplished by applying a chemical etch to the surface that removes several microns of glass as shown in Fig. 3.12b. The duration of this etching step can be increased to provide longer protrusions of microwires, which reduce the electrode impedance by increasing the metal microwire surface area in contact with the saline environment of the eye.

3.5.3 *Supporting microelectronics*

In all likelihood, any high resolution retinal prosthesis will include microelectronics based on silicon CMOS technology (Gerrish et al., 2005). CMOS is ideally suited to ultra-low power applications and has a vast commercial technology base which has been intensely developed over the past 50 years. Commercial digital electronics strive for advantages such as speed and low cost memory, neither of which of is necessary for a retinal prosthesis device. However, the evolution of microelectronics has followed Moore's law in terms of more densely packed circuitry leading to greater device complexity and expanding functionality. For high resolution retinal prosthesis, future trends will be smaller electrodes and pixels on the size of neurons or smaller with more on-chip image processing.

For future high resolution, large area retinal prosthesis devices, a major challenge will be achieving low power dissipation while at the same time providing adequate electrical current to simulate retinal neurons. For example, it has been argued that other neural prosthesis applications such as cochlear implants require voltage supplies as high as 14 Volts (Weiland et al., 2005) which may not be compatible with many advanced microelectronic fabrication processes. For example, submicron CMOS design rules typically require voltages of approximately 1 Volt. However, research at the Salk Institute indicates that threshold currents can be as low as 1 µA for dense electrode arrays with small electrodes in close proximity to the retinal ganglion cells (Sekirnjak et al., 2008). Recent development of prototype high density electrode arrays using CMOS electronics hybridized to curved microwire glass arrays as (as discussed above) has shown that voltages of a few hundred millivolts can drive biphasic current pulses of 1 µA per pixel with an arrays size of 80 x 40 array (Scribner et al., 2007). This same research also demonstrated that thermal energy from the microelectronics can be kept to a safe level with respect to heating the retina (European standards require that the surface of an implant not exceed body temperature by more than 1 degree C).

3.5.4 *Integration and packaging*

An important requirement for an implantable retinal prosthesis will be encapsulation to protect all microelectronics from corrosive biological fluids. In the case of related prosthetic devices such as pacemakers, all microelectronics and batteries are packaged and sealed in metal cans. Considering that no FDA-approved designs exist for a commercial retinal prosthesis device, it is not possible to state what techniques will be used to achieve reliable encapsulation. Nevertheless, it is expected that any system design with a large number of electrical feed-throughs will be prone to failures. Furthermore, many types of welding and sealants tend to leak over time, are not biocompatible, and are expensive (Weiland et al., 2005).

An alternative approach to hermetic packaging of electronics in a hard shell case is to simply coat the electronics with thin film of protective material. Weiland has discussed the two categories of thin film encapsulations, organic and inorganic materials (Weiland et al., 2005). Organic materials include epoxies, silicones, and polymers. These are generally flexible and easy to deposit, but not reliable over the long time periods required by chronic implants. Inorganic materials that are used to overcoat silicon microelectronics include silicon nitride, silicon carbide, and polycrystalline diamond. The major advantage of these inorganic films is that the packaged microelectronics is no larger than the size of the original chip. A major consideration is choosing a thin film process is that it must not exceed any temperature constraints of the original microelectronics – for example, some diamond coating can require deposition temperatures of several hundred degrees C.

3.6 Conclusions

The hope of restoring vision to the blind is now believed to be a real possibility using neural prosthetics. However, many technical problems remain and many engineering issues must be resolved before complete clinical success is achieved. Not the least of these problems will be obtaining a better understanding of the visual pathways and the plasticity of the nervous system with respect to artificial electrical stimulation.

Other issues that will require great attention are long term biocompatibility and reliability - devices will be implanted and expected to function without degradation for decades. Assuming that these basic challenges are met, the demand for high resolution devices will grow. Then biomedical engineers will employ advanced technologies, like those discussed above, to develop retinal prosthesis devices that will allow blind patients to perform normal tasks like reading and facial recognition.

Ultimately, the true measure of success will be the acceptance of retinal prosthesis by the blind community. Hopefully this will parallel the success of the cochlear implant that, although initially slow, continues to grow exponentially each year and is now a fully commercialized medical product.

3.7 References

Ameri, H., Guven, D. and Freda, R. (2005). Surgical Implantation of Epiretinal Prosthesis With Spring–Mounted Electrodes. *Invest. Ophthalmol. Vis. Sci*, pg. 46.

Bebek, C. J. et al. (2004). Development of fully depleted back-illuminated charge-coupled devices. In *Proceedings of SPIE*. pp. 140-150.

Blanche, T. J. et al. (2005). Polytrodes: High-Density Silicon Electrode Arrays for Large-Scale Multiunit Recording. *J. Neurophysiol*, 93(5), pp. 2987-3000.

Brindley, G. S. (1965). The number of information channels needed for efficient reading. *J Physiol*, 177, pg. 44.

Bullara, L. et al. (1983). A microelectrode for delivery of defined charge densities. *Journal of Neuroscience Methods*, 9(1), pp. 15-21.

Cha, K., Horch, K. and Normann, R. A., (1992). Simulation of a phosphene-based visual field: Visual acuity in a pixelized vision system. *Annals of Biomedical Engineering*, 20(4), pp. 439-449.

Chow, A. Y. et al. (2004). The Artificial Silicon Retina Microchip for the Treatment of Vision Loss From Retinitis Pigmentosa. *Arch. Ophthalmol.*, 122(4), pp. 460-469.

Chyu, K. and Shah, P.K., 2007. Choking off Plaque Neovascularity: A Promising Atheroprotective Strategy or A Double-Edged Sword? *Arterioscler. Thromb. Vasc. Biol.*, 27(5), pp. 993-995.

Cogan, S. F. et al. (2004). Over-pulsing degrades activated iridium oxide films used for intracortical neural stimulation. *Journal of Neuroscience Methods*, 137(2), pp. 141-150.

Culurciello, E. and Andreou, A. G. (2004). 16/spl times/16 pixel silicon on sapphire CMOS digital pixel photosensor array. *Electronics Letters*, 40(1), pp. 66-68.

Dagnelie, G. et al. (2006). Paragraph Text Reading Using a Pixelized Prosthetic Vision Simulator: Parameter Dependence and Task Learning in Free-Viewing Conditions. *Invest. Ophthalmol. Vis. Sci.*, 47(3), pp. 1241-1250.

Fish, A., Yadid-Pecht, O. and Culurciello, E. (2007). Responsivity of Gated Photodiode in SOS Technology. *Sensors, 2007 IEEE*, pp. 527-530.

Friedman, D. (2002). Vision problems in the US. National Eye Institute Report

Field, G. D. and Chichilnisky, E. J. (2007). Information Processing in the Primate Retina: Circuitry and Coding. Available at: http://arjournals.annualreviews.org/doi/abs/10.1146/annurev.neuro.30.051606.0 94252 [Accessed December 8, 2008].

Gekeler, F. and Zrenner, E. (2005). Status of the subretinal implant project. An overview. *Ophthalmologe*, 102(10), pp. 941-949.

Gekeler, F. et al. (2007). Compound subretinal prostheses with extra-ocular parts designed for human trials: successful long-term implantation in pigs. *Graefe's Archive for Clinical and Experimental Ophthalmology*, 245(2), pp. 230-241.

Gerrish, P. et al. (2005). Challenges and constraints in designing implantable medical ICs. *IEEE Transactions on Device and Materials Reliability*, 5(3), pp. 435-444.

Grumet, A. E., Wyatt J. L., and Rizzo, J. F. (2000). Multi-electrode stimulation and recording in the isolated retina. *Journal of Neuroscience Methods*, 101(1), pp. 31-42.

Guenther, E. et al., (1999). Long-term survival of retinal cell cultures on retinal implant materials. *Vision Research*, 39(24), pp. 3988-3994.

Güven, D. et al. (2006). Implantation of an inactive epiretinal poly (dimethyl siloxane) electrode array in dogs. *Experimental Eye Research*, 82(1), pp. 81-90.

Heetderks, W. (1988). RF powering of millimeter- and submillimeter-sized neural prosthetic implants. *IEEE Trans. Biomed. Engin.*, 35(5), pp. 323-327.

Hetke, J. et al. (1994). Silicon ribbon cables for chronically implantable microelectrode arrays. *IEEE Trans. Biomed. Engin.*, 41(4), pp. 314-321.

Hetling, J. R. and Baig-Silva, M. S. (2004). Neural prostheses for vision: Designing a functional interface with retinal neurons. *Neurological Research*, 26(1), pp. 21-34.

Hornig, R. et al. (2005). A method and technical equipment for an acute human trial to evaluate retinal implant technology. *J. Neural. Eng.*, 2(1), pp. S129-S134.

Humayun, M. S. et al. (1999). Pattern electrical stimulation of the human retina. *Vision Research*, 39(15), pp. 2569-2576.

Humayun, M. S. et al. (1996). Visual perception elicited by electrical stimulation of retina in blind humans. *Archives of Ophthalmology*, 114(1), pp. 40-46.

Ito, A. et al. (2005). Construction and delivery of tissue-engineered human retinal pigment epithelial cell sheets, using magnetite nanoparticles and magnetic force. *Tissue Engineering*, 11(3-4), pp. 489-496.

Jacobs, A. L. and Werblin, F. S. (1998). Spatiotemporal Patterns at the Retinal Output, *J. Neurophysiol.*, 80, pp. 447-451.

Janders, M. et al. (1996). Novel thin film titanium nitride micro-electrodes with excellentcharge transfer capability for cell stimulation and sensing applications. In *Engineering in Medicine and Biology Society, 1996. Bridging Disciplines for*

Biomedicine. Proceedings of the 18th Annual International Conference of the IEEE, pp. 245-247.

Jensen, R. J. and Rizzo, J. F. (2006). Thresholds for activation of rabbit retinal ganglion cells with a subretinal electrode. *Experimental Eye Research*, 83(2), pp. 367-373.

Johnson, L. et al. (2007). Impedance-based retinal contact imaging as an aid for the placement of high resolution epiretinal prostheses. *Journal of Neural Engineering*, 4(1), pp. S17-S23.

Johnson, L. J. et al. (2002). Low Charge Density Stimulation Of Isolated Retina With Microchannel Glass Electrodes. *Invest. Ophthalmol. Vis Sci.*, 43, ARVO E-Abstract, pg. 4480.

Kolb, H. (1994). The architecture of functional neural circuits in the vertebrate retina. Invest. Ophthal. Vis Sci., 35(5), pp. 2385-2404.

Kubota, A. et al. (2006). Transplantable retinal pigment epithelial cell sheets for tissue engineering. *Biomaterials*, 27(19), pp. 3639-3644.

Laing, P. G., Ferguson Jr, A. B. and Hodge, E. S. (1967). Tissue reaction in rabbit muscle exposed to metallic implants. *J Biomed Mater Res*, 1(1), pp. 135-49.

Mahadevappa, M. et al. (2005). Perceptual thresholds and electrode impedance in three retinal prosthesis subjects. *IEEE Transactions on Neural Systems and Rehabilitation Engineering*, 13(2), pp. 201-206.

Majji, A. B. et al. (1999). Long-Term Histological and Electrophysiological Results of an Inactive Epiretinal Electrode Array Implantation in Dogs. *Investigative Ophthalmology and Visual Science*, 40(9), pp. 2073-2081.

Makhdoum, M. J. A., Snik, A. F. M. and van den Broek, P. (2007). Cochlear Implantation: A Review of the Literature and the Nijmegen Results. *The Journal of Laryngology and Otology*, 111(11), pp. 1008-1017.

Marc, R. E. et al. (2003). Neural remodeling in retinal degeneration. *Progress in Retinal and Eye Research*, 22(5), pp. 607-655.

Margalit, E. et al. (2000). Bioadhesives for intraocular use. *Retina*, 20(5), pg. 469.

Margalit, E. et al. (2002). Retinal Prosthesis for the Blind. *Survey of Ophthalmology*, 47(4), pp. 335-356.

McCreery, D. et al. (1990). Charge density and charge per phase as cofactors in neural injury induced by electrical stimulation. *IEEE Trans. Biomed. Engin.*, 37(10), pp. 996-1001.

McHardy, J. et al. (1980). Electrical stimulation with pt electrodes. IV. Factors influencing Pt dissolution in inorganic saline. *Biomaterials*, 1(3), pp. 129-134.

Okandan, M. et al. (2003a). MEMS conformal electrode array for retinal implant. In: *Transducers, 12th International Conference on Solid State Sensors, Actuators and Microsystems,* pp. 1643-1646.

Okandan, M. et al. (2003b). Micromachined conformal electrode array for retinal prosthesis application. In *Proceedings of SPIE*. pg. 45.

Palanker, D. et al. (2005). Design of a high-resolution optoelectronic retinal prosthesis. *J Neural Eng*, 2(1), pp. S105-S120.

Panigrahi, D. et al. (2005). *Surgical Approach and Initial Histological Results of an Implantable High Resolution Epiretinal Stimulation Array in the Porcine Model, Invest. Ophthalmol. Vis Sci.,* 46, ARVO E-Abstract, pg. 1532.

Peachey, N. S. and Chow, A. Y. (1999). Subretinal implantation of semiconductor-based photodiodes: progress and challenges. *Low Vision and Blindness: Research And Development*, 36(4), pp. 371-376.

Peterman, M. C., Bloom, D. M. et al. (2003). Localized Neurotransmitter Release for Use in a Prototype Retinal Interface. *Invest. Ophthalmol. Vis. Sci.*, 44(7), pp. 3144-3149.

Peterman, M. C., Mehenti, N. Z. et al. (2003). The Artificial Synapse Chip: A Flexible Retinal Interface Based on Directed Retinal Cell Growth and Neurotransmitter Stimulation. *Artificial Organs*, 27(11), pp. 975-985.

Peyman, G. et al. (1998). Subretinal semiconductor microphotodiode array. *Ophthalmic Surg Lasers*, 29(3), pp. 234-41.

Pudenz, R. H., Bullara, L. A., Dru, D. et al. (1975). Electrical stimulation of the brain II. Ei ects on blood barrier. *Surg. Neurol*, 4, pp. 265-270.

Pudenz, R. H., Bullara, L. A., Jacques, S. and Hambrecht, F. T. (1975). Electrical stimulation of the brain. III. The neural damage model. *Surg Neurol*, 4(4), pp. 389-400.

Pudenz, R. H., Bullara, L. A. and Talalla, A. (1975). Electrical stimulation of the brain. I. Electrodes and electrode arrays. *Surg Neurol*, 4(1), pp. 37-42.

Rattay, F. and Resatz, S. (2004). Effective electrode configuration for selective stimulation with inner eye prostheses. *IEEE Trans. Biomed. Engin.*, 51(9), pp. 1659-1664.

Rizzo, J. F. et al., (2001). Accuracy and reproducibility of percepts elicited by electrical stimulation of the retinas of blind and normal subjects. *Invest. Ophthalmol. Vis. Sci.*, 42, pg. 5045.

Rizzo, J. F. et al. (2003). Perceptual Efficacy of Electrical Stimulation of Human Retina with a Microelectrode Array during Short-Term Surgical Trials. *Invest. Ophthalmol. Vis. Sci.*, 44(12), pp. 5362-5369.

Robblee, L. and Rose, T. (1990). The Electrochemistry Of Electrical Stimulation. In *Engineering in Medicine and Biology Society, 1990., Proceedings of the Twelfth Annual International Conference of the IEEE.* pp. 1479-1480.

Robblee, L. and Rose, T. (1990). Electrochemical guidelines for selection of protocols. Agnew, W. F., and McCreery, D. B., eds., *Neural prostheses: fundamental studies,* Prentice Hall, Biophysics and Bioengineering Series, Englewood Cliffs, New Jersey, pp. 25-66.

Rose, T. and Robblee, L. (1990). Electrical stimulation with Pt electrodes. VIII. Electrochemically safe charge injection limits with 0.2 ms pulses (neuronal application). *IEEE Trans. Biomed. Engin.*, 37(11), pp. 1118-1120.

Scribner, D. et al. (2007). A Retinal Prosthesis Technology Based on CMOS Microelectronics and Microwire Glass Electrodes. *IEEE Transactions on Biomedical Circuits and Systems*, 1(1), pp. 73-84.

Sekirnjak, C. et al. (2008). High-resolution electrical stimulation of primate retina for epiretinal implant design. *The Journal of Neuroscience: The Official Journal of the Society for Neuroscience*, 28(17), pp. 4446-4456.

Shire, D., Rizzo, J. and Wyatt, J., 2001. *Chronically implantable retinal prosthesis*, US Patent 6,324,429.

Stieglitz, T., Schuettler, M. and Koch, K. P. (2004). Neural prostheses in clinical applications--trends from precision mechanics towards biomedical microsystems in neurological rehabilitation. *Biomed Tech (Berl)*, 49(4), pp. 72-77.

Suzuki, S. et al. (2004). Comparison of Electrical Stimulation Thresholds in Normal and Retinal Degenerated Mouse Retina. *Japanese Journal of Ophthalmology*, 48(4), pp. 345-349.

Troyk, P. and Schwan, M. (1992). Closed-loop class E transcutaneous power and data link for MicroImplants. *IEEE Trans. Biomed. Engin.*, 39(6), pp. 589-599.

Wang, K. et al. (2006). Neural stimulation with a carbon nanotube microelectrode array. *Nano. Lett.*, 6(9), pp. 2043-2048.

Weiland, J. D., Liu, W. and Humayun, M. S. (2005). Retinal Prosthesis. In: *Annual Review of Biomedical Engineering*, 7, 361-401.

Weiland, J. and Anderson, D. (2000). Chronic neural stimulation with thin-film, iridium oxide electrodes. *IEEE Trans. Biomed. Engin.*, 47(7), pp. 911-918.

Weiland, J., Anderson, D. and Humayun, M., (2002). In vitro electrical properties for iridium oxide versus titanium nitride stimulating electrodes. *IEEE Trans. Biomed. Engin.,* 49(12), pp. 1574-1579.

West, D. C. and Wolstencroft, J. H., 1983. Strength-duration characteristics of myelinated and non-myelinated bulbospinal axons in the cat spinal cord. *The Journal of Physiology*, 337(1), 37-50.

Winter, J. O. et al. (2008). Tissue engineering applied to the retinal prosthesis: Neurotrophin-eluting polymeric hydrogel coatings. *Materials Science and Engineering C*, 28(3), pp. 448-453.

Wise, K., Angel, H., and Starr, A. (1970). An integrated-circuit approach to extracellular microelectrodes. *IEEE Trans. Biomed. Engin.*, 17, pp. 238-246.

Yamauchi, Y. et al. (1992). Comparison of electrically evoked cortical potential thresholds generated with subretinal or suprachoroidal placement of a microelectrode array in the rabbit. *IEEE Trans. Biomed. Engin.*, 39, pp. 424-426.

Yanai, D. et al. (2007). Visual performance using a retinal prosthesis in three subjects with retinitis pigmentosa. *Amer. J. Ophthalmol.*, 143(5), pp. 820-827.

Zrenner, E. et al. (1999). Can subretinal microphotodiodes successfully replace degenerated photoreceptors? *Vis. Res.*, 39(15), pp. 2555-2567.

Zrenner, E., (2002). Will retinal implants restore vision? *Science*, 295(5557), pp. 1022-1025.

3.8 Review Questions

Q3.1 Retinitis Pigmentosa (RP) and Age-Related Macular Degeneration (AMD) are both serious eye diseases that progress with aging. Which disease is more prevalent? Which disease is more likely to lead to total blindness?

Q3.2 What are the implications for retinal prosthesis pertaining to each disease (RP and AMD)?

Q3.3 Retinal prosthesis devices are generally designed based on the following principle:

A. epiretinal devices are safer and less invasive than subretinal devices.

B. biocompatibility is a minor consideration because extensive testing in humans has shown this is not an issue.

C. in advanced stages of retinal diseases, the inner retinal layers of the retina remain viable for long periods of time - by stimulating these remaining functional retinal layers, it may be feasible to restore visual perception.

D. to design a prototype device, start with an exact replica of the cochlear implant and proceed from there.

Q3.4 True or false. A basic strategy for any neural prosthesis is to intervene in the central nervous system at a point that is closest to the damaged or diseased area. This is especially true for retinal prosthesis because it would also take advantage of the spatially organized neural structure of the retina.

Q3.5 From a systems engineering perspective there are many important considerations that need to be made when designing an epiretinal prosthesis device. Of the four statements below, which one is NOT true:

A. the distance between any electrode array and the retina should be minimized to reduce the electrical charge needed to cause cell firing and thus save power.

B. the distance between any electrode array and the retina should be minimized to reduce diffusion of electrical charge which would lead to "blurring" of the perceived image.

C. the minimum level of electrical charge needed to stimulate retinal cells and the maximum level of electrical charge that can cause cell damage differ by four orders of magnitude.

D. powering an intraocular retinal prosthesis device using electromagnetic inductive coupling is practical approach.

Q3.6 The development a high resolution retinal prosthesis device for the blind appears feasible, but the path forward is limited by which of the following:

A. new advances in microelectronics and nanotechnology research at universities and commercial companies.

B. the ability of scientists and biomedical engineers to learn from the cochlear implant.

C. the lack of knowledge of how the human eye-brain system will adapt to artificial electrical stimulation.

Chapter 4

Models of Myopia Development

Andrew J. Fiedler, B.S.[1], Jimo Liu, B.S.[1], George K. Hung, Ph.D.[1], and Kenneth J. Ciuffreda, O.D., Ph.D.[2]

[1] Dept. of Biomedical Engineering, Rutgers University
599 Taylor Rd., Piscataway, NJ 08854, USA
PH: 732-445-4500, ext. 6306; FX: 732-445-3753; EM: shoane@rci.rutgers.edu

[2] Dept. of Vision Sciences, State University of New York, State College of Optometry, 33 West 42nd St. New York, NY 10036; PH: (212) 780-5132, FX: 212-780-5124; EM: kciuffreda@sunyopt.edu

4.1 Introduction

As one of our most used senses, clear vision is a crucial prerequisite for our ability to observe and interact with our environments. In the United States, 25% of the adult population is affected by myopia (Sperduto, et al., 1983) and up to 75% of the adult population in Taiwan is affected (Lin et al., 1996). While refractive errors can be corrected by spectacles or surgery, both have drawbacks. Surgery is expensive (Grosvenor and Goss, 1999) and may lead to long term side effects while spectacles can limit vocational pursuits.

For years, scientists have been trying to understand the biological basis for the development of refractive errors. It has long been postulated that excessive "nearwork," or performing tasks up close to the eyes such as reading or computer work, is a significant contributory factor to the development of refractive errors. In addition, there is some evidence of a genetic basis for the development of refractive errors that compounds the influence of nearwork.

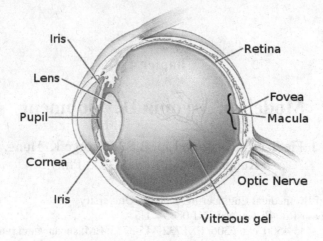

Figure 4.1. Basic anatomy of the eye. National Eye Institute.

Because there is an observed relation between nearwork and the development of refractive errors, the scientific community has devoted significant resources towards understanding and explaining this link. With a better understanding of the underlying mechanisms involved, the hope is that we can understand and mitigate the effects of nearwork in our technology and information-driven society, and thus improve our ocular health.

In this chapter, we survey the literature of previous models and theories relating to the development of refractive errors, examining them in light of new experimental results in the field of refractive error development. Building upon the previous literature, we also present a new homeomorphic, biomechanically-based model of the development of refractive errors.

4.1.1 *Basic anatomy of the eye*

The tunic of the eye is formed by three principle layers: the cornea and sclera, the choroid, and the retina. The sclera is a collagenous layer with elastic fibers and proteoglycans that provides structural integrity for the rest of the eye (Rada, et al., 1997 and Moses, et al., 1978). In the visible anterior portion, it is the "white" part of the eye. Experimental studies have shown that the composition and biomechanical properties of the sclera depend greatly on the visual environment (Rada, et al. 2000). For example, there is a decreased level of proteoglycans in the sclera after induced myopia (Rada, et al, 2000) or form-deprived vision (Troilo, et al., 1987), which weakens the sclera and results in vitreous cavity elongation.

The cornea is the transparent portion of the outer covering of the eye that is structurally continuous with the sclera. It consists of a superficial, thin layer of regenerating cells exposed to the environment, moistened by a tear film which helps to maintain its optical quality. Deeper, there are layers of collagen providing rigidity, and finally a layer of endothelium which provides the majority of glucose transport to the other corneal layers. The cornea is responsible for the majority of the refractive power of the eye (Ehlers and Hjortdal, 2006).

Below the sclera lies the pigmented choroid. The choroid has extensive vascularization and provides nourishment to the retina. It consists primarily of blood vessels, but also contains non-vascular layers where it meets the sclera and the retina. In addition to supplying blood to the retina, the choroid plays a role in the maintenance of intraocular pressure and temperature regulation (Kiilgaard and Jensen, 2006).

The inner-most layer of the eye is the light-sensitive retina. The retina is comprised of three layers of nerve cells: the photoreceptor, bipolar cell, and ganglion cell layers. Interposed between the photoreceptor and the bipolar cell layers are the horizontal cells, and interposed between the bipolar and ganglion cell layers are the amacrine cells. The photoreceptors respond to light input and send signals to the bipolar cells, which relay the signal to the ganglion cells. The ganglion cells produce action potentials, which are sent to higher visual centers via the optic nerve. The horizontal and amacrine cells modulate the signal through a center-surround mechanism to process contrast and change in contrast, respectively.

Light rays entering the eye pass through the two primary refractive regions, the cornea and lens, to reach the retina. If the light rays are not focused on the retina (e.g., focused beyond on the retina), the eye is able to adjust the power of the optical system through the accommodative reflex by changing the shape of the lens. It accomplishes this by contracting the ciliary muscles, which reduces the tension on the zonular fibers attached to the lens. This causes the lens to assume a more spherical shape, increasing the optical power of the eye to focus on the nearby object. However, excessive difference between the optics and the axial length of the eye, developed either genetically or through environmental experience, may cause more permanent changes in the shape of the eyeball that result in a refractive error.

4.1.2 *The development of refractive errors*

There are two main types of refractive error: hyperopia and myopia. Hyperopia, or farsightedness, occurs under the condition in which the combined optical power of the cornea and the un-accommodated lens is less than that needed for the axial length of eye, so that the light rays entering the eye are overly-diverged. Consequently, the image is focused beyond the retina. Conversely, myopia, or nearsightedness, occurs under the condition in which the combined optical power exceeds that required for the axial length of the eye. Light rays entering the eye are over-converged, and the image is focused in front of retina.

During normal ocular development, the growth of eye must closely match its optics to ensure that images are properly focused. If the eye grows too fast, the image will be focused in front of the retina. In this case, subsequent eye growth will tend to be slower (Bennet and Rabbetts, 1989; Grosvenor and Goss, 1998). If the eye grows too slowly, the image will be focused behind the retina, tending to increase the rate of eye growth. This continuous process that balances optical power and axial growth of the eye is called emmetropization (Yackle and Fitzgerald, 1999). Under repeated exposure to abnormal or more severe optical situations—such as excessive near-work, form deprivation, or defocus—the axial growth rate may exceed the capability of the system to attain an emmetropized state. This will result in the development of a refractive error.

By exposing animals to these abnormal optical situations, researchers have developed a better understanding of the environmental factors that can disrupt the emmetropization process and cause the development of myopia or hyperopia.

Two main mechanisms for which myopia has been induced in animals are form deprivation and optical defocus. Experimentalists can induce form deprivation by the application of translucent occluders over an animal's eyes or by surgically fusing the animal's eyelids closed. For example, using occlusion foils to induce form deprivation has been shown to produce axial elongation and myopia in monkeys (Hung and Smith, 1995). Similar results in chickens have been reported with occluders (Gottlieb et al, 1987 and Napper et al, 1995). In addition to occluders, researchers have shown that optical defocus can induce both myopic and hyperopic refractive errors. For example, optical defocus induced by spectacle lenses has been shown to affect the emmetropization process in young monkeys. For small, lens-induced refractive errors (with low powered lenses), ocular growth was able to compensate and minimize the refractive errors in monkeys while for larger refractive errors, the eyes were not able to compensate. Compensation took place for both negative lenses (myopic growth) and positive lenses (hyperopic growth) (Hung and Smith, 1995; Kee et al., 2007). Hyperopic refractive errors have also been induced in monkeys by less-severe diffusion (Bradley, et al, 1995) and by removing the crystalline lens (Wilson, et al, 1987).

Many different theories have been proposed to explain the emmetropization process as experimental evidence has added to knowledge of how eye growth responds to environmental stimulus. An early notion was that higher centers in the visual system were responsible for controlling emmetropization, but experimental results showed that the process is localized to the eye (Wilsoet and Pettigrew, 1988). And, since emmetropization is a local process, the challenge for modelers in the past has been to understand how the growth rates of various sections across the retina can synchronize and grow the eye into the correct shape. Modelers have long believed that the size of the blur circle on any given point in the retina provides necessary information to determine ocular growth, based on research showing that changing the amount of contrast with occluders or lenses affects the growth of the eye. (Smith and Hung, 2000; Gottlieb et al, 1987; and Hung, et al, 1995). However, the size of the blur circle alone does not provide sufficient information on the directionality of the refractive error (both an over- and under-focused image could have the same blur circle). Additionally, because no higher-level neural process is involved, there must be a mechanism that detects both magnitude and directionality of retinal defocus.

4.2 Previous Models of the Development of Refractive Errors

We examine a few models and theories developed to explain the development of refractive errors, and discuss how they address the concept of emmetropization. See Hung and Ciuffreda (2002) for a more detailed review.

4.2.1 *Modeling the time-course of refractive error development*

An early study by Medina and Fariza (1993) proposed a model which generated a simulated output curve to match the experimental refractive error development time-course (Fig. 4.2). The time constant, k, was selected to fit the refractive error vs. age curve. Although the model lacked homeomorphic correspondence with underlying physiology associated with refractive error development and emmetropization process, the curve fitting mechanism illustrated the exponential development of refractive error and inability of the eye to self correct in some cases.

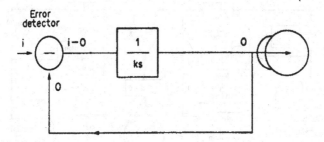

Figure 4.2. Feedback system proposed by Medina and Fariza (1993). The refractive error is controlled by a feedback mechanism where there is a command refraction level i, and an output refraction level O. The refractive error is i-O. Reprinted from Medina and Fariza (1993) with permission of Elsevier Science.

4.2.2 *Accommodative and retinal feedback loop model*

Schaeffel and Howland (1988) proposed a model in which two independent mechanisms were assumed to regulate eye growth (Fig. 4.3). The first mechanism, an accommodative loop, operated under crystalline lens optical power feedback; the second mechanism, the retinal loop operated under local retinal feedback without accommodation. The simulation results concluded that the accommodative feedback loop was responsible for the imposed-lens experimental results and also for the transient hyperopia observed after sectioning the optic nerve and lesioning of the Edinger – Westphal nucleus; on the other hand, the retinal feedback loop was responsible for form-deprivation myopia, myopia in restricted retinal areas, myopia after optic nerve section, and recovery from form-deprivation myopia with lesioning of the Edinger-Westphal nucleus. However, the model did not provide for the interaction that is significantly important between accommodation and retinal feedback.

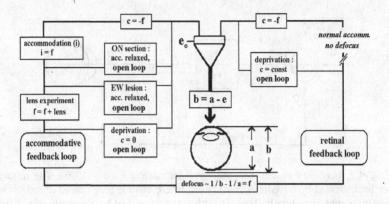

Figure 4.3. Model of refractive error developed by Schaeffel and Howland (1988). This model consists of two feedback loops; to the left is a feedback loop modeling the accommodative reflex. To the right is a loop modeling feedback from the retina. Symbols: a = control or reference axial length, b = current axial length, c = correction signal derived from either accommodative or retinal feedback, e0 = initial difference between control and current axial length, EW = Edinger-Westphal nucleus, f = refractive state of the eye, lens = imposed lens optical power, ON section = optic nerve section, i = average amount of accommodation due to hyperopic defocus. Reprinted from Schaeffel and Howland (1988) with permission of Optical Society of America.

4.3 The Incremental Retinal-Defocus Theory

While experimentalists have published numerous studies on stimuli that cause refractive errors (Troilo et al, 1987; Smith and Hung, 1999, 2000; Wildsoet and Collins, 2000), theorist have long striven to develop a unifying theory that explains the experimental results. One such theory is the Incremental Retinal-Defocus Theory (IRDT) developed by Hung and Ciuffreda (2000a-c).

The IRDT is based on two key insights. First, local retinal-defocus magnitude is critical in the development of environmentally-induced refractive error. Second, development of refractive error occurs during the growth and maturation period. These two key insights led to the main thrust of the IRDT, namely, that during the genetically-preprogrammed growth period, this naturally-occurring change in axial length provides the information to distinguish between hyperopic and myopic defocus, and in turn provides the directionality control for emmetropization.

The main connection between natural eye growth and environmentally-induced eye growth are the neuromodulators. These are neurochemicals, such as dopamine, serotonin, and neuropeptides, that act over long periods of time to modulate cellular processes. In the retina, neuromodulators are continually being released from certain retinal cells to serve as the baseline control of scleral matrix formation. Environmental factors such a change in retinal defocus provides a signal for modulation of neuromodulator release, with the direction of change in retinal-defocus magnitude determining the direction of change in neuromodulator release rate. The details of this process as proposed by the IRDT are provided below.

Hung and Cuiffreda (2000a-c) propose a feedback regulation mechanism whereby amacrine cells in the inner plexiform layer release dopamine onto horizontal cells in the outer plexiform layer, resulting in synaptic changes. This, in turn, alters the retinal sensitivity to center-surround input and shifts the steady-state sensitivity to retinal defocus. By this mechanism, the eye is sensitive to changes in retinal defocus without the need for a higher-center "memory" mechanism that stores the previous retinal defocus levels. Instead, this information is encoded in the retinal-neuron's normal response to change in retinal defocus.

Research has also shown that changes in neuromodulator release cause changes in the structure of the sclera via modulation of proteoglycan synthesis (Troilo, et al., 2006). An increase in proteoglycan synthesis results in greater structural integrity of the sclera. This reduces the sclera's growth rate in that region because greater structural integrity is able to resist the outward forces of internal ocular pressure.

Hung and Cuiffreda (2000a-c) theorize that genetics set a predetermined neuromodulator release rate that is associated with a normal growth rate (by setting a normal structural integrity of the sclera). In an increment of genetically predetermined growth, the visual environment determines the actual changes in blur circle magnitude, and through this, the changes in neuromodulator release rate.

For example, under normal conditions, there is no change in retinal-defocus magnitude, hence no change in neuromodulator release rate, no change in proteoglycan synthesis rate, and no change in scleral structural integrity. This results in normal axial growth (Fig. 4.4a). If a large minus lens is imposed in front of the eye during an increment of genetically-predetermined growth, there is a decrease in retinal-defocus magnitude, and hence a decrease in neuromodulator release rate, a decrease in proteoglycan synthesis rate, and a decrease in scleral structural integrity. This results in increased axial growth rate (Fig. 4.4b). If a large plus lens is imposed in front of the eye during an increment of genetically-predetermined growth, there is an increase in retinal-defocus magnitude, and hence an increase in neuromodulator release rate, an increase in proteoglycan synthesis rate, and an increase in scleral structural integrity. This results in a decrease in axial growth rate (Fig. 4.4c).

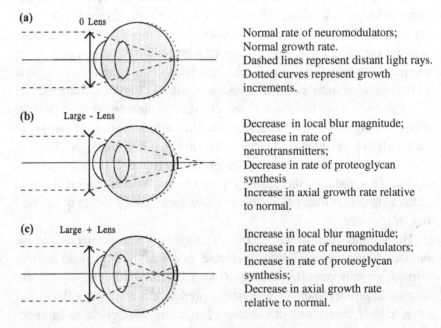

(a) 0 Lens

Normal rate of neuromodulators;
Normal growth rate.
Dashed lines represent distant light rays.
Dotted curves represent growth increments.

(b) Large - Lens

Decrease in local blur magnitude;
Decrease in rate of neurotransmitters;
Decrease in rate of proteoglycan synthesis
Increase in axial growth rate relative to normal.

(c) Large + Lens

Increase in local blur magnitude;
Increase in rate of neuromodulators;
Increase in rate of proteoglycan synthesis;
Decrease in axial growth rate relative to normal.

Figure 4.4. Effect of imposed lenses on axial growth rate. Reprined from Hung and. Ciuffreda (2000c), with permission of Bull. Math. Biol.

The IRDT theory can also be applied to recent experimental results on the effect of graded diffusers in monkeys (Smith and Hung, 2000). Although a diffuser can have complex optical effects (Smith and Atchison, 1997), its primary effect is to disperse or scatter the rays of light that are transmitted through the diffuser. This is schematically represented by cones of light emanating from the diffuser..For simplicity, only the two lines emanating from points at the outer boundaries of the diffuser are shown (Fig. 4.5a-c). The angle of the cone, representing the amount of dispersion, increases with increasing diffuser strength. The combined dispersion of these cones of light from a diffuser is to effectively converge at a point beyond the retina. With increasing diffuser strength, the point of convergence occurs further beyond the retina. The overall effect is an effective increase in hyperopic defocus with increasing diffuser strength. Therefore, based on the concept discussed above regarding hyperopic defocus (see Fig. 4.4b), the axial growth rate would be expected to increase with increasing strength of the diffuser. This is consistent with experimental results in animals (Smith and Hung, 2000).

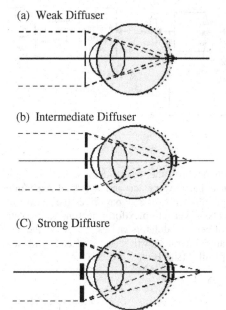

(a) Weak Diffuser

(b) Intermediate Diffuser

(C) Strong Diffusre

Figure 4.5. Note that the diffuser increases the dispersion of any ray of light, resulting in increasing amounts effective hyperopic defocus. Dashed lines represent distant light rays. Dotted curves represent growth increments. See text for details. Reprinted from Hung and Ciuffreda (2000c) with permission of Bull. Math. Biol.

4.3.1 *(Model 1) Matlab/Simulink quantitative model*

Hung and Ciuffreda (2002) presented a model of the IRDT as a MATLAB and Simulink program, shown as a conceptual block diagram in Figure 4.6. It is based on the principle that the magnitude of retinal defocus can be represented by the difference in center and surround excitation. A <u>change</u> in this signal, and thus a change in retinal-defocus magnitude, provides the requisite sign for modulating ocular growth. The sensitivity to local retinal-image contrast is maintained at a relatively constant level by means of feedback regulation of horizontal cell gain provided by the interplexiform neurons. This precludes the need for a "memory mechanism" (Norton, 1999) for storing information regarding the immediately previous level of retinal-defocus magnitude, so that its change can be discerned. The release of neuromodulator in turn results in changes in the rate of scleral proteoglycan synthesis, which causes a change in scleral growth rate. This relative growth rate is added to the ongoing and normal genetically-programmed ocular growth rate to provide the overall axial length growth.

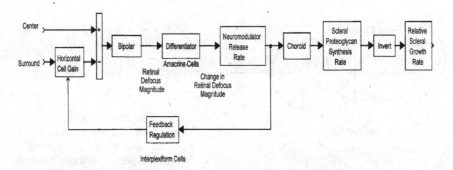

Figure 4.6. Conceptual block diagram model of the retinal-defocus pathway for regulating sclera growth. The difference between center and surround excitation provides the retinal-defocus signal. The derivative of the signal drives the release of neuromodulators, which provides the feedback via interplexiform neurons to regulate horizontal cell gain. In addition, release of neuromodulators causes changes in the rate of proteoglycan synthesis, and in turn relative scleral growth rate. Adapted from Hung and Ciuffreda (2000c), with permission of Bull. Math. Biol.

The detailed model is shown in Fig. 4.7. The sustained pathway consists of the photoreceptor, bipolar, and <u>sustained</u> ganglion cells. It is modulated by surround signals via horizontal cells in the outer plexiform layer to provide local steady-state or sustained contrast information. The transient pathway also consists of photoreceptor, bipolar, and transient ganglion cells. However, it is modulated by surround signals via amacrine cells in the inner plexiform layer to provide information regarding local change or <u>transients</u> in contrast information. Feedback regulation is provided locally by the interplexiform neurons that receive signals for neuromodulator release in the inner plexiform layer and modulate the gain of horizontal cells in the outer plexiform layer to maintain a relatively constant sensitivity to change in local contrast. The center bipolar cell receives a signal derived from the difference between center and summed surround inputs, which represents the summated amount of retinal-image defocus across the overlapping, spatially-contiguous center and surround receptive field area. This signal is differentiated by neural circuitry in the inner plexiform layer, which most likely contains amacrine cells. This change is rectified, so that the "envelope" of the signal, which represents the overall change in retinal-defocus magnitude, drives the rate of neuromodulator release. The neuromodulator, or a cascade of neurochemicals related to the release of the neuromodulator (Wallman, 1997), passes through the choroid to reach the sclera. The transit of the neuromodulator through the choroid may result, at least in the monkey, in a volume change that is observed as a change in choroidal thickness (Curtin, 1985; Cheng et al, 1992; Wildsoet and Wallman, 1995; Marzani and Wallman, 1997; Hung et al, 2000b,c; Troilo et al, 2006*)*. This may explain why, as expected, choroidal thickness changes in the monkey are correlated with changes in retinal-defocus magnitude, but the optical change associated the thickness change is too small to account for any significant contribution towards full emmetropization (Hung et al, 2000b.c; Troilo et al, 2006). On the other hand, the neuromodulator that reaches the sclera modifies proteoglycan synthesis to result in changes in ocular growth that does provide nearly full emmetropization, as described in the schematic model (Fig. 4.6).

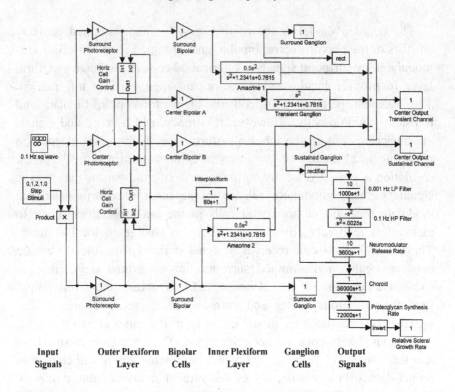

Figure 4.7. Detail block diagram model depicting the regulation of scleral growth rate. The retinal layers (outer to inner) are arranged from left to right: photoreceptor, outer plexiform, bipolar, inner plexiform, and ganglion. The sustained pathway consists of center photoreceptor, center bipolar B, and sustained ganglion cell. Horizontal cell, whose gain is regulated by feedback via interplexiform cells, relays surround information to modify sustained ganglion output. The transient pathway consists of center photoreceptor, center bipolar A, and transient ganglion cell. Amacrine cell relay change in surround information to modify transient ganglion output. Center bipolar B signal consists of retinal-defocus information and passes through a rectifier, lowpass filters, and elements representing neuromodulator release, the choroid, and proteoglycan synthesis. This is inverted to provide relative scleral growth rate relative to normal. Reprinted with permission of Bull. Math. Biol.

Model simulation responses to center and surround stimuli are shown in Figs. 4.8a-d. The center stimulus representing sharp focus consists of a ± 1 amplitude (in arbitrary units representing change in luminance relative to the background level) peak-to-peak, 0.1 Hz, square-wave signal. The surround stimuli, representing varying degrees of retinal-image defocus, consists of the same square wave but modulated by different step levels over the time span of the simulation. Figure 4.8a shows the various steps of modulation of the surround amplitude (solid) and the feedback-regulated change in gain of the horizontal cells. As noted above, this provides relatively constant sensitivity to changes in retinal-defocus magnitude. The pulse-like responses for the rates of neuromodulator release (solid) and proteoglycan synthesis (dashed) are shown in Figure 4.8b. The change in proteoglycan synthesis rate in turn

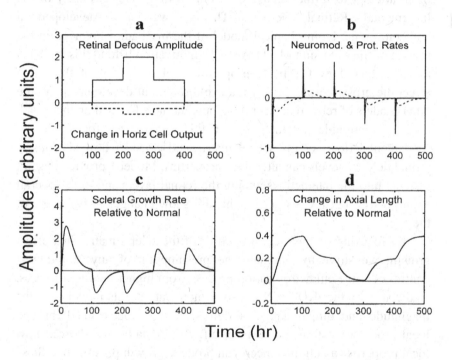

Figure 4.8. (a) Envelope of surround stimulus representing various levels of defocus (solid). Changes in horizontal cell output, which are regulated by interplexiform neuronal feedback, shows a complementary response to surround defocus (dashed). (b) Pulses of rates of neuromodulator release (solid) and proteoglycan synthesis (dashed) occur at the transitions of surround stimulus (see Fig. 4.8a). (c) Rate of scleral growth relative to normal follows the pulses in the rate of proteoglycan synthesis (see Fig. 4.8b). (d) Integration of scleral growth rate provides the change in axial length relative to normal. The direction of change is consistent with experimental findings and with the analysis provided by the schematic model. Reprinted with permission of Bull. Math. Biol.

causes changes in the scleral growth rate relative to normal (Figure 4.8c). Finally, the cumulative change in axial length relative to normal is shown in Figure 4.8d. These results clearly demonstrate that the model is able to simulate the bi-directional aspects of choroidal and scleral axial length changes found experimentally.

4.3.2 (Model 2) *A homeomorphic biomechanical model of the Incremental Retinal-Defocus Theory*

In an attempt to further analyze the implications and feasibility of the Incremental Retinal Defocus Theory, we have developed a homeomorphic, biomechanical model of the mechanics involved in the growth of the eye using MATLAB. The motivation behind this model is to understand how the IRDT-proposed local properties of the retina affect the gross morphology of the eye throughout development. While other models of refractive error development have focused on the broad, ocular-system-wide interactions, in this model we focus on the fundamental fibers of the scleral matrix and consider how changes in retinal defocus levels can alter their properties. Model 1 provided useful insights into the interactions among the retinal layers and to the overall axial growth, but it does not graphically show changes in the shape of the eye.

By focusing on the local properties of the scleral matrix that affect growth, we strive to eliminate the presumption of any "top-down" control over the emmetropization process from higher neural processes, as dictated by the IRDT. We also demonstrate in this model both the magnitude and directionality of defocus can be determined through local processes within the retina itself. Additionally, we showed how local properties acting in concert can produce growth patterns like those observed in experimental situations.

4.3.2.1 *Basic assumptions and simplifications*

The scleral matrix is a deformable, elastic structure that is supported by the outward force of the intraocular pressure. The matrix provides surface tension by the adhesion of interlocking filaments, thereby counterbalancing the pressure force acting outwards with an elastic, resistive force acting inwards. Histological studies of the eye have revealed that the sclera is comprised of a dense layer of fibers, primarily parallel to the surface and crossing in all directions. In the posterior pole of the eye, these fibers are aligned like meshwork around a balloon which expand with increased intraocular pressure (Wolff, 1968). The stress-strain relationship of the sclera has been investigated, thus revealing that the posterior pole has about 60% of the stiffness of the anterior sclera (Friberg and Lace, 1988).

To model this system, we have reduced the scleral matrix to a ring of springs in two dimensions. Each spring has an internal spring force proportional to its length that acts on its two neighboring springs. This corresponds to the scleral matrix of the eye where filaments produce a tensile force as they are stretched by the internal pressure forces in the eye. The internal pressure force is modeled as a force vector acting normal to and outwards from the ring of springs. We add this force vector into the modeling at each spring-to-spring connection, which we call a "node" (see Fig. 4.9).

We have, however, neglected visco-elastic properties of the actual scleral matrix because the time course of ocular growth is very long, with changes in the axial length of the viterious chamber possible even into adulthood (McBrien and Adams, 1997). Additionally, in ocular growth, there are typically no rapid dynamics, which would leave us to believe that the viscoelasticity of the scleral matrix plays a relatively small role in long-term ocular growth. We have also made the simplification of configuring in two dimensions to reduce the complexity in the model simulation and for ease of visualization, while in actuality there are complex three-dimensional mechanics at work which may be an area of future research and modeling.

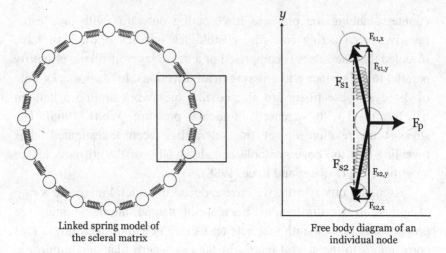

Linked spring model of
the scleral matrix

Free body diagram of an
individual node

Figure 4.9. Linked-spring model of the scleral matrix. The left image shows the ring of linked springs we use to model the scleral matrix. Sixteen springs are shown, but upwards of 30 are used in actual modeling. The right image shows a free body diagram of one node in the linked spring model. Each node has forces $F_{s,1}$ and $F_{s,2}$ from it's two attached springs as well as F_p, an internal ocular pressure force which acts normally to the surface.

4.3.2.2 *Fundamental equations and constraints*

This model is a long-term time-course model, where we use the internal forces in the system along with the previous locations of the components to calculate the location and shape of the system in the subsequent time periods. The motion and shape of the model eyeball is determined by moving the individual nodes based on the sum of forces acting on each node. Each node has the following forces as shown in Figure 4.9:

1. The force from each adjacent spring, with the net spring force acting inward
2. The intraocular pressure force, acting outward

In the x-direction, the sum of forces on a node (see Fig. 4.9) can be written as Eq. 4.1.

$$\sum F_x = F_p - F_{s1,x} - F_{s2,x} \tag{4.1}$$

The net force acting on the node is determined by summing all the forces. This net force vector changes the direction and magnitude of the node's acceleration and in turn the location of the node in the next time period. We used a simple, two-step Euler's integration algorithm to predict the subsequent positions of the nodes based on the previous position and speed. For each dimension (x and y), there are two integration steps to determine the next position. Using the x-dimension as an example, the total force in the x-direction is calculated. Then, we use this force with an assumed node mass of $m = 1$ to find the node's acceleration at time t, $\ddot{x}_t$, as shown in Eq. 4.2. Using the acceleration and the node's previous velocity in the x-direction, we approximate the new velocity by Eq. 4.3, where $\Delta t = t_n - t_{n-1}$ is a small increment in time.

$$\ddot{x}_t = \frac{1}{m} \sum F_{x,t} \tag{4.2}$$

$$\dot{x}_t = \dot{x}_{t-1} + \ddot{x}_t \Delta t \tag{4.3}$$

The next integration step uses the newly calculated node velocity (i.e., the movement of the node's corresponding mass), $\dot{x}$, with the previous node position to determine the new position. While in reality the time course of ocular growth is long and the instantaneous movement of any given point on the sclera matrix is minute, the node's velocity here can be thought of as the current baseline rate of axial elongation or contraction. Thus, this baseline rate of axial growth times an increment of time gives a change in position of a point on the sclera, as shown in Eq. 4.4:

$$x_t = x_{t-1} + \dot{x}_t \Delta t \tag{4.4}$$

In addition to the integration method above, we also subject the nodes to constraints in their motion, so that the system remains well-formed. As the nodes move, we check to insure that the nodes remain in their relative positions and furthermore that none of the springs intersect. Also, we constrain the motion of the nodes so that no nodes create indentations (i.e., deflect backwards towards the center of the eyeball). This can happen if, for example, the surface is nearly flat in some portion of the scleral matrix. Both of these constraints were needed to maintain the consistency within the model so as not to introduce errors that would propagate through the subsequent steps of the numerical integration.

4.3.2.3 *Modeling the optical interactions*

To simulate the effect of retinal defocus on neuromodulator release and the subsequent change in scleral matrix integrity, the stiffness of the spring is dependent on the changes in defocus. The homeomorphic, time-course mapping will change the shape of the eye to something that resembles the observed refractive errors in experiments using similar optical defocus conditions. The starting point for this is the calculation of the blur circle size, which is then used to adjust the spring constants.

In reality, the optical system of the eye is very complex with an accommodating intraocular crystalline lens comprised of layers of material with many different refractive indicies. For this model, we simplify this system so that each node in a specific "retina region" has a lens assigned to it. This corresponds to the photosensitive region in the actual eye that responds to changes in blur circle size. For each node in this region, a conceptual lens is placed outside of the eye to refract light from a conceptual distant object onto the node. Because infants are born hyperopic, we set the focal length of the conceptual lens so that light entering the lens is focused just beyond that lens's node. The normal, genetically preset growth pattern for the eye ball is to increase in axial length as the child matures. We model this as an initial intraocular pressure force acting outwards that is greater than the spring forces (sclera tension) acting inwards. As the axial length of the eye increases due to the large outward force of the intraocular pressure, individual nodes will move outwards, reducing the initial hyperopia as they move closer to the focal plane. This will create a decreasing level of retinal defocus, measured as the size of the blur circle where the light cone crosses the retina, as shown in Fig. 4.10. We can also adjust the model by artificially decreasing the focal lengths of the conceptual lenses so that the incoming light is focused far in front of the nodes in the retina region. In this case, an increment in outward movement of the nodes (caused by the high intraocular pressure forces) will result in an increase in the size of the blur circle, as shown in Fig. 4.10.

To modulate the strength of the sclera matrix, we use the change in blur circle size caused by incremental movements of the nodes. The biological analog to this process is the baseline level of neurotransmitters released by the amacrine cells of the retina. This baseline is determined by the level of contrast at that location in the retina. As the contrast level changes, this baseline level of neurotransmitter release is modulated. This change in neurotransmitter levels alters the stiffness of the scleral matrix by increasing or decreasing the proteoglycan synthesis rate. In our model, a change in blur circle size at an individual node causes a proportional change in the spring constants of the two springs attached to that node. This, in turn, affects the spring forces acting on the node, resulting in a net increase in spring force for a positive change in blur circle size or a net decrease in spring force for a negative change in blur circle size.

In effect, the change in blur circle size during an increment of genetically pre-programmed growth is providing information on the directionality of retinal defocus. An increase in blur circle size will occur if the focal point lies in front of the retina, signaling that the light cone is diverging and that axial length of the eye ball is too long for accurate focus. The local retinal response to this is an increase in proteoglycan synthesis, which leads to a stiffening of the retina and retarded axial growth. Conversely, a decrease in blur circle size signals an excessively short axial length, and results in the opposite local retinal response causing an increase in the axial growth rate.

Myopic Defocus

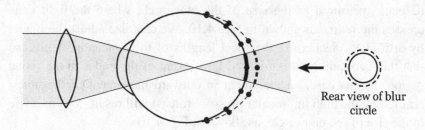

Rear view of blur circle

Hyperopic Defocus

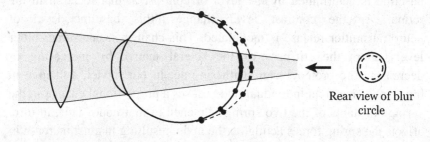

Rear view of blur circle

━━━━━ Original Boundary
▃▃▃▃▃ Boundary after an increment in growth

Figure 4.10. Changes in blur circle size for increments in retinal growth. The solid eye ball boundary indicates the original boundary of the sclera, the dashed boundary indicates the boundary after an increment in ocular growth. Dots on the boundaries indicate the positions of nodes in the retina region. Only one conceptual lens is shown for a node; however, the simulation uses conceptual lenses for all nodes in the retina region. For *myopic defocus* (focal plane located in front of the retina), incremental changes in growth result in *increased* blur circle size at nodes in the retina region. For *hyperopic defocus* (focal plane located behind the retina), incremental changes in growth result in *decreased* blur circle size. Based on the principles of the IRDT, myopic defocus will cause hyperopia due to retarded axial growth, while hyperopic defocus will cause myopia due to excessive axial growth.

4.3.2.4 *Simulation results*

Eye growth was simulated for three cases of retinal defocus comprised of: normal growth, or growth where the image is focused on the retina; myopic growth, or growth where the image is focused behind the retina (hyperopic defocus due to imposed minus lens); and hyperopic growth, or growth where the image is focused in front of the retina (myopic defocus due to imposed plus lens). Here the distinction must be made between hyperopic growth and hyperopic defocus (and likewise myopic growth versus myopic defocus). Hyperopic defocus refers to an optical environment where the image is focused *behind* the retina. This causes myopia or myopic growth. Myopic defocus refers to an optical environment where the image is focused *in front of* the retina. This leads to hyperopia or hyperopic growth. By adjusting the level of retinal defocus, the model responds with different growth patterns similar to growth patterns observed in laboratory experiments.

For these simulations, all other variables remained constant (such as internal pressure force magnitude, initial spring constants, and the size of the deformable region). A few simplifications were made for plotting clarity, including the use of dashed lines to indicate relative weakening and thickened lines to indicate relative strengthening of the sclera. Also, the boundaries of the lens light-cone are plotted to help visualize the blur circle and location of the focal points. Figure 4.11 shows the freeze-frame simulation results taken throughout the growth of the eye.

For hyperopic growth (left), light entering the eye is focused in front of the retina, with increments in growth causing an increase in blur circle size and in turn a relative strengthening of the posterior sclera. The stiffer posterior sclera creates a stronger force offsetting the internal ocular pressure, thus resulting in relatively reduced axial elongation and a more oblate spheroid shape (Singh et al., 2006). In the case of myopic growth (right), the situation is reversed, where light entering the eye is focused far behind the retina, causing increments in growth to reduce the blur circle size. This, in turn, weakens the posterior sclera, resulting in less resistance to internal ocular pressure and an increase in axial length, and a more prolate spheroid shape (Singh et al., 2006). This is consistent with previous experimental results (Smith and Hung, 1999).

Time course simulation of refractive error development

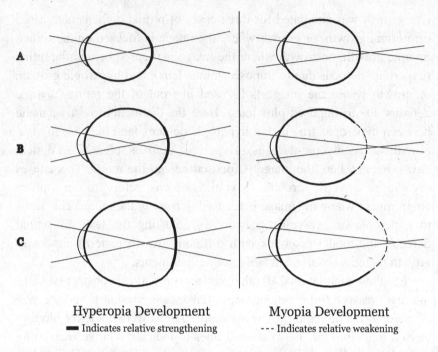

Hyperopia Development
■ Indicates relative strengthening

Myopia Development
--- Indicates relative weakening

Figure 4.11. Simulated hyperopic and myopia development, exported from our MATLAB simulation. Frames A, B, and C show time course simulation of eye growth. For hyperopic growth (left), light entering the eye is focused in front of the retina, with increments in growth causing an increase in blur circle size and in turn a relative strengthening of the posterior sclera. The stiffer posterior sclera creates a stronger force offsetting the internal ocular pressure, thus resulting in retarded axial elongation. In the case of myopic growth (right), the situation is reversed, where light entering the eye is focused far behind the retina, causing increments in growth to reduce the blur circle size. This, in turn, weakens the posterior sclera, resulting in less resistance to internal ocular pressure and an increase in axial length.

4.4 Clinical Treatment for Myopia

The models above have provided a better understanding of the underlying mechanisms of myopia development. This can serve as a basis for improved clinical treatment for prevention and reduction of myopia. Over the past several decades, there have been numerous clinical approaches to the treatment of myopia (Ong and Ciuffreda, 1997; Rosenfield and Gilmartin, 1998). These have included pharmacological intervention, corneal refractive surgery, corneal molding with hard contact lenses, ergonomically-applied nearwork modifications, vision therapy, and near-point lenses. It is the last two aspects that are most relevant for clinical application of the models, as they represent the most common therapeutic approaches. In both cases, the goal is to reduce the chronic retinal defocus, which is purported to be myopigenic (Ong and Ciuffreda, 1997; Hung and Ciuffreda, 2007). In addition, and more recently, they appear to provide an optimal oculomotor feedback control "balance" between the accommodative and vergence systems to minimize their respective errors (i.e., retinal defocus and fixation disparity). (Jiang et al., 2008; Liu, et.al. 1979).

Vision Therapy. Vision therapy, or "VT", refers to specific sequences of oculomotor training procedures, in actuality neurological "oculomotor learning" (Ciuffreda, 2002), that help to establish concordant and time-optimal ("efficient") motor patterns for the accommodative and vergence systems and their mutual interactions. We speculate that this may be due to increased synchronicity of oculomotor neural firing within, and then between, both systems with training. This would result in improved timing and increased neural response amplitude (i.e., gain). Thus, with successful training, there would be more accurate focus and precise bifoveal alignment, with both responses being attained in a rapid, time-optimal manner. The presumption is that with accurate accommodation, primarily via blur and vergence-drive, the reduced accommodative error (i.e., retinal defocus) will prevent/reduce the onset and/or progression of myopia, respectively.

Near-point lenses. Similar to the above, the approach here is to use plus lenses at near that minimize the potentially myopigenic retinal defocus. These lenses would also minimize the steady-state vergence error (i.e., fixation disparity). Although recent evidence by Jiang and colleagues (2008) has demonstrated that the addition of specific plus lenses at near cannot simultaneously reduce both system errors to zero, an optimal "balance" lens does exist to minimize their system errors, with emphasis on the steady-state accommodative error, that is dependent on viewing distance. For example, for a 40 cm adult working distance, a +0.75 D lens functions in this dual manner. For children with a shorter working distance, the lens might be either +1.00 or +1.25 D.

Thus, a simple and practical clinical solution for the treatment, and perhaps prevention, of myopia has been proposed. The vision therapy acts to establish and reinforce new and more effective oculomotor neural patterns and correlated oculomotor responses, while the near-point lenses act to maintain this relationship over extended periods of sustained near work.

4.5 Summary and Conclusions

Early modeling of refractive errors focused on explaining the exponential nature of the time-course development of refractive errors through feedback mechanisms (Medina and Fariza, 1993). Additionally, some components of ocular physiology were incorporated, such as the accommodative reflex and retina feedback loops (Schaeffel and Howland, 1988). As more experimental research has been conducted, researchers developed a better understanding of the importance of defocus in the emmetropization process (Smith and Hung, 2000 and Hung, et al, 1995) as well as its localized nature (Wilsoet and Pettigrew, 1988). Expanded research into the biomechanical properties and make-up of the sclera, including modulators of proteoglycan synthesis (Rada, et al, 2000) has led to further improvements in theories and models of ocular growth.

Emmetropization now appears to be governed by a relatively simple mechanism, which has been described by our newly proposed Incremental Retinal-Defocus Theory (Hung and Ciuffreda, 2000a-c).

The theory states that the rate of change of retinal defocus determines the rate of release of neuromodulators, which modulates rate of proteoglycan synthesis, and in turn regulates the rate of scleral growth. The critical point is that the detection mechanism does not depend on the sign of the blur, but rather on the change in blur magnitude that is either environmentally-induced or results from an increment of genetically-programmed ocular growth. Thus, this unifying theory provides an understanding of the basic underlying retinal mechanism for detecting blur magnitude, and furthermore explains how the neurochemical signal is processed to modulate the rate of eye growth, and in turn the resultant development of axial myopia.

Building upon previous models of the development of refractive errors and on the IRDT, we have developed a new homeomorphic, biomechanical model of the emmetropization process that responds to changes to the optical environment (Model 2). Model 2 uses a linked-spring model of the scleral matrix, with spring constants that can be changed to simulate stiffening or weakening of the scleral matrix based on changes in the size of the blur circle at different regions of the retina. This model is able to reflect experimental results showing elongation of the axial length of the eye when the focused image falls behind the retina and shortening of the axial length of the eye when the focused image is in front of the retina. Finally, simple and practical clinical techniques, based on understanding of the underlying principles provided by the models, have been proposed for the treatment and perhaps prevention of myopia development.

4.6 References

Bennett, A. G., and Rabbetts, R. B., (1989). *Clinical Visual Optics,* pg. 75.

Bradley, D. V., Fernandes, A., Tigges, M., and Boothe, R. G. (1996). Diffuser Contact Lenses Retard Axial Elongation in Infant Rhesus Monkeys. *Vis. Res.*, 36, pp. 509-514.

Cheng, H.-M., Omah, S.S., and Kwong, K. K., (1992). Shape of the myopic eye as seen with high-resolution magnetic resonance imaging, *Optom. Vis. Sci.*, 36, pp. 698-701.

Ciuffreda, K. J. (2002) The scientific basis for and efficacy of optometric vision therapy in non-strabismic accommodative and vergence disorders. *Optometry*, 73, pp. 735-762.

Curtin, B. J. (1985). The etiology of Myopia, in: The Myopias: Basic Science and Clinical Management, pp. 61-151.

Ehlers, N. and Hjortdal, J. (2006). The cornea: epithelium and stroma. *Advances in Organ Biology*, 10, pp. 83-111.

Friberg, T. R. and Lace, J. W. (1988). A comparison of the elastic properties of human choroids and sclera. *Exp. Eye Res.*, 47, pp. 429-436.

Gottlieb, M. D., Fugate-Wentzek, L. A. & Wallman, J. (1987). Different visual deprivations produce different ametropias and different eye shapes. *Invest. Ophthalmol. Vis. Sci.*, 28, pp. 1225-1235.

Grosvenor, T., and Goss, D. A., (1998). *Clinical Management of Myopia.* pp. 49-62.

Hung, G. K., and Ciuffreda, K. J. (2000a). Differential retinal-defocus magnitude during eye growth provides the appropriate direction signal. *Med. Sci. Monitor.* 6, pp. 791-795.

Hung, G. K., and Ciuffreda, K. J., (2000b). Quantitative analysis of the effect of near lens addition on accommodation and myopigenesis, *Cur. Eye. Res.*, 20, pp. 293-312.

Hung, G. K., and Ciuffreda, K. J., (2000c). A unifying theory of refractive error development , *Bull. Math. Biol.* 62, pp. 1087-1108.

Hung, G. K., and Ciuffreda, K. J. (2002). Models of Refractive Error Development, in G. K. Hung and K. J. Ciuffreda (Eds.) *Models of the Visual System.* Kluwer Academic/Plenum Publishers, pp. 643-677.

Hung, G. K. and Ciuffreda, K. J., (2007). Incremental retinal-defocus theory of myopic development --- schematic analysis and computer simulation. *Comput. Biol. Med.,* 37, pp. 930-946.

Hung, L. F., Crawford, M.L.J., and Smith, E. L. (1995). Spectacle lenses alter eye growth and the refractive status of young monkeys. *Nature Med.*, 1, pp. 761-765.

Jiang, B. C., Bussa, S., Tea, Y. C., and Seger, K. (2008). Optimal dioptric value of near addition lenses intended to slow myopic progression. *Optom. Vis. Sci.*, 85, pp. 1100-1105.

Kee, C.-S., Hung, L. F., Qiao-Grider, Y., Ramamirtham, R., Winawer, J., Wallman, J., and Smith, E. III. (2007). Temporal constraints on experimental emmetropization in infant monkeys. Invest. Ophthal. Vis. Sci., 48, pp. 957-962.

Kiilgaard, J. F. and Jensen, P. K. (2006). The choroid and optic nerve head. *Advances in Organ Biology*, 10, pp. 273-290.

Lin, L. L. K., Shih, Y. F., Hung, P. T., and Hou, P. K. (1996). Changes in ocular refraction and its components among medial students-a 5-Year longitudinal study, *Optom. Vis. Sci.*, 73, pp. 495-498.

Liu, J. S., Lee, M., Jang, J., Ciuffreda, K. J., Wong, J. H., Grisham, D., and Stark, L. (1979). Objective assessment of accommodation orthoptics: 1.dynamic insufficiency. *Am. J. Optom, Physiol. Opt.*, 56, pp. 285-294.

Marzani, D., and Wallman, J. (1997). Growth of the two layers of the chick sclera is modulated reciprocally by visual conditions, *Invest. Opthal. Vis. Sci.*, 38, pp. 1726-1739.

McBrien, N.A., and Adams, D. W. (1997). A longitudinal investigation of adult-onset and adult-progression of myopia in an occupational group: Refractive and biometric findings. *Invest. Ophthal. Vis. Sci.*, 38, pp. 3211-333.

Medina, A., and Fariza, E. (1993). Emmetropization as a first-order feedback system, *Vis. Res.*, 33, pp. 21-26.

Moses, R.A., Grodzki W.J., Starcherd, B.C., and Galione, M.J. (1978). Elastic content of the scleral spur, trabecular meshwork, and sclera. *Invest. Ophthalmol. Vis. Sci.*, 17, pp. 817-818.

Napper, G. A., Brennan, N. A., Barrington, M., Squires, M. A., Vessey, G. A., and Vingrys, A. J. (1995). The duration of normal visual exposure necessary to prevent form deprivation myopia in chicks. *Vision Res.*, 35, pp. 1337-1344.

Norton, T. T. (1999). Animal Models of Myopia: Learning How Vision Controls the Size of the Eye, *J. Insitut. Lab. Anim. Res.*, 40(2).

Ong, E. and Ciuffreda, K. J. (1997). *Accommodation, Nearwork, and Myopia.* Optometric Extension Program Foundation, Santa Ana, CA.

Rada, J. A., Achen, V. R., Penugonda, S., Schmidt R. W., and Mount, B. A. (2000). Proteoglycan Composition in the Human Sclera During Growth and Aging, *Invest Ophthalmol Vis Sci.* 41, pp. 1639-1648.

Rada J. A., Achen V. R., Perry, C. A., and Fox, P. W. (1997). Proteoglycans in the human sclera: evidence for the presence of aggrecan. *Invest Ophthalmol. Vis. Sci.*, 38, pp. 1740-1751.

Rada, J. A., Nickla, D. L., and Troilo, D. (2000). Decreased Proteoglycan Systhesis Associated with Form Deprivation Myopia in Mature Primate Eyes. *Invest. Ophthalmol. Vis. Sci.*, 41, pp. 2050-2058.

Rosenfield, M. and Gilmartin, B. (eds) (1998) *Myopia and Nearwork*, Butterworth-Heinemann, Boston, MA.

Schaeffel, F., and Howland, H.C. (1988). Mathematical model of emmetropization in the chichen, J. Opt. Soc. Am. A, 5, pp. 2080-2086.

Siegwart, J. T. Jr., and Norton, T.T. (1999). Regulation of the mechanical properties of tree shrew sclera by the visual environment, *Vis. Res.*, 39, pp. 387-407.

Singh, K. D., Logan, N. S., and Gilmartin, B. (2006). Three-dimensional modeling of the human eye based on magnetic resonance imaging. *Invest. Ophthal. Vis. Sci.*, 47, pp. 2272-2279.

Smith, E. L., and Hung, L. F. (1999). The role of optical defocus in regulating refractive development in infant monkeys, *Vis. Res.* 39, pp. 1415-1435.

Smith, E. L., Hung, L. F. (2000). Form-deprivation in monkeys is a graded phenomenon. *Vision Res.*, 40, pp. 372-381.

Smith, G., and Atchison, D. A. (1997). *The Eye and Visual Optical Instruments*, Cambridge Univ. Press, United Kingdom, pp. 274, 796.

Sperduto, R. D., Seigel, D., Robers, J., and Rowland, M. (1983). Prevalence of myopia in the United States, *Arch. Ophthalmol.*, 101, pp. 405-407.

Trier, K. (2006). The sclera. *Advances in Organ Biology*, 10, pp. 353-373.

Troilo, D., Gottlieb, M. D., and Wallman, J. (1987). Visual Deprivation causes myopia in chicks with optic nerve section, *Cur. Eye Res.*, 6, pp. 993-999.

Troilo, D., Nickla, D. L., Mertz, J. R., and Rada, J. A. (2006). Change in the Synthesis Rates of Ocular Retionoic Acid and Scleral Glycosaminoglycan during Experimentally Altered Eye Growth in Marmosets, *Invest. Ophthalmol. Vis. Sci.*, 47(5), pp. 1768-1777.

Wallman, J. (1997). Can myopia be prevented? 14th Biennial Research to prevent *Blindness Science Wirters Seminar in Ophthalmology* , pp. 52-52.

Wildsoet, C. F. and Collins, M. J. (2000). Competing defocus stimuli of opposing sign produce opposite effects in eyes with intact and sectioned optic nerves in the chick. *Invest. Ophthalmol. Vis. Sci.*, 41, S738.

Wildsoet, C. F., and Pettigrew, J. D. (1988). Experimental myopia and anomalous eye growth patterns unaffected by optic nerve section in chickens: Evidence for local control of eye growth , Clin., *Vis. Sci.,* 3, pp. 99-107.

Wildsoet, C. F., and Wallman, J. (1995). Choroidal and cleral mechanisms of compensation for spectacle lenses in chicks, *Vis. Sci., 35, 1175-1194.*

Wilson, J.R., Fernandes, A., Chandler, C. V., Tigges, M., Boothe, R.G., and Gammon, J. A. (1987). Abnormal Development of the axial length of aphakic monkey eyes. *Invest. Ophthalmol. Vis. Sci.*, 28, pp. 2096-2099.

Wolff, E. (1968). *Anatomy of the Eye and Orbit*, pp. 49-67. W. B. Saunders & Co., Philadelphia, PA.

Yackle, K., and Fitzgerald, D. E. (1999). Emmetropization: an overview, *J. Behav. Optom.,* 10, pp. 38-43.

4.7 Review Questions

Q4.1 The innermost retinal cell layer (closest to the vitreous fluid) is:

A. Inner plexiform cell layer

B. Photoreceptor cell layer

C. Ganglion cell layer

D. Bipolar cell layer

Q4.2 ____ defocus tends to cause axial ____ in the eyeball, resulting in ____ in the long-term if the subject is exposed to the abnormal defocus for extended periods of time.

A. Myopic; elongation; myopia

B. Hyperopic; elongation; myopia

C. Myopic; shortening; myopia

D. Hyperopic; shortening; hyperopia

Q4.3 Describe the theoretical mechanism of emmetropization in the Incremental Retinal Defocus Theory.

Q4.4 Early refractive error modeling attempts presumed ____, which was later disproved by laboratory experiments.

A. control over emmetropization from higher neural centers

B. genetic pre-programming

C. change in defocus provided necessary information to control emmetropization

D. the importance of environmental causes

Q4.5 In the IRDT Model 2, describe the forces acting on one node in the retinal region.

Q4.6 Blur circle size on one portion of the retina alone does not provide enough information to determine the directionality (hyperopic or myopic) of retinal defocus because ____.

A. the eye must integrate blur circle sizes from the entire retina

B. the eye must combine blur circle size with zonular fiber tension and lens shape

C. both hyperopic and myopic defocus can cause equal–size blur circles

D. blur circle size is static as the eye grows

Q4.7   What steps make up the procedure IRDT Model 2 uses in determining the location of the nodes in the each frame?

Q4.8   Which of the following claims about the scleral matrix is false?

    A. The cornea is structurally continuous with the sclera

    B. The sclera has elastic but not viscoelastic properties

    C. The posterior sclera is has less stiffness than the anterior sclera

    D. The visual environment affects the stiffness of the sclera by augmenting proteoglycan synthesis

III

EAR

Chapter 5

Advances in the Design of Hearing Aids

Ian C. Bruce, Ph.D.[1]

[1] Dept. of Electrical & Computer Engineering, McMaster University
1280 Main St. W., Hamilton, Ontario L8S 4K1, Canada
PH: 905-525-9140, ext. 26984; FX: 905-521-2922; EM: ibruce@ieee.org

5.1 Introduction

For at least four centuries, human ingenuity has been applied to developing devices that amplify sounds for the purpose of alleviating hearing loss. From the mechanical devices of the 17th century such as ear trumpets and horns, through the carbon and vacuum-tube electronic amplifiers of the first half of the 20th century, to the solid-state analog electronics of the latter half of the 20th century, the main focus has been on finding and refining technologies that can produce sufficient amplification gain over a satisfactory range of acoustic frequencies without introducing detrimental noise or distortion. Parallel with these advances in the efficacy of the devices has been the miniaturization of hearing aid components, bringing increased wearer comfort, more pleasing aesthetics, and reduced power consumption.

Despite this technological progress, analog hearing aids are unable to compensate fully for the effects of hearing loss in most individuals, particularly in difficult listening environments. However, with the introduction of digital hearing aids at the end of the 20th century, an avenue has opened for much more sophisticated sound processing and amplification, producing the potential to compensate more fully for the effects of hearing loss. Some advances have already been made in applying sound processing algorithms that help attenuate background noise sources or optimally adjust the amplifier gain for different listening environments. Many further innovations should result from our rapidly increasing knowledge of how the ear and brain normally process and represent sounds and how hearing impairment leads to degradation of the neural representation of sounds.

5.1.1 *Anatomy & physiology of the ear*

The human ear can be divided into the three major anatomical sections illustrated in Fig. 5.1: the outer, middle and inner ears. Each of these anatomical divisions has a corresponding functional role: the outer ear funnels sound waves into the eardrum, the middle ear provides a mechanical coupling between the low-impedance air within the ear canal

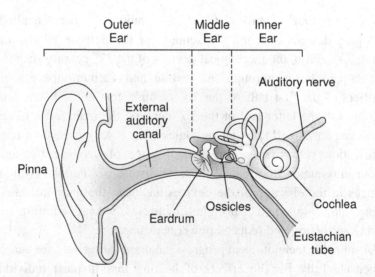

Figure 5.1. Anatomy of the human ear, showing the division of the outer, middle and inner ears. Modified with permission from Clark (2003), © Springer Science+Business Media.

and the high-impedance fluid within the cochlea, and the inner ear transduces sound waves into neural activity. Understanding the details of how each section of the ear processes sounds will assist in appreciating how the normal perception of sound is generated, how pathologies of the ear result in hearing loss, and what types of amplification strategies can be used in hearing aids to compensate for hearing loss.

The pinna of the outer ear is shaped in such a way as to reflect sounds into the external auditory canal (meatus). Consequently, the ear is able to collect sounds impinging on the head over a larger area than the canal itself. Furthermore, the interaction of the reflected sounds causes the pinna to acts as a direction-dependent filter, referred to as the head-related transfer function (HRTF). The effects of the HRTF on the frequency spectrum of incoming sounds is monitored by the brain to estimate the elevation of sound sources and determine whether the sound is coming from in front of the listener or from the rear.

The eardrum (tympanic membrane) and ossicles of the middle ear transfer the sound vibrations from the ear canal to the oval window of the cochlea. The lever action of the three ossicles (the malleus, the incus and the stapes) and the relative sizes of the eardrum and the footplate of the stapes on the oval window act together to transform the higher-velocity, lower-pressure vibrations of the eardrum to lower-velocity, higher-pressure vibrations of the oval window. Without this transformation, sound waves in the low-impedance air would be largely reflected at the oval window, rather than being transmitted into the high-impedance cochlear fluids, producing a substantial hearing loss.

The cross section of the human cochlea illustrated in Fig. 5.2 shows that the cochlea is longitudinally divided by two membranes to form three compartments: the scala tympani, the scala media and the scala vestibuli. Sitting on the basilar membrane within the scala media is the organ of Corti, which performs the transduction of sound wave vibrations within the cochlea into neural impulses (also referred to as *action potentials*, *spikes* or *discharges*) in the auditory nerve fibers that innervate the auditory brainstem.

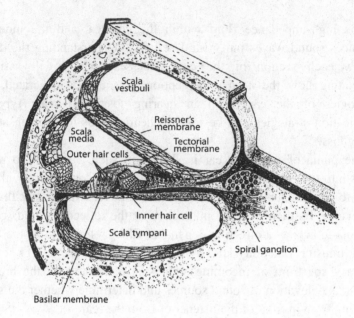

Figure 5.2. A cross section of the human cochlea. Reprinted with permission from Nolte (1993), © Elsevier.

Figure 5.3A illustrates the process by which vibrations at the oval window generate neural impulses in particular auditory nerve fibers along the length of the cochlea. Sound waves travel through the cochlear fluids from the base of the cochlea (i.e., closest to the stapes) towards the apex. However, the resonant properties of the basilar membrane vary continuously from the base to the apex, such that vibrations propagate to different positions along the basilar membrane depending on their frequency: high-frequency vibrations reach their maximum amplitude near the base of the cochlea and low-frequency vibrations near the apex. This spatial representation of vibration frequency illustrated in Figure 5.3B is referred to as "tonotopy." Inner hair cells in the organ of Corti have small hair-like stereocilia extending from their apical surface into the scala media, with the tips of the tallest stereocilia reaching up to the tectorial membrane. The motion of the basilar membrane relative to the tectorial membrane and the fluid trapped under the tectorial membrane

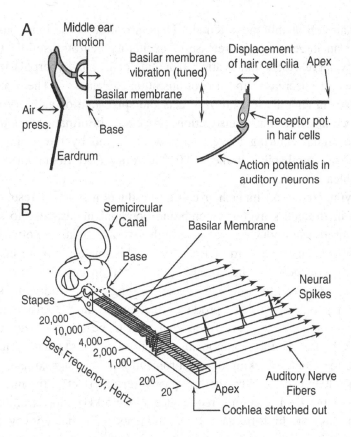

Figure 5.3. A. Schematic summarizing the transduction process in the mammalian cochlea, from air pressure fluctuations impinging on the eardrum to action potentials in primary auditory neurons that innervate the brainstem. Reprinted with permission from Sachs et al. (2002), © Biomedical Engineering Society. B. Illustration of the tonotopic organization of the cochlea. Adapted with permission from Zweig et al. (1976), © Acoustical Society of America.

causes bending of the stereocilia and the opening and closing of potassium (K^+) transduction channel gates within the stereocilia. Endolymph, the fluid within the scala media, has a higher concentration of K^+ ions and a higher electrical potential (endocochlear potential) than the inner hair cell's cytoplasm. Thus, opening or closing of the transduction channels affects the influx of K^+ into the hair cell and subsequently produces depolarization or hyperpolarization, respectively, of the hair cell membrane potential. Depolarization of the inner hair cell leads to an increase in the release of excitatory neurotransmitter to the auditory nerve fibers innervating that hair cell, and hyperpolarization produces a decrease in neurotransmitter release. The rate of neurotransmitter release in turn affects the spike rate of auditory nerve fibers, completing the transduction process. Information about the acoustic signal entering the ear is now conveyed by the timing (and number) of neural spikes in the ~30,000 auditory nerve fibers innervating the cochlea.

Asymmetry in an inner hair cell's transduction function results in a change in the cell's average membrane potential in response to sound wave vibrations, producing a change in the average spike rate of auditory nerve fibers synapsing onto that hair cell. This tonotopic representation of sound frequencies by the average spike rate in different auditory nerve fibers is referred to as "rate-place" coding. In addition, sound frequencies below ~5 kHz produce fluctuations in the instantaneous spike rate of auditory nerve fibers that tend to be synchronized to the positive phase of the component waveform. This phenomenon is referred to as phase locking or synchronization. The approximate upper limit of 5 kHz is created by the low-pass filtering effect of the inner hair cell's membrane. For sound frequencies above 5 kHz, slower amplitude modulations of high-frequency components can be conveyed by fluctuations in the spike rate synchronized to the modulations. Representing sound component frequencies or modulation frequencies in the instantaneous spike rate is a form of temporal coding.

From the description of cochlear processing above, it can be seen that the auditory periphery can be roughly approximated as a bank of bandpass filters. However, it is important to note that the filterbank is not linear. One group of nonlinearities is referred to as the "cochlear amplifier". The cochlear amplifier behavior is thought to be caused primarily through the action of outer hair cells in the organ of Corti (Robles and Ruggero, 2001). Outer hair cells, like inner hair cells, exhibit fluctuations in their membrane potential in response to bending of their stereocilia by basilar membrane vibration. However, rather than affecting neurotransmitter release, changes in the membrane potential of outer hair cells induce length and stiffness changes in the cell wall, a phenomenon known as electromotility (Brownell et al., 1985). The cochlear amplifier locally boosts small vibrations of the basilar membrane to increase the cochlea's sensitivity and frequency selectivity at low sound pressure levels. As sound levels increase, the gain of the cochlear amplifier is reduced, producing a form of compression in the basilar membrane response. The cochlear amplifier gain can also be reduced by off-frequency sound components, giving rise to suppression of responses to an on-frequency sound component. Additionally, the inner hair cell, the synapse and the spike generation mechanism of the auditory nerve fibers all exhibit further nonlinearities that affect the neural representation of sounds (Sachs et al., 2002; Bruce et al., 2003; Zilany and Bruce, 2006), as will be discussed in Section 5.2.

5.1.2 *Auditory pathways of the brain*

Auditory nerve fibers split as they enter the cochlear nucleus in the auditory brainstem. As shown in Fig. 5.4, the auditory nerve fibers innervate the dorsal cochlear nucleus (DCN), the anteroventral cochlear nucleus (AVCN), and the posteroventral cochlear nucleus (PVCN) in parallel. The DCN is thought to be involved in detecting spectral notches that result from the HRTF (Oertel and Young, 2004) and consequently provides information about the elevation of sound sources and whether they are in the front or the rear. Outputs from the AVCN bilaterally innervate the medial (MSO) and lateral (LSO) nuclei of the superior olive, which are involved in processing interaural timing and intensity cues, respectively, providing information about sound source location in azimuth. Outputs from the brainstem all pass through the inferior colliculus (IC) in the auditory midbrain and the medial geniculate body (MGB) of the thalamus, before reaching the auditory cortex. The integration of information from the different brainstem nuclei produces quite complex and varied response properties in the IC and above. Some of this integration is likely to involve fusion of the different spatial location cues received from the DCN, MSO and LSO. More specific tuning to sound features such as frequency, amplitude and duration also begin to emerge in the IC. An interesting feature of many cortical neurons is that they appear to be tuned to specific spectrotemporal modulations, which Shamma and colleagues have proposed could be the fundamental cortical representation of sounds for tasks such as speech perception (e.g., Elhilali et al., 2003). It is important to note that the tonotopic representation of sound frequencies set up in the cochlea is preserved in the auditory nuclei of the brainstem and the primary nuclei of the auditory midbrain, thalamus and cortex.

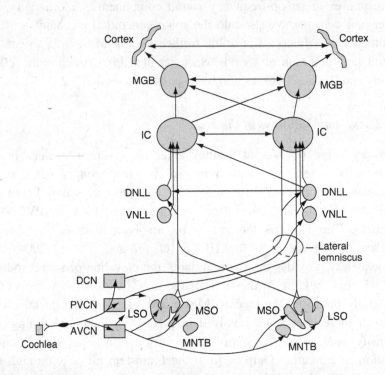

Figure 5.4. Schematic of the major ascending auditory pathways of the mammalian brain. Abbreviations: Dorsal cochlear nucleus (DCN); posteroventral cochlear nucleus (PVCN); anteroventral cochlear nucleus (AVCN); lateral nucleus of the superior olive (LSO); medial nucleus of the superior olive (MSO); medial nucleus of the trapezoid body (MNTB); ventral nucleus of the lateral lemniscus (VNLL); dorsal nucleus of the lateral lemniscus (DNLL); inferior colliculus (IC); medial geniculate body of the thalamus (MGB). Reprinted with permission from Pickles (2008), © Emerald Group Publishing Limited.

5.1.3 *Hearing loss*

Hearing loss is normally classified as conductive or sensorineural. The former refers to impairment of sound conduction by the outer and/or middle ear, which may result from disease, injury or abnormal development of the anatomical structures. The latter refers to impairment within the cochlea and/or the auditory nerve. The two most frequent causes of sensorineural impairment in the adult population are aging and exposure to loud sounds. Other causes that occur commonly in children as well as adults are disease, genetic disorders, head injury and ototoxic drugs.

The most obvious effect of both conductive and sensorineural hearing loss is the loss of audibility. The degree to which audibility is impaired for different sound frequencies is quantified by hearing thresholds for pure tones presented in a quiet listening environment. The hearing threshold at a certain frequency is defined as the minimum sound pressure level for a tone that is audible to the listener. Hearing thresholds are typically reported using a decibel scale relative to the hearing thresholds of normal hearing listeners, referred to as decibel hearing level (dB HL). An audiogram shows hearing thresholds plotted as a function of tone frequency, typically with −10 dB HL at the top and ~110 dB HL at the bottom. Four example audiograms are given in Fig. 5.5. By convention, the hearing thresholds for the left ear (LE) are plotted as Xs and those for the right ear (RE) as Os.

A number of different schemes have been developed over the years to provide a simple categorization of the degree of hearing loss. Typically these schemes are based on the pure tone average (PTA), which is the average of the hearing thresholds at 500, 1000 and 2000 Hz. A widely-used classification scheme for adults is:

0 to 25 dB HL;	normal limits
25 to 40 dB HL:	mild loss
40 to 55 dB HL:	moderate loss
55 to 70 dB HL:	moderate-to-severe loss
70 to 90 dB HL:	severe loss
90+ dB HL:	profound loss

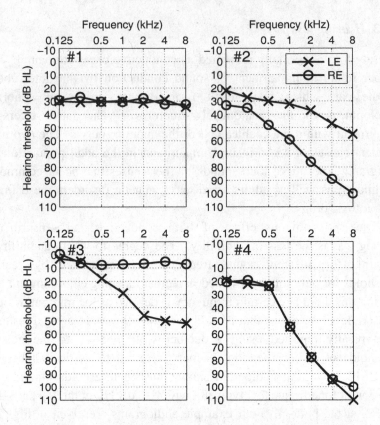

Figure 5.5. Four example audiograms showing hearing thresholds for the left ear (LE) and right ear (RE) of four individual with different patterns of hearing loss. See the text for a description of how these different audiograms are categorized.

In addition to categorizing the degree of hearing loss, the general shape of the audiogram is usually reported (e.g., flat, low-frequency, high-frequency, sloping) and any major differences between the two ears are noted (e.g., unilateral if there is hearing loss in one ear only, asymmetrical if the loss is bilateral but the thresholds are very different in the two ears). For example, audiogram #1 in Fig. 5.5 shows a symmetrical, flat, mild hearing loss (PTA = ~30 dB HL). Audiogram #2 illustrates an asymmetrical hearing loss, with a mild high-frequency sloping loss in the left ear (PTA = ~33 dB HL) and a moderate-to-severe high-frequency sloping loss in the right ear (PTA = ~61 dB HL).

Audiogram #3 depicts a unilateral, high-frequency sloping mild hearing loss in the left ear (PTA = ~31 dB HL). Audiogram #4 shows a bilateral, symmetrical moderate high-frequency hearing loss (PTA = ~52 dB HL). Audiograms such as #4 with a flat loss at low frequencies and a steep slope at high frequencies are sometimes referred to as "ski-slope" losses.

From the standard audiogram it is not possible to determine how much of the hearing loss is conductive and how much is sensorineural. A bone-conduction audiometer must be used to identify conductive losses. This device delivers sounds via a small vibrator placed on the skull, rather than through airborne sound waves. The vibrations propagate through the skull and directly into the cochlea, bypassing the outer and middle ears. As is the case for the standard audiogram, bone-conduction thresholds in the listener are compared to the average bone-conduction thresholds from normal hearing listeners to give threshold shifts in dB HL. If the bone-conduction thresholds in a listener are normal, then the hearing loss must be entirely conductive. If the bone-conduction threshold shifts are the same as the threshold shifts from the standard audiogram, then the loss is completely sensorineural. The hearing loss is referred to as "mixed" if the bone-conduction threshold shifts only account for some of the hearing loss.

The outer and middle ears are fairly linear systems, and subsequently, conductive hearing loss typically produces a simple linear reduction in the amplitude of acoustic signals as they are transmitted to the inner ear: loud sounds become quieter and quiet sounds may become inaudible. In the case of a purely conductive loss, the audiogram provides a direct estimate of the reduction in signal amplitude experienced at different frequencies. In the case of sensorineural hearing loss, the specific cochlear impairments contributing to the threshold shifts cannot be determined directly from the audiogram. However, for sound-induced hearing loss, the elevation of hearing thresholds are likely explained by the loss of auditory nerve sensitivity with dysfunction of both the inner and outer hair cells (Liberman and Dodds, 1984; Bruce et al., 2003; Zilany and Bruce, 2006). Figure 5.6 compares the appearance of normal inner and outer hair cell stereociliar bundles (panels A & B) with those in a cochlea exposed to very loud sound (panels C & D). In the noise-exposed cochlea, many stereociliar bundles are in disarray

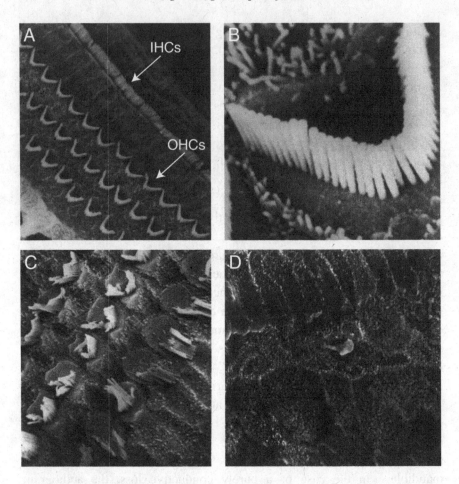

Figure 5.6. Scanning electron micrographs of inner hair cell (IHC) and outer hair cell (OHC) stereociliar bundles in normal-hearing and noise-exposed ears. A. Surface of the normal organ of Corti. B. Close-up view of the stereocilia of a normal OHC. C. Changes in the stereocilia 30 minutes after exposure to a 120 dB SPL (i.e., dB re. 20 µPa) broadband noise for 150 minutes. This ear showed a 45–50 dB temporary threshold shift at 2, 4 and 8 kHz. D. Changes in the apical surface of the organ of Corti 80 days after noise exposure. This ear had a 30–35 dB permanent threshold shift at 2 and 4 kHz. Note the surface was devoid of both stereocilia and hair cells. Reprinted with permission from Gao et al. (1992), © Elsevier.

(panel C) and in some cases a large fraction of the OHC hair bundles can be missing entirely (panel D). The hair cells themselves may die as a result of noise-exposure and the auditory nerve fibers innervating them subsequently degenerate.

Presbycusis (progressive age-related hearing loss) may result from a mix of gradual noise exposure, hair cell death and reduction of the endocochlear potential (Suryadevara et al., 2001). All of these are likely to contribute to a mix of outer and inner hair cell dysfunction, similar to noise-induced hearing loss. Psychophysical estimates of outer and inner hair cell contributions to threshold shifts show a range of outer and inner hair cells contributions in different listeners with sensorineural hearing loss (Moore et al., 1999). In cases of severe and profound hearing loss, the inner hair cells may be mostly dysfunctional or dead in an entire region of the cochlear, which is consequently referred to as a "dead region" (Moore et al., 2001). Additionally, some anti-cancer drugs are preferentially more toxic to inner or outer hair cells. Furthermore, congenital sensorineural hearing loss may result from abnormalities of the other cell types of the cochlea in addition to the hair cells.

Some consequences of sensorineural hearing impairment are not captured by the audiogram and need to be evaluated by more sophisticated psychophysical tests. Typical changes in psychophysical performance include reduction in the dynamic range of hearing, decreased frequency resolution, and decreased temporal resolution (Moore, 2003). The majority of the perceptual impairments can be explained from the direct effects of damaged inner and outer hair cells on the transduction process, but the effects of sensorineural hearing loss on the central auditory pathways of the brain must also be considered. Examples of central effects include changes in synaptic strengths and neurotransmitter expression, reorganization of tonotopic maps, and aberrant patterns of neural activity that may generate tinnitus, the phantom perception of sound (Eggermont, 2007).

A particular case of interest for hearing aids is the reduction in the dynamic range of loudness for a hearing impaired listener, usually referred to as "loudness recruitment." In this phenomenon, the hearing threshold is elevated at a frequency experiencing hearing loss, but the sound level at which a tone at that frequency becomes uncomfortably loud is relatively normal. That is, there is an abnormally steep growth of loudness with stimulus level between threshold and uncomfortable loudness. It is widely assumed that loudness recruitment is a result of more rapid growth of auditory nerve spike rates with sound level because of loss of cochlear compression. However, recent physiological data dispute this theory and suggest that temporal aspects of auditory-nerve responses and/or central mechanisms may be necessary to explain loudness recruitment (Heinz et al., 2005).

5.1.4 *Historical approaches to hearing aid amplification*

From the advent of electronic hearing aids, much effort has been expended in determining the optimal amplification strategy to compensate for an individual's hearing loss. Throughout this history, a major constraint in obtaining "optimal" amplification has been the capability of hearing aid technologies to amplify sounds over a wide enough frequency range and a large enough intensity range, without introducing undue distortion, extraneous noise or time delay to the acoustic signal. However, a perhaps equally important constraint has been a lack of complete understanding of how hearing loss affects the neural representation (and consequently the perception) of sounds.

From the beginning it was understood that the gain of the amplifier should vary as a function of frequency in a way that provides more amplification at frequencies where there is more hearing loss. If the ear performed only linear processing and hearing loss resulted only in linear attenuation of sounds, then it would make sense to provide 1 dB of gain at each frequency for each 1 dB of hearing loss at that frequency, as measured by the audiogram. However, this approach, often referred to as "mirroring the audiogram," was found only to be satisfactory for individuals with purely conductive hearing losses. The applicability of this tactic makes sense given that the middle ear is in the most part linear. Nevertheless, it has since been determined that in most cases providing linear gain of around 75% of any purely conductive loss is preferable to providing 100% gain.

For individuals with mixed or purely sensorineural losses, it was found that mirroring the audiogram excessively amplified loud sounds.

Consequently, it was suggested by several researchers that the gain should be reduced by a constant amount, perhaps dependent on measurements of most comfortable loudness levels as a function of frequency. Lybarger suggested the alternative "half gain rule," that 0.5 dB of gain should be applied for each 1 dB of hearing loss (Lybarger 1944). This approach has been further refined in modern amplification prescription formulas through extensive experimental testing. One example is the NAL-R prescription from the National Acoustic Laboratories of Australia, which is appropriate for individuals with mild to moderate hearing loss listening to speech at comfortable levels. The NAL-R formula prescribes the target gain G_i in the ith frequency band as:

$$G_i = X + 0.31 \cdot H_i + k_i, \qquad (5.1)$$

where X is equal to 0.15 times the 3-tone pure tone average (as defined in Section 5.1.3 above), H_i is the hearing loss in dB in the ith frequency band, and k_i is a frequency-dependent (and hearing-loss-independent) factor with the values given in Table 5.1.

Table 5.1. Frequency-dependent, hearing-loss-independent gain factors in the NAL-R formula (Eq. 5.1).

Freq (kHz)	0.25	0.5	1	2	3	4	6
k_i (dB)	−17	−8	1	−1	−2	−2	−2

A comparison of audiogram mirroring, the half-gain rule and the NAL-R prescription is given in Fig. 5.7 for the right ears of audiograms #1 and #2 from Fig. 5.5. It can be observed that the main difference between the NAL-R gains and the half-gain rule is that NAL-R prescribes substantially-reduced gains for frequencies below 1 kHz and somewhat reduced gains for frequencies above 1kHz. The advantage of reducing the gains away from 1 kHz is thought to be that it lessens the masking of the most important frequencies for speech (around 1 kHz) by lower and higher frequency components. See Dillon (2001) for a more extensive comparison of modern hearing aid gain prescription formulas.

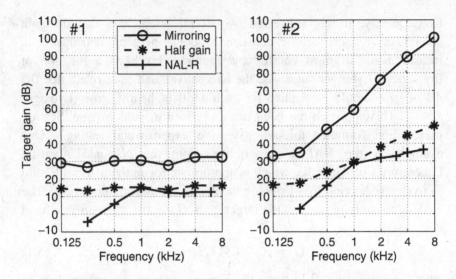

Figure 5.7. Comparison of three different amplification prescription formulae: audiogram mirroring, the half-gain rule and the NAL-R prescription, appropriate for the right ears of audiograms #1 and #2 from Figure 5.5.

Although the NAL-R formula and other linear amplification schemes work well for normal levels of conversational speech, because of loudness recruitment they still provide too much gain for loud sounds. Additionally, waveform peak clipping can occur in the amplifier or receiver at high input sound levels. Consequently, many hearing aids utilize automatic gain controls (AGCs) to vary the amplifier gain as a function of time and the input or output signal, thus producing nonlinear amplification. Reduction of the amplifier gain as a function of the input or output signal level via a fast-acting AGC is referred to as compression; slow-acting AGC can be used as an automatic volume control. In compression limiting, the gain is reduced so that the output level does not exceed the level at which peak clipping begins to occur. Compression that acts over the normal range of speech sound levels is referred to as wide-dynamic-range compression (WDRC). An example input/output curve for a compression system is shown in Fig. 5.8, with the gain versus input level shown in panel B. Here, a gain of 40 dB is

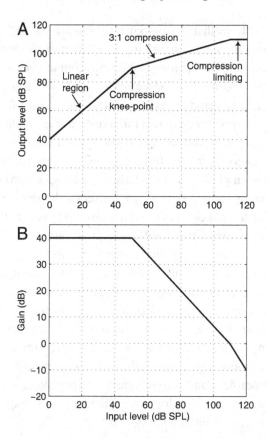

Figure 5.8. Example static characteristics of a compression system. A) Input/output curve for a system with wide-dynamic-range compression (WDRC) with a 3:1 compression ratio for input levels above 50 dB SPL and compression limiting at an output level of 110 dB SPL. B) The amplifier gain versus input-level function required to achieve the compression characteristics described in panel A.

applied for all input signals that are lower than 50 dB SPL, the knee-point (threshold) of the WDRC. Above 50 dB SPL, the gain of the amplifier is reduced by 10 dB for each 15 dB increase in the input level. This compresses input levels over a range of 60 dB into an output range of 20 dB, producing a compression ratio of 3:1. At an input level of 110 dB SPL, the gain has consequently been reduced to 0 dB, i.e., no amplification is applied. Compression limiting is applied for input levels above 110 dB SPL so that the output level cannot exceed 110 dB SPL. In addition to the static input/output characteristics, an important property of compression schemes is the time-course over which the gain is changed. The time it takes for a compressor to react to an increase in the signal level is referred to as the attack time, and the release time corresponds to the time taken to react to a decrease in signal level.

The parameters of the compression system can be set to avoid distorted and uncomfortably loud signals, to reduce the intensity differences between phonemes or syllables, to provide automatic volume control, to increase sound comfort, to normalize loudness, to maximize intelligibility, or to reduce background noise. However, the parameter sets required to achieve these different goals are very different, and consequently any one compression scheme tends to provide benefit in some but not all aspects of compensating for hearing impairment. Evidently, nonlinear amplification is required to compensate for the nonlinear effects of sensorineural hearing loss on the representation of sounds in the brain, but the optimal form of nonlinear processing appears to be something beyond what can be achieve by simple compression schemes. Consequently, the following section will explore the biomedical principles and engineering methodologies that will be required in order to develop amplification schemes that better compensate for sensorineural hearing loss.

5.1.5 *Biomedical principles for improving hearing aids*

A major biomedical consideration for hearing aid devices is the placement of the microphone, the amplifier package and the receiver (the miniature loudspeaker) in or near the ear. Figure 5.9 shows the range of styles of typical modern hearing aids, including behind-the-ear (BTE), in-the-ear (ITE), in-the-canal (ITC) and completely-in-the-canal (CIC) hearing aids. Each of these styles places different constraints on the size of the components and consequently the achievable performance of those components. In addition, the physical placement of the microphone and receiver will influence the input signal to the amplifier and the achievable frequency response at the ear drum, respectively.

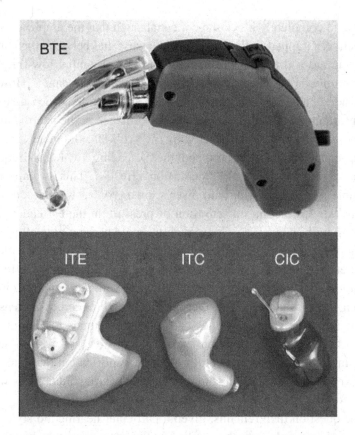

Figure 5.9. Modern hearing aid styles: behind-the-ear (BTE); in-the-ear (ITE); in-the-canal (ITC); completely-in-the-canal (CIC). Not shown is the earmold that connects to the BTE ear-hook via a tube to deliver amplified sounds to the ear canal. Reprinted with permission from Dillon (2001).

A particular issue for hearing aids is the fitting of the earmold or the aid in the ear canal. Of significant concern is achieving a comfortable and secure fit. However, the resulting acoustics of the ear canal and hearing aid can be of even greater importance for the operation of the hearing aid. In particular, any acoustic pathways for amplified sounds to return to the microphone can lead to an unstable feedback loop, causing a loud squeal or whistling sound. Thus, in order to minimize the possibility of acoustic feedback, it is desirable to have the earmold or hearing aid completely block the ear canal, such that the amplified sound in effectively trapped in the section of the ear canal between the earmold or hearing aid and the ear drum. In addition, substantial low-frequency gain can only be obtained in a blocked or *occluded* ear canal. However, an occluded ear canal also traps moist air and earwax, which can cause discomfort and potentially hamper the performance of the hearing aid. In addition, sounds that are conducted by the skull into the inner section of the ear canal can also be trapped there, leading to a low-frequency resonance referred to as the "occlusion effect". This is particularly noticeable for the hearing aid user's own voice, which can sound "boomy", and sometimes a sensation of pressure in the ear canal can be felt along with the sound. Consequently, most hearing aids allow some venting of air through the earmold or hearing aid, and a balance must be made between reducing acoustic feedback and reducing the effects of occlusion. Feedback can also be reduced by increasing the distance between the receiver and the microphone, which becomes increasingly more difficult the smaller the device. Modern methods for dealing with such difficulties in conventional hearing aids are explored in Section 5.3.3. In addition, approaches to providing amplification that attempt to circumvent some of the limits of conventional hearing aid designs will be discussed in Section 5.4.2.

The question then remains, given a particular hearing aid style, what biomedical principles can be applied to improve how that hearing aid amplifies and processes sounds? The ultimate goal is undoubtedly to fully restore the normal neural representation of all types of sounds at every level of processing within the auditory systems of the brain (Edwards, 2007). Through human testing and trial-and-error, some progress has been made in reaching this goal. However, an impediment has clearly been our incomplete understanding of how the ear and brain normally process and represent sounds and what effect hearing loss has on these. Therefore, Sachs and colleagues proposed that an intermediate goal might be to attempt to restore the neural representation of at least speech sounds at the level of the auditory nerve (Sachs et al., 2002). This approach seems achievable given the insights obtained from recent physiological and modeling studies into the effects of sensorineural hearing loss on the auditory nerve's representation of speech sounds. In

Section 5.2, the normal and impaired neural representation of sounds will be reviewed. State-of-the-art approaches to compensating for the effects of hearing loss on the peripheral and central auditory system will be examined in Section 5.3. Finally, future directions in hearing aid design from a biomedical perspective will be considered in Section 5.4.

5.2 Normal and Impaired Neural Representation of Sounds

To begin to tackle the problem of restoring near-normal auditory nerve representation of sounds in an impaired ear, it is necessary to understand in more detail how acoustic features are encoded in the spike patterns of the auditory nerve and how cochlear impairment leads to degradation of the neural representation. First the encoding of simple acoustic features will be examined, and then studies of the neural representation of speech stimuli will be reviewed.

5.2.1 *Fundamental acoustic features*

Any acoustic stimulus can be considered to consist of one or more frequency components with a particular time duration, amplitude and phase. Therefore, to appreciate how acoustic stimuli in general are represented by neural spike patterns, it is instructive to begin with the response of neurons to simple sinusoidal stimuli, referred to as "pure tones" because they contain only one frequency component, and work towards stimuli with more complicated sets of frequency components.

Figure 5.10 shows the response of a cat auditory nerve fiber to a 25-ms, 600 Hz tone, this fiber's preferred or *best frequency* (BF; also known as the *characteristic frequency* or CF). The response is quantified by a peri-stimulus time (PST) histogram, i.e., the number of neural spikes recorded in consecutive 0.1-ms time bins for 200 repetitions of the stimulus. Each panel of Fig. 5.10 shows the response to the stimulus presented at the sound pressure level indicated. Included in the bottom panel is the stimulus waveform delayed in time to align it with the phase of the neural response. It can be seen that at all SPLs the spikes tend to synchronize to the stimulus waveform. Because of rectification in the IHC transduction, there is also increase in the average stimulus-driven

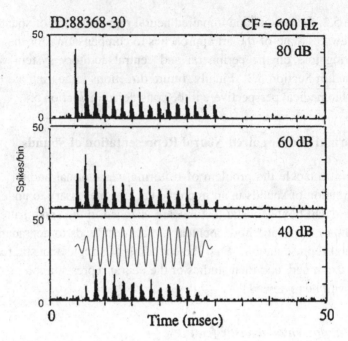

Figure 5.10. Response of AN fiber with CF = 600 Hz to a 25-ms 600-Hz tone presented at three different sound pressure levels. The tone waveform is shown within the bottom panel. Reprinted with permission from Zhang et al. (2001), © Acoustical Society of America.

spike rate above the spontaneous spike rate of this fiber. At 40 dB SPL, the average spike rate remains fairly constant throughout the response. When the presentation level is increase to 60 dB SPL, the onset response grows larger, but the response adapts over time such that the steady-state response is similar to that seen at 40 dB SPL. At 80 dB SPL, the onset response continues to grow, while the steady-state response remains saturated.

If the responses of a population of AN fibers to tones with varying frequency and SPL are recorded, the frequency-tuning properties of the cochlea (as illustrated in Fig. 5.3) are seen to be inherited. Figure 5.11A illustrates how the tuning properties of a single fiber are measured and quantified. Tuning curves in normal ears exhibit a narrow "tip" at the BF, which is determined by the location along the cochlea of the IHC

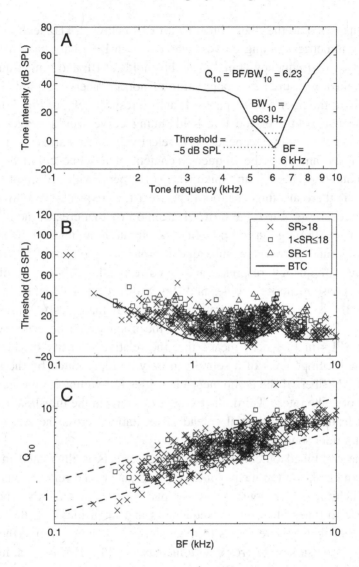

Figure 5.11. A. Example single-fiber threshold tuning curve. The fiber threshold, best frequency (BF) and tuning quality (Q_{10}) are calculated as illustrated, where BW_{10} is the tuning curve bandwidth 10 dB above threshold. B. Cat AN fiber thresholds at BF for a population of normal fibers with different spontaneous rates (SRs). BTC indicates the best threshold curve. C. Q_{10} values plotted versus BF. The dashed lines indicate the 5th and 95th percentiles of the data. Panels B & C reprinted with permission from Miller et al. (1997), © Acoustical Society of America.

that synapses onto the fiber. Fibers with BFs below ~2 kHz tend to have fairly symmetrical tuning curves, whereas high-BF fibers have a high-intensity, low-frequency "tail." The thresholds at BF and tuning quality (Q_{10}) values measured in a population of normal fibers are plotted as a function of the fiber's BF in panels B and C, respectively, of Fig. 5.11.

The narrow tip of the threshold tuning curve would suggest that auditory nerve fibers respond very selectively to a narrow range of frequencies, and thus the frequency content of a sound could be well represented by the mean spike rate of fibers with different BFs. However, there are three factors that affect the frequency resolution of the AN response. First, the OHC electromotility that creates the narrow and sensitive tuning curve tip begins to saturate at around 30 dB above threshold, and there is a subsequent broadening of the BM filter's magnitude-frequency response and a corresponding flattening of the relative phase response (Robles and Ruggero, 2001). That is, the tuning of the BM is broader for suprathreshold sounds than it is for threshold sounds. Second, the saturation in the mean spike rate observed at the higher SPLs in Fig. 5.10 means that the relative intensity of different frequency components of a sound can only be represented by the spike rate of AN fibers if the component intensities fall within the unsaturated region of spike rates. Third, the existence of tails in the threshold tuning curves leads to a substantial spread of excitation across the AN in the case of louder sounds.

The combined outcome of these three effects is illustrated in Fig. 5.12, which shows the mean spike rate (top panel) and relative phase of the synchronized response (bottom) panel for a single AN fiber in response to tones of different frequencies and intensities. At the lower SPLs, the fiber only responds to tones with frequencies around the BF, and the mean spike rate grows with increasing SPL. However, at higher SPLs the spike rate at the BF saturates, and the fiber starts to respond strongly to frequencies away from BF, particularly on the low frequency side. This indicates that the mean spike rate representation of sounds may be compromised at higher SPLs, whereas the spike-timing information in the synchronized response appears to be more robust to changes in presentation level and background noise (Young, 2008).

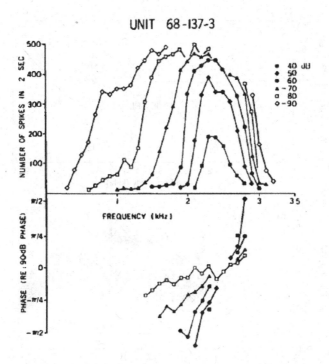

Figure 5.12. Intensity-dependent spike rate and phase responses for a fiber with BF of 2.3 kHz. Rates were computed from the sustained responses to 100 repetitions of a 50 ms tone burst. The phase for each response was referenced to the phase in response to that frequency at 90 dB SPL. Reprinted with permission from Anderson et al. (1971), © Acoustical Society of America.

Noise exposure, presbycusis and ototoxicity, amongst other forms of cochlear hearing loss, will alter the mechanics of the BM vibrations (because of impairment of OHC electromotility) and the transduction process (because of IHC impairment), leading to changes in the AN's representation of sounds. The effects of noise exposure on cat AN fiber threshold tuning curves is shown in Fig. 5.13. It is observed that noise exposure leads to elevation of thresholds in the region of hearing loss (panel B), resulting from the combined effects of OHC and IHC impairment, and to broadened tuning (indicated by the reduced Q_{10} values in panel C), arising primarily from OHC impairment (Liberman

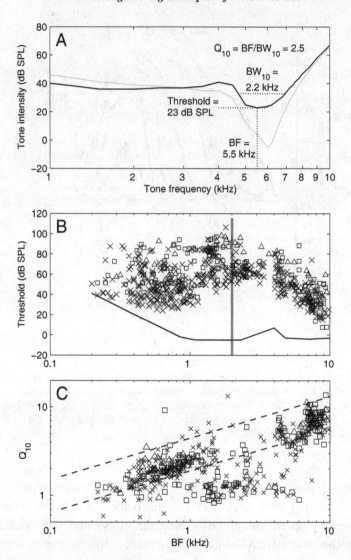

Figure 5.13. Threshold tuning curve characteristics [calculated as shown in panel A] for fibers in a pool of impaired cats produced by noise exposure. Cats were anesthetized and exposed to a 50 Hz wide band of noise centered at 2 kHz for 2 h at levels between 110–115 dB SPL (the vertical gray bar in panel B). (B) Thresholds and (C) Q_{10} for fibers recorded after noise exposure. The gray line in panel A shows the normal tuning curve from Fig. 5.11A. The dashed lines in panel C indicate the 5th and 95th percentiles of the normal Q_{10} data from Fig. 5.11C. Panels B & C reprinted with permission from Miller et al. (1997), © Acoustical Society of America.

and Dodds, 1984; Bruce et al., 2003; Zilany and Bruce, 2006). Thus, AN fibers in an impaired ear lose their sensitivity to quieter sounds and their frequency selectivity. Along with the broadening of tuning at threshold comes a flattening of the phase-frequency response, as occurs at higher SPLs in the normal ear (see the bottom panel of Fig. 5.12). In addition to the changes to the threshold tuning properties, impairment of the OHCs leads to loss of the compressive and suppressive nonlinearities of the cochlear response that are created by the OHC electromotility (Sachs et al., 2002).

While the loss of frequency selectivity and nonlinearity may somewhat degrade the representation of tones, its biggest effect is seen for broadband sounds. In the next section we will look specifically at the neural representation of speech sounds in the normal ear and at the effects of hearing loss on this representation.

5.2.2 *Speech*

Just as features of simple acoustic stimuli are represented by changes in the mean spike rate and spike timing of AN fibers, so too are features of complex stimuli such as speech. The narrowband filtering properties of the normal ear produce fluctuations in the mean spike rate of AN fibers that reflect fluctuations in the speech envelope for frequencies around each fiber's CF (see Fig. 5.14A). This mean-rate representation is limited by the rate spread/saturation phenomenon depicted in Fig. 5.12, but there is a class of low-spontaneous-rate/high-threshold AN fibers (see Fig. 5.11B), which do not exhibit strong saturation. In addition, the suppression effects created by the cochlear amplifier tend to preserve the rate-place representation at higher presentation levels (Young, 2008). Subsequent processing of AN responses to speech by neurons in the cochlear nucleus (see Fig. 5.14B) and inferior colliculus (see Fig. 5.14C) produces spike patterns that maintain the representation of the narrowband envelope fluctuations in the speech in a robust fashion.

In addition to the rate-place representation, voiced speech segments (such as vowels) produce a tonotopic representation of the harmonic components of the stimulus in the synchronized (i.e., phase-locked) response of the AN. Fig. 5.15A shows the spectrum of the synthetic

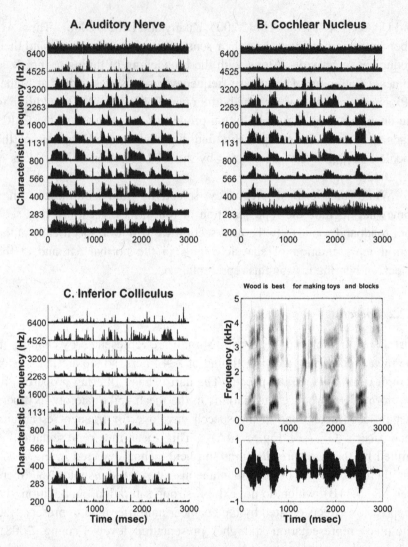

Figure 5.14. Neural response to the speech utterance "Wood is best for making toys and blocks" for populations of neurons in the AN, CN, and IC. Neural responses (A–C) are shown as "neurograms", where each trace represents the average PST histogram for all neurons whose CF was contained in one of 11 ½-octave bands. The center frequency of each band is shown at the left. The bottom right panels show the waveform and broadband spectrogram of the utterance. Reprinted with permission from Delgutte et al. (1998), © John Wiley & Sons Limited.

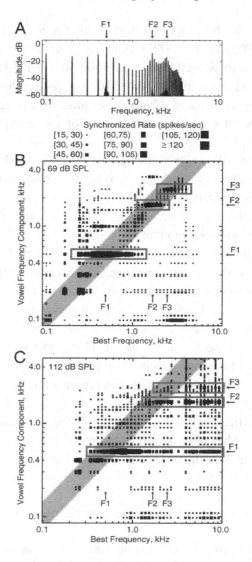

Figure 5.15. A. Spectrum of the vowel /ɛ/. B. AN synchronized vowel responses in normal ears. C. Synchronized responses in ears with noise-induced hearing loss similar to that of Fig. 5.13. The magnitude of the synchronized response of an AN fiber with a particular BF (along the abscissa) to a particular vowel frequency component (along the ordinate) is indicated by the size of the filled box, according to the scale given above panel B. The gray shaded area along the diagonal denotes the region where the synchronization frequency is within one octave of the BF. Panels B & C reprinted with permission from Schilling et al. (1998), © Elsevier.

vowel /ɛ/ that has been widely studied in physiological experiments (Sachs et al., 2002; Young, 2008). Fig. 5.15B depicts the magnitude of the synchronized response (according to the size of the filled boxes) in the normal ear as a function of AN fiber BF (along the abscissa) and vowel frequency component (along the ordinate). Strong synchronized responses to the first three spectral peaks (or formants) of the vowel, indicated by F1, F2 & F3, are observed in the correct tonotopic place, i.e., the matching BF region (indicated by the gray shaded area). This spike-timing representation of speech tends to be more robust than the rate-place representation (Young, 2008).

In ears suffering from hearing loss, both the rate-place and synchronized-response representations of speech are degraded because of the broadened tuning and loss of suppression (Sachs et al., 2002; Young, 2008). Fig. 5.15C depicts the synchronized AN response to the vowel /ɛ/ in ears suffering from noise exposure as shown in Fig. 5.13. Note that the presentation level has been increased to make the vowel audible in the impaired ear. A marked spread to higher BFs is observed in the synchronized response to each formant, along with an increase in the synchrony to non-formant frequency components of the vowel.

Such substantial degradation in the neural representation of speech sounds, even without the additional burden of background noise, indicates the difficult job that a hearing aid faces in compensating for hearing loss. The next section describes the latest advances in amplification and speech processing strategies to be applied in hearing aids.

5.3 Recent Advances in Hearing Aid Algorithms and Device Designs

The introduction of digital hearing aids has enabled sophisticated amplification and processing of sound, well beyond what was achievable in analog hearing aids. A primary goal of such algorithms is to compensate for the ways in which an impaired ear deviates from the normal processing and transduction of sounds. Advances have been made in developing schemes to counteract the direct peripheral effects of hearing loss, as discussed below. However, an algorithm (or set of algorithms) that fully counteracts the effects of peripheral hearing loss has not been found to date. Consequently, speech processing strategies have also been created to help the central auditory system cope better with the degraded input that it receives from an impaired ear. In addition, device designs have continued to evolve, bringing further improvements to the performance of hearing aids.

5.3.1 *Compensating for peripheral effects of hearing loss*

The current standard in amplification schemes is multiband WDRC (Souza, 2002). While simple forms of multiband WDRC were available on analog hearing aids, the signal processing capabilities of digital hearing aids facilitate much greater flexibility in approaches to compression and consequently allow for more efficient and effective application of compressive amplification (Kates, 2005). In particular, many digital hearing aids utilize compression with a large number of frequency channels (>4). Such real-time, multi-channel processing is made possible by dedicated filterbank and fast Fourier transform (FFT) circuitry on the hearing aid processing chip, instead of having to implement these algorithms entirely in software. An enduring concern with WDRC is that the optimal temporal dynamics of compression (i.e., the attack and release times) vary depending on the listening conditions and on whether the goal is to maximize listening comfort or to maximize speech intelligibility (Dillon, 2001; Souza, 2002).

An alternative form of nonlinear amplification scheme that has gained widespread use in recent years is Adaptive Dynamic Range Optimization (ADRO; Blamey, 2005, 2006). ADRO departs from the standard approach to compression and instead uses a set of fuzzy-logic rules to set gains in each frequency band (out of 16, 32 or 64, depending on the implementation), as illustrated in Fig. 5.16. The gain in each channel is based on a statistical analysis of the output of each channel, according to the following four rules:

1. The "comfort rule" ensures that sustained sounds are not uncomfortably loud. It reduces gain in a channel if the output level exceeds the "comfort target" (comfortable threshold) more than 10% of the time.

2. The "audibility rule" ensures that sustained sounds are not too soft. It increase the gain in a channel if the output level is below the "audibility target" (audibility threshold) more than 30% of the time.
3. The "hearing protection rule" prevents damage and uncomfortably loud sounds. A maximum output level limit is applied to each channel.
4. The "background noise rule" prevents low-level background noise from high-level amplification. It limits the maximum gain in each channel.

Adjustments to the gain based on the comfort and audibility rules are made slowly (3 to 6 dB/s, depending on user preference), such that most of the time ADRO is performing linear amplification, whereas the hearing protection rule acts instantaneously. In several speech perception studies, ADRO was found to provide better speech intelligibility than linear and WDRC schemes in some listening conditions, and the majority of subjects preferred listening with the ADRO scheme (Blamey, 2005).

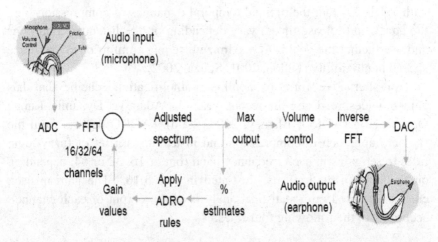

Figure 5.16. Flow diagram of signal processing by the Adaptive Dynamic Range Optimization (ADRO) nonlinear amplification scheme. Reprinted with permission from Blamey (2006).

5.3.2 *Compensating for central effects of hearing loss*

The inability of hearing aid amplification schemes to fully compensate for the peripheral effects of hearing loss is indicated by the difficulty that hearing aid users experience in complex listening environments.   These difficulties include not only poorer speech perception in background noise or reverberant environments but also increased listening effort in directing attention, problems with localizing sound sources and annoyance by background sounds (Moore, 2003; Edwards, 2007).   This is not surprising, given that much of the processing of the neural representation of sounds that occurs in the subcortical and cortical auditory nuclei relies on the time-frequency analysis that is performed by the normal cochlea.   In the case of impairment of the AN representation of the time-frequency content of acoustic signals because of sensorineural hearing loss, it is to be expected that the subsequent neural processing in the central auditory system will be compromised.   An example of this is the processing that the dorsal cochlear nucleus (DCN) neural circuitry performs to extract information about sound source elevation.   This circuit includes excitatory and inhibitory inputs from auditory nerve fibers with specific CF ranges, such that it is sensitive to spectral notches caused by the outer ear (Oertel and Young, 2004).   However, in animals with noise-induced hearing loss, the response properties of the neurons in the DCN circuitry are very different to those in a normal-hearing ear (Ma and Young, 2006).   One would expect sound source elevation estimation to be greatly impaired as a consequence.

Given the listening difficulties that hearing-aid users experience with conventional amplification schemes, there has been substantial interest in hearing aid features that improve listening comfort and ease. One simple approach to attenuating low-intensity background sounds that may cause attentional distraction is to incorporate an expansive gain region at low SPLs in compression schemes. This effectively turns down the hearing aid's gain for very low-intensity sounds, many of which will be background noises. Digital signal processing can also be used to obtain more sophisticated background noise reduction (Bentler and Chiou, 2006). Methods that do not make use of any directional information about the target sound source and background sounds are referred to as single-microphone noise reduction algorithms. These techniques attempt to characterize some features of background noise signals and attenuate them.

Another aid to attending to a specific sound source is the use of directional microphones, which is becoming widespread in hearing aids. Typically the hearing aid allows the user to switch between directional and non-directional microphone modes, depending on the user's present listening environment. A more advanced form of directionality can be achieved via adaptive beamforming algorithms. These signal processing techniques attempt to detect and cancel sounds that do not arrive from the preferred direction, normally to the front of the listener. In contrast to single-microphone noise reduction schemes, directional noise reduction approaches are capable of achieving increases in speech intelligibility, in addition to increased listening comfort. However, the efficacy of adaptive beamforming algorithms currently used in hearing aids depends greatly on the types and positions of interfering sound sources (Kim and Barrs, 2006).

5.3.3 *Device improvements*

Hearing aids making use of an earmold that keeps the ear canal mostly unblocked, referred to as an "open fitting", have gained in popularity in recent years (Kim and Barrs, 2006). The primary aim of an open fitting is to avoid the occlusion effect. Open fittings were not feasible in most analog hearing aids because of acoustic feedback, but the acoustic feedback cancellation algorithms that are available in digital aids enable sufficient gain to be achieved for many hearing aids users in an open fitting without producing feedback (Edwards, 2007; Levitt, 2007). However, sufficient gain without acoustic feedback in an open fitting is often not achievable in individuals with severe or profound hearing loss. In addition, the acoustics of an open fitting are such that substantial gain cannot be obtained at low frequencies. On the other hand, the open fitting does allow a relatively unimpeded acoustic path for low-frequency sound components to reach the ear drum from outside the ear. Thus, an open fitting is only suitable for individuals with high-frequency hearing loss and near-normal low-frequency hearing.

In some BTE devices with an open fitting, instead of using a tube to deliver the sound from the BTE package to the ear canal, the receiver (i.e., the miniature loudspeaker) itself is placed in the ear canal, with wires connecting the receiver to the BTE aid. Such devices are referred to as receiver-in-the-ear (RITE) hearing aids. In addition, recent improvements in receiver design enable greater gain to be applied in the region from 5 to 10 kHz than was previously possible, but the benefits of additional high-frequency gain depend on the form of the hearing loss (Ricketts et al., 2008).

Many hearing aid users have a bilateral hearing loss and consequently wear a hearing aid in each ear, with each hearing aid acting independently. With the more sophisticated processing now available on digital hearing aids, many devices allow for manual or automatic switching between preprogrammed sets of hearing aid algorithm parameters, commonly referred to as "programs". However, in a bilateral fitting, the program in each hearing aid needs to be manually switched or will experience independent automatic switching. To alleviate this problem, low-power wireless links are now being added to some hearing aids to allow for coordinated programming and program switching. Wireless links can also be used to receive audio signals from a device such as a cellphone in some newer hearing aids.

5.4 Future Directions in Hearing Aid Design

This chapter has described many of the advances that have been made in hearing aid design over the last century. In the 1990s, user satisfaction with hearing aids was only around 59% (Kochkin, 2002). With the further improvements in hearing aids described in the previous section, user satisfaction has grown to around 78% in recent years (Kochkin, 2005). While this progress in the benefits obtained by hearing aid users is encouraging, modern hearing aids still do not fully compensate for all the effects of hearing loss. Consequently, further improvements in the efficacy of conventional hearing aids are being pursued by means of innovative amplification and speech processing algorithms. In addition, some of the difficulties faced by conventional hearing aids are being tackled by the introduction of implantable hearing aid components or complete systems.

5.4.1 *Amplification & speech processing*

While compression schemes aim to compensate for the loss of compression in basilar membrane vibrations within the impaired ear, they do not deal with the accompanying loss of frequency selectivity. Consequently, several groups have proposed speech processing schemes that apply spectral sharpening, but improvements in speech intelligibility have been generally minor (Moore, 2003). One new form of nonlinear processing that includes spectral enhancement is companding i.e., a compressing-and-expanding strategy (Turicchia and Sarpeshkar, 2005). This scheme simultaneously produces multiband compression, spectral sharpening and reduction of low-level background noise. Promising results have been found using companding in processing for cochlear implants, but the benefits for hearing aid processing remain to be seen.

Physiological experiments and models have lead to several new ideas for amplification schemes. Contrast-enhancing frequency shaping (CEFS) is a form of spectral sharpening aimed at restoring the neural representation of voiced speech formants (Miller et al., 1999; Sachs et al., 2002; Bruce, 2004). Instead of attempting to sharpen all spectral peaks, as is typically done in spectral enhancement algorithms, CEFS tracks the voiced speech formants over time and adjusts the relative amplitudes of the formants to produce a more normal AN response to the formants. Recently, Shi and colleagues (2006) have proposed an algorithm designed to compensate for the changes in the phase response of the impaired cochlea.

The recent development of faster and more accurate computational models of the normal and impaired auditory periphery has prompted several groups to investigate direct use of these models in hearing aid speech processing algorithms—see Bruce (2006) and Edwards (2007) for reviews. These model-based approaches hold the promise of more faithful compensation for the physiological effects of hearing loss than *ad hoc* nonlinear schemes such as WDRC and ADRO.

As described previously, several schemes for single- and multiple-microphone noise reduction make use of manipulations in gain over time in order to filter out background noise while preserving the target sound (Bentler and Chiou, 2006). A recent study by Anzalone and colleagues (2006) showed that in order for such noise reduction scheme to improve speech intelligibility the speech/noise detection algorithm must be at least 90% accurate in discriminating between the speech and noise components of the signal and the gain changes must be made on the order of 15 ms or faster. Such requirements are very challenging for current speech/noise detection algorithms, motivating research into more accurate methods for detecting speech components in noisy signals.

A high bit-rate wireless link between bilateral hearing aids that allowed for high-fidelity audio streaming would open up the possibility of implementing sophisticated binaural signal processing strategies in a pair of hearing aids (Rohdenburg et al., 2007), but present low-power wireless links cannot achieve transmission at such high bit rates. It has also been proposed that algorithms could be developed to deal more directly with the perceptual and cognitive difficulties faced by hearing aid users, beyond simple noise-reduction schemes (Edwards, 2007). Such algorithms would likely require binaural processing facilitated by a wireless link.

5.4.2 *Implantable components*

The clinical success of cochlear implants (see Chapter 6) over the last three decades has generated interest in developing implantable components for hearing aids. Conventional hearing aids with components placed on the external ear are subject to environmental wear, and components in the ear canal can produce discomfort and occlusion and may be hampered by earwax buildup. The aim of implanting hearing aid components is to eliminate these drawbacks by moving components away from the outer ear and ear canal.

A primary focus has been development of mass-transducers to directly drive the ossicular chain in the middle ear, instead of providing acoustic amplification (Kim and Barrs, 2006; Jenkins et al., 2007). Various forms of mass-transducer have been investigated, including piezoelectric drivers, electromagnetic drivers and electromechanical drivers. Such hearing aids are now referred to as implantable middle-ear hearing devices. If the microphone and speech processor are worn externally, then the device is referred to as semi-implantable, whereas fully-implantable devices have all components implanted, an example of which is shown in Fig. 5.17. The benefit gained over conventional hearing aids must be substantial enough to justify the surgery that is required to implant middle-ear hearing devices, and consequently further clinical evaluations of these types of devices are required to prove their efficacy (Kim and Barrs, 2006; Jenkins et al., 2007).

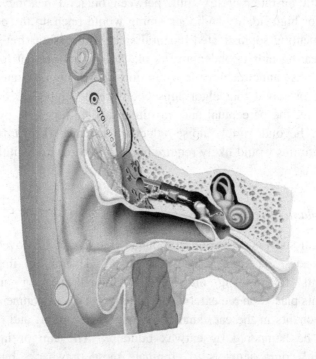

Figure 5.17. Example of the placement of a fully implantable middle-ear hearing device, the Otologics Fully-Implantable MET Ossicular Stimulator.

For individuals with conductive hearing loss that cannot be rectified with surgery, bone-anchored hearing aids (BAHAs) are an alternative to conventional acoustic-amplifier hearing aids (Kim and Barrs, 2006). This device utilizes a screw implanted into the skull, just behind the ear, to transmit vibrations in the skull that then propagate to the cochlea and produce cochlear excitation. Another hearing aid making use of an implantable component is the RetroX, which achieves an open fitting by transmitting sound to the ear canal from a BTE hearing aid via a titanium tube implanted in the skull behind the ear (Garin et al., 2004).

5.5 Summary

Hearing aids confront the difficult task of compensating for degradation and loss of information about acoustic stimuli in impaired ears. However, with recent advances in device design, the power of digital signal processing, and continuing progress in our understanding of the human auditory system, the future appears promising for restoring near-normal hearing to the many who suffer from hearing loss in our society.

5.6 References

Anderson, D. J., Rose, J. E., Hind, J. E. and Brugge, J. F. (1971). Temporal position of discharges in single auditory nerve fibers within the cycle of a sine-wave stimulus: frequency and intensity effects, *J. Acoust. Soc. Am.*, 49(4B), pp. 1131–1139.

Anzalone, M., Calandruccio, L., Doherty, K. and Carney, L. (2006). Determination of the potential benefit of time-frequency gain manipulation, *Ear Hear.* 27, pp. 480–492.

Bentler, R. and Chiou, L. K. (2006). Digital noise reduction: an overview, *Trends Amplif.*, 10(2), pp. 67–82.

Blamey, P. J. (2005). Adaptive dynamic range optimization (ADRO): A digital amplification strategy for cochlear implants and hearing aids, *Trends Amplif.*, 9(2) , pp. 77–98.

Blamey, P. J. (2006). Adaptive dynamic range optimization for hearing aids, Presented at *9th Western Pacific Acoustics Conference (WESPAC IX)*, June 26–28, Seoul, Korea.

Brownell, W. E., Bader, C. R., Bertrand, D. and de Ribaupierre, Y. (1985). Evoked mechanical responses of isolated cochlear outer hair cells, *Science*, 227(4683), pp. 194–196.

Bruce, I. C. (2004). Physiological assessment of contrast-enhancing frequency shaping and multiband compression in hearing aids, *Physiol. Meas.*, 25, pp. 945–956.

Bruce, I. C. (2006). Physiological insights into hearing loss and optimal amplification, *Canadian Hearing Report* 1(2), pp. 20–21.

Bruce, I. C., Sachs, M. B. and Young, E. D. (2003). An auditory-periphery model of the effects of acoustic trauma on auditory nerve responses, *J. Acoust. Soc. Am.*, 113(1), pp. 369–388.

Clark, G. M. (2003). *Cochlear Implants: Fundamentals and Applications.* Springer-Verlag, New York, NY.

Delgutte, B., Hammond, B. M. and Cariani, P. A. (1998). Neural coding of the temporal envelope of speech: relation to modulation transfer functions. In *Psychophysical and Physiological Advances in Hearing*, A. R. Palmer, A. Rees, A. Q. Summerfield and R. Meddis, eds., Whurr Publishers, London, UK, pp. 595–603.

Dillon, H. (2001). *Hearing Aids*. Thieme Medical Publishers, New York, NY.

Edwards, B. (2007). The future of hearing aid technology, *Trends Amplif.* 11(1), pp. 31–46.

Eggermont, J. J. (2007). Pathophysiology of tinnitus, *Prog. Brain Res.*, 166, pp. 19–35.

Elhilali, M., Chi, T. and Shamma S. (2003). Intelligibility and the spectrotemporal representation of speech in the auditory cortex, *Speech Commun.*, 41, pp. 331–348.

Garin, P., Genard, F., Galle, C. and Jamart, J. (2004). The RetroX auditory implant for high-frequency hearing loss, *Otol. Neurotol.*, 25(4), pp. 511–519.

Gao, W. Y., Ding, D. L., Zheng, X. Y., Ruan, F. M. and Liu, Y. J. (1992). A comparison of changes in the stereocilia between temporary and permanent hearing losses in acoustic trauma, *Hear. Res.*, 62(1), pp. 27–41.

Heinz, M. G., Issa, J. B., Young, E. D. (2005). Auditory-nerve rate responses are inconsistent with common hypotheses for the neural correlates of loudness recruitment, *JARO*, 6(2), pp. 91–105.

Jenkins, H. A., Atkins, J. S., Horlbeck, D., Hoffer, M. E., Balough, B., Arigo, J. V., Alexiades, G. and Garvis, W. (2007). U.S. Phase I preliminary results of use of the Otologics MET Fully-Implantable Ossicular Stimulator, *Otolaryngol. Head Neck Surg.*, 137(2) , pp. 206–212.

Kates, J. M. (2005). Principles of digital dynamic-range compression, *Trends Amplif.* 9(2), pp. 45–76.

Kim, H. H. and Barrs, D. M. (2006). Hearing aids: A review of what's new, *Otolaryngol. Head Neck Surg.*, 134(6), pp. 1043–1050.

Kochkin, S. (2002). MarkeTrak VI: 10-year customer satisfaction trends in the US hearing instrument market, *The Hearing Review*, 9(10), pp. 14–25.

Kochkin, S. (2005). MarkeTrak VII: Customer satisfaction with hearing instruments in the digital age, *Hear J.*, 58, pp. 30–42.

Levitt, H. (2007). A historical perspective on digital hearing aids: How digital technology has changed modern hearing aids, *Trends Amplif.* 11(1), pp. 7–24.

Liberman, M. C. and Dodds, L. W. (1984). Single-neuron labeling and chronic cochlear pathology. III. Stereocilia damage and alterations of threshold tuning curves, *Hear. Res.*, 16, pp. 55–74.

Lybarger, S. F. (1944). US Patent Application SN 543,278.

Ma, W. L. and Young, E. D. (2006). Dorsal cochlear nucleus response properties following acoustic trauma: response maps and spontaneous activity, *Hear Res.*, 216–217, pp. 176–188.

Miller, R. L., Schilling, J. R., Franck, K. R. and Young, E. D. (1997) Effects of acoustic trauma on the representation of the vowel /ɛ/ in cat auditory-nerve fibers, *J. Acoust. Soc. Am.*, 101, pp. 3602–3616.

Miller, R. L., Calhoun, B. M. and Young, E. D. (1999). Contrast enhancement improves the representation of /ɛ/-like vowels in the hearing-impaired auditory nerve, *J. Acoust. Soc. Am.*, 106, pp. 2693–2708.

Moore, B. C. J. (2003). Speech processing for the hearing-impaired: Successes, failures, and implications for speech mechanisms, *Speech Commun.*, 41(1), pp. 81–91.

Moore, B. C. J., Glasberg, B. R. and Vickers, D. A. (1999). Further evaluation of a model of loudness perception applied to cochlear hearing loss, *J. Acoust. Soc. Am.*, 106(2), pp. 898–907.

Moore, B. C. J., Huss, M., Vickers, D. A. and Baer, T. (2001). Psychoacoustics of dead regions, In *Physiological and Psychophysical Bases of Auditory Function*, D. J. Breebaart, A. J. M. Houtsma, A. Kohlrausch, V. F. Prijs and R. Schoonhoven, eds., Shaker, Maastricht, pp. 419–429.

Nolte, J. (1993). The Human Brain: An Introduction to its Functional Anatomy, 3rd Ed. Mosby, St. Louis, MO.

Oertel, D. and Young, E. D. (2004). What's a cerebellar circuit doing in the auditory system? *Trends Neurosci.*, 27(2), pp. 104–110.

Pickles, J. O. (2008). *An Introduction to the Physiology of Hearing*, 3rd Ed. Emerald Group Publishing Ltd, Bingley, UK.

Ricketts, T. A., Dittberner, A. B. and Johnson, E. E. (2008) High-frequency amplification and sound quality in listeners with normal through moderate hearing loss, *J. Speech Lang. Hear. Res.*, 51(1), pp. 160–172.

Robles, L. and Ruggero, M. A. (2001). Mechanics of the mammalian cochlea, *Physiol. Rev.*, 81, pp. 1305–1352.

Rohdenburg, T., Hohmann, V. and Kollmeier, B. (2007). Robustness analysis of binaural hearing aid beamformer algorithms by means of objective perceptual quality measures, In *Proceedings of 2007 IEEE Workshop on Applications of Signal Processing to Audio and Acoustics*, pp. 315–318.

Sachs, M. B., Bruce, I. C., Miller, R. L. and Young, E. D. (2002). Biological basis of hearing-aid design, *Ann. Biomed. Eng.*, 30, pp. 157–168.

Schilling, J. R., Miller, R. L., Sachs, M.B. and Young, E.D. (1998). Frequency shaped amplification changes the neural representation of speech with noise-induced hearing loss, *Hear. Res.*, 117, pp. 57–70.

Shi, L., Carney, L. H. and Doherty, K. A. (2006). Correction of the peripheral spatio-temporal response pattern: A potential new signal-processing strategy, *J. Speech Lang. Hear. Res.*, 49, pp. 848–855.

Souza, P. E. (2002). Effects of compression on speech acoustics, intelligibility, and sound quality, *Trends Amplif.* 6, pp. 131–165.

Suryadevara, A. C., Schulte, B. A., Schmiedt, R. A. and Slepecky, N. B. (2001). Auditory nerve fibers in young and quiet-aged gerbils: morphometric correlations with endocochlear potential, *Hear. Res.*, 161(1–2), pp. 45–53.

Turicchia, L. and Sarpeshkar, R. (2005). A bio-inspired companding strategy for spectral enhancement, *IEEE Trans. Speech Audio Process.*, 13, pp. 243–253.

Young, E. D. (2008). Neural representation of spectral and temporal information in speech, *Phil. Trans. R. Soc. B*, 363(1493), pp. 923–945.

Zhang, X., Heinz, M. G., Bruce, I. C. and Carney, L. H. (2001). A phenomenological model for the responses of auditory-nerve fibers. I. Nonlinear tuning with compression and suppression, *J. Acoust. Soc. Am.*, 109, pp. 648–670.

Zilany, M. S. A. and Bruce, I. C. (2006). Modeling auditory-nerve responses for high sound pressure levels in the normal and impaired auditory periphery, *J. Acoust. Soc. Am.*, 120(3), pp. 1446–1466.

Zweig, G., Lipes, R. and Pierce, J. R. (1976). The cochlear compromise, *J. Acoust. Soc. Am.*, 59, pp. 975–982.

5.7 Review Questions

Q5.1 Why are hearing aids better able to compensate for conductive hearing loss than sensorineural hearing loss?

Q5.2 The transduction of sound wave vibrations in the cochlea to neural activity in the auditory nerve is performed by:

A. the inner hair cells

B. the outer hair cells

C. the ossicles

D. medial geniculate body

Q5.3 What is the frequency range for human hearing?

Q5.4 An individual starts experiencing some hearing loss at mid-frequencies and visits an audiologist. Their audiogram shows a threshold shift of 15 dB HL at 4 kHz. How much greater in amplitude (i.e., sound pressure in units of Pascal) does a 4 kHz tone need to be for this individual to hear it, relative to the normal-hearing population?

Q5.5 Classify the degrees of hearing loss for the three audiograms given in the following table:

F (kHz)	0.25	0.5	1	2	3	4	6
H_i #1 (dB HL)	62	59	73	81	98	111	104
H_i #2 (dB HL)	15	10	20	22	25	31	29
H_i #3 (dB HL)	42	43	47	51	67	66	71

Q5.6 Calculate the hearing aid gains G_i prescribed by the NAL-R formula (Eq. 5.1) for the three audiograms given in the table above.

Q5.7 What are the motivations for utilizing compression algorithms in hearing aids?

Q5.8 How does damage of the outer hair cells affect neural threshold tuning curves, and how does this compare to the effects of inner hair cell impairment?

Q5.9 A normal auditory nerve fiber has a BF of 3 kHz and a Q_{10} of 5. What is the bandwidth of this fiber's tuning curve 10 dB above the minimum threshold? Subsequent to noise exposure, this fiber's BF shifts downwards by ½ octave and its bandwidth 10 dB above the minimum threshold increases by a factor of 3.5. What are the impaired BF and Q_{10} values for this fiber?

Q5.10 What are the advantages and disadvantages of miniaturization of hearing aids?

Q5.11 An "open fitting" of a hearing aid is most likely to be suitable for an individual with:

A. a severe, low-frequency sensorineural hearing loss

B. a profound, flat sensorineural hearing loss

C. a moderate, high-frequency sensorineural hearing loss

, D. a profound, conductive hearing loss

Q5.12 What are the advantages and disadvantages of implantable hearing aid components or systems?

Chapter 6

Restoration of Hearing by Electrical Stimulation of the Human Cochlea, Brainstem, and Midbrain

Robert V. Shannon, Ph.D.[1]

[1] House Ear Institute, 2100 W. Third St., Los Angeles, CA 90057
PH: 213-353-7020; FX: 213-413-0950; EM: shannon@hei.org

6.1 Introduction

When cochlear implants were in an early stage of development in the 1970s most auditory neuroscientists were highly skeptical that electrical stimulation of the cochlea could ever produce useful auditory sensations. The scientists predicted that patients might hear "beeps and boops" but would never be able to understand complex auditory patterns like speech. It was unthinkable at the time that a small number of electrodes stimulating broad regions of neurons could provide functional replacement for the complex nonlinear hydrodynamics of the cochlea and the highly complex pattern of neural responses by more than 30,000 stochastically independent nerves. The initial devices did provide mostly sound awareness and rudimentary sound discrimination. However, improvements in electrode arrays and signal processing have resulted in steady improvements over time. Figure 6.1 shows a meta-analysis of average levels of word and sentence recognition by cochlear implants from published clinical studies. The initial bars on the left were from single channel cochlear implants in the early 1970s and the rightmost bars are recent results from the latest implant technology. As of 2008 the average postlingually deaf adult cochlear implant recipient can understand about 96% of sentences and 64% of isolated single words using only the sound from their implant (Spahr and Dorman, 2006). This level of performance is easily good enough to converse normally on the telephone. People with cochlear implants can now converse with people so effortlessly that many people cannot believe that they are really deaf. How could the auditory neuroscientists of the 1970s have been so wrong? How can a small number of electrodes so successfully replace the function of the cochlea and its 30,000 hair cells? In this chapter we will explore the technological and scientific discoveries that contributed to this amazing improvement in function. First let us review the history of this technology and its variations.

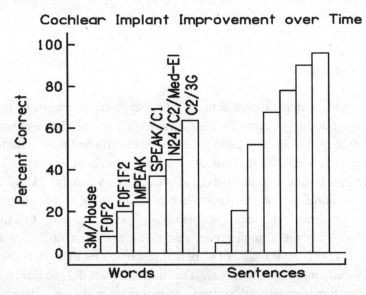

Figure 6.1. Cochlear implant outcomes over time. The results shown are derived from clinical studies reporting word and sentence recognition of postlingually deafened adults across evolving signal processing strategies. The earliest signal processing strategies (left-most bars) were single-channel and occurred in the early 1970s and the latest results are from the newest signal processing strategies (C2 and 3G) reported by Spahr and Dorman (2006).

6.2 Brief History of Cochlear Implants

Volta may have been one of the first people to experience electrical stimulation of hearing. It is reported that he charged up a glass rod and shoved it in his ear canal. He described a sound like "thick boiling soup". It's not clear if he was hearing the sounds of the dc current electrolysis of his inner ear fluids or some electrophonic activation of his inner ear, but he found the experience unpleasant and did not pursue it.

The first scientific study of electrical stimulation of hearing was performed by a French engineer Andre Djourno and the surgeon Charles Eyries. They implanted a simple coil in the auditory nerve of two deaf volunteers in 1957. While the devices provided rudimentary sound sensations, the devices failed in a short time and personal disagreements between the two men halted the project (Eisen, 2003).

Modern cochlear implants started with single-channel devices in the 1960's (House and Urban, 1973; Michelson et al., 1973; Simmons, 1966). While these devices did not provide recognizable speech they were highly useful as communication aids and patients were highly enthusiastic. Multichannel devices were developed simultaneously by several research groups (Eddington et al., 1978; House and Edgerton, 1982; Merzenich et al., 1979; Clark et al., 1990; Simmons et al., 1981; Chouard, 1980; Hochmair-Desoyer et al., 1983). Some of these early devices evolved into the modern implants while others were abandoned.

The auditory system consists of the external ear (pinna) and ear canal, the middle ear (ear drum and middle ear bones), and inner ear (cochlea). Sound vibration enters the outer ear and is transduced into the fluids of the inner ear by the vibration of the ear drum and bones of the middle ear (ossicles). The vibrations within the inner ear (cochlea) convert the sound from vibrational energy into nerve impulses to the brain. The cochlea contains some 30,000 tiny cells, called hair cells, which transduce the vibrations into nerve impulses. Most types of deafness are caused by the loss of these fragile hair cells. In this case the hydrodynamic vibration of the cochlea is still intact and the nerve is still intact, but the connection between the two is lost so sound energy does not reach the brain. Cochlear implants are intended to replace the hair cells and activate the nerves directly. An array of electrodes is inserted into the cochlea (Fig. 6.2) and electrical stimulation is delivered which stimulates the nerves. The normal cochlea separates sounds by frequency, called a tonotopic representation, with high frequency sounds represented near the base of the cochlea and low-frequency sounds represented near the apex. The multiple electrodes of the cochlear implant are designed to activate different pitch regions to reconstruct the frequency combinations of sound. While the hearing ear contains about 30,000 hair cells, implants have 16-22 electrodes distributed along a region that would normally respond to acoustic frequencies of 500 - 8000 Hz. Figure 6.3 shows a modern cochlear implant inserted into a clear acrylic model of a human cochlea. The electrode is designed to lie along the inner wall of the chamber, which is closest to the stimulable neurons.

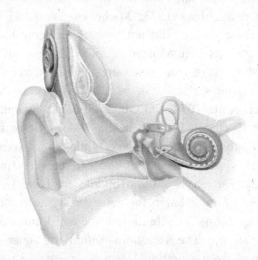

Figure 6.2. Illustration of a cochlear implant. The cochlear implant consists of an external portion, and an implantable portion. The external portion (brown) contains a microphone, signal processor, and rf transmitter. The implanted portion contains an rf antenna receiver, a signal decoder, and a stimulus generator. The cochlear implant electrode array, containing 12-22 stimulating sites, is inserted into the scala tymapni of the cochlea (blue). Acoustic signals are received at the microphone, processed and transmitted to the internal electronics. The received signal is then decoded and sent to the appropriate electrodes in the cochlea.

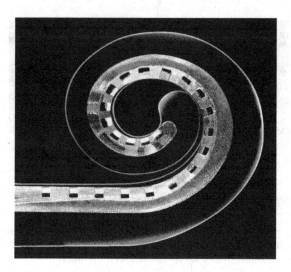

Figure 6.3. The cochlear implant electrode array is designed to be inserted more than one full turn into the scala tympani of the cochlea. This picture shows the ideal placement of the cochlear implant electrode array in an acrylic model of a human cochlea.

6.2.1 *Auditory brainstem implants*

Some people don't have an auditory nerve that can be stimulated by a cochlear implant. The auditory nerve can be damaged by head trauma, severe ossification, or tumors. The most common cause of VIII nerve damage is from neurofibromatosis type 2 (NF2), a genetic condition resulting from a mutation on chromosome 22 (Baser et al., 2003). NF2 produces schwannomas on the vestibular branch of the VIII nerve. Removal of these tumors usually damages the VIII nerve and results in complete deafness. A cochlear implant is of no use to these patients since there is no auditory nerve. An auditory brainstem implant (ABI) was developed for these patients (Fig. 6.4).

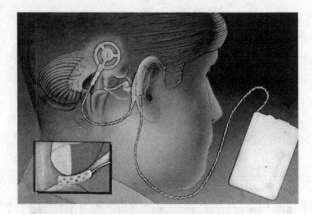

Figure 6.4. A schematic representation of the auditory brainstem implant (ABI). The exterior microphone and signal processing are similar to that of a cochlear implant. The implanted package is also similar except for the electrode array.

The first auditory brainstem imlant (ABI) was done in 1979 by William House and William Hitselberger in Los Angeles (Edgerton et al., 1982; Eisenberg et al., 1987). They placed a ball electrode into the region of the cochlear nucleus complex in the brainstem during a surgery to remove a vestibular schwannoma (VS) in a patient with NF2. That first ABI is still functioning in 2008 and the patient wears the device every waking hour. From 1979 to 1990 the ABI progressed slowly from a single electrode to a three electrode model (Fig. 6.5), with successive electrodes designed in collaboration with the Huntington Medical Research Institute in Pasadena. The array was designed with a mesh backing to encourage ingrowth of a fibrotic tissue reaction. Unlike a cochlear implant, where the electrode array is inserted into a bony chamber, the ABI is placed in the lateral recess of the IV ventricle and is not strongly attached to the brainstem. The mesh backing allows the natural foreign body fibrotic reaction to fix the electrode to the brainstem.

In 1992 Cochlear Corporation, the leading manufacturer of cochlear implants, collaborated with the House Ear Institute and HMRI to develop a commercial multichannel ABI (Brackmann et al., 1993; Shannon et al.,

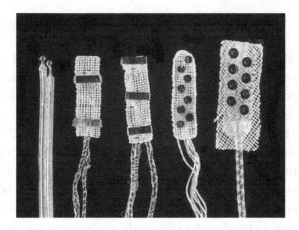

Figure 6.5. The evolution of ABI electrode design. The first ABI was a single pair of ball electrodes. Subsequent designs incorporated a woven mesh to encourage fibrous ingrowth to fix the array in place.

1993). The initial design contained 8 electrodes on a silicone substrate. Later the number of electrodes was increased to 21 to take advantage of the stimulation capabilities of their system. Figure 6.6 shows the present commercial ABI system. The implanted portion of the device contains

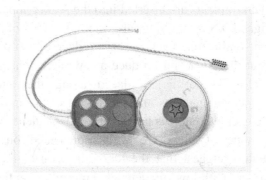

Figure 6.6. The ABI implantable system consists of a receiving antenna, a hermetically sealed electronics package that receives and decodes the signal, and a current source stimulator, and the electrode array.

the electrode array and the hermetically sealed receiver/stimulator package. This implanted unit received signals transmitted across the skin, decodes the signal, and presents a biphasic current-controlled pulse to the appropriate electrode. The external unit contains a microphone, digital sound processor, and rf transmitter circuitry. The external transmitter coil and the internal receiver coils are aligned by magnets.

The ABI was approved for clinical use by the Food and Drug Administration in 1996 and has now been implanted in more than 700 patients worldwide. The average level of performance is not as high as that observed in cochlear implant recipients. Most ABI listeners receive sound awareness, sound differentiation, some recognition/discrimination of environmental sounds, and help with lipreading (Otto et al., 2002). On average ABI listeners can understand 30% more speech when using the ABI in conjunction with lipreading than with lipreading alone. But overall, most ABI patients are not able to understand speech with only the sound from their implant. Average ABI performance is similar to the early single-channel cochlear implants, represented by the leftmost bars in each cluster in Fig. 6.1.

The reasons for the rather limited performance with the ABI are not clear. It was thought that the surface electrodes on the cochlear nucleus were not making good contact with the tonotopic axis of the auditory system. Cochlear implants are inserted into the scala tympani where they are nicely aligned with the normal tonotopic axis of the cochlea; electrodes at one end activate nerves that produce a high pitch sensation and electrodes at the other end produce a low pitch sensation. But the surface ABI electrode array is placed along the outside of the posteroventral cochlear nucleus and the dorsal cochlear nucleus in the brainstem. The cochlear nucleus has several independent representations of pitch and none of them are well represented on the surface. Anatomical studies suggest that the tonotopic axis of the PVCN runs deep to the surface, with low frequencies represented on the surface and high frequencies represented deep to the surface (Moore, 1987).

It was thought that it would be necessary to use penetrating microelectrodes to access the tonotopic organization of the auditory brainstem (McCreery et al., 1998). Under an NIH contract electrodes were developed and safety studies verified that such a device was feasible. Microelectrodes were 50 micron diameter iridium shafts insulated with parylene. The tip of each electrode was etched into a conical shape with a final tip diameter of 6 microns. Repeated insertion studies in cat spinal chord showed these electrodes to produce minimal tissue and vascular injury. The first human patients were implanted in 2004 (Fig. 6.7) and the evaluation continues (Otto et al., 2008). At the present time it is clear that the penetrating microelectrodes are implanted correctly in the cochlear nucleus and that they produce highly selective activation of the tonotopic dimension of the CN. However, it is not clear at present if this improved spectral selectivity will result in improved speech recognition over the surface electrode ABI.

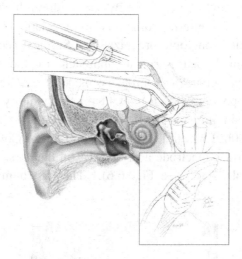

Figure 6.7. Illustration of the penetrating auditory brainstem implant. Top insert shows the electrode insertion tool and the lower insert shows the optimal placement of the penetrating microelectrodes into the ventral cochlear nucleus.

A new development in ABI results throws doubt on the original reason for developing penetrating microelectrodes. It was thought that surface electrodes were limiting performance because of their poor connection to the tonotopic dimension of the auditory brainstem.

However, some patients were observed who could obtain high levels of speech recognition with the normal surface electrode ABI - performance that was similar to that seen in cochlear implants (Colletti and Shannon, 2005). This result shows that excellent speech recognition is possible with surface electrode stimulation of the brainstem and suggests that the pathology associated with NF2 is responsible for limiting performance, not the device design or placement.

6.2.2 *Auditory midbrain implants*

If the ABI can produce excellent speech recognition, but NF2 patients cannot achieve this result due to localized damage to the brainstem, then a better outcome might be possible by stimulating a higher level of the auditory system. The inferior colliculus (IC) is a large midbrain nucleus with a well-studied tonotopic organization. Surgical access is possible using a traditional neurosurgical approach to the midbrain: the infratentorial supracerebellar approach (Fig. 6.8). At the present time there are two approaches to an implant for the auditory midbrains: the Auditory Midbrain Implant (AMI) using a penetrating electrode array (Lenarz et al, 2006; Lim et al, 2006) and the Inferior Colliculus Implant (ICI) using a surface electrode array placed on the dorsal surface of the IC (Colletti et al., 2007; see Fig. 6.6). The first human patient was

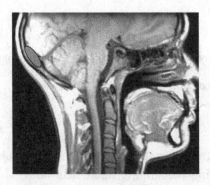

Figure 6.8. Schematic diagram of the placement of the ICI on the surface of the Inferior Colliculus. Surgical access was via the infratentorial supracerebellar approach.

implanted with the ICI in 2005 and the first patient with the AMI was implanted in 2006. It is still too early to know how well these approaches will work relative to cochlear implants and ABIs. The initial results of the ICI and AMI show auditory sensations and different pitch percepts across the electrode array but relatively poor speech recognition ability (Colletti et al., 2007; Lim et al., 2007, 2008a, b). For patients whose cochlea and brainstem are damaged from NF2 and other pathologies these implants may provide the only possibility for auditory function. But the higher in the system we stimulate the more intrinsic neural processing is bypassed. At some point we will likely reach the "point of diminishing returns", where stimulation is not useful in terms of speech. The excellent speech recognition in non-NF2 ABI patients shows that the CN is not too central. It is not yet clear whether the IC is still peripheral enough that prosthetic activation can still provide useful pattern recognition.

6.3 Safety of Electrical Stimulation

Useful hearing sensations would not be as desirable if the prosthetic devices caused damage to the stimulated neurons that eventually reduced their effectiveness. What do we know about the long-term safety and stability of electrical stimulation of neurons? Firstly, we know that cochlear implants have been in use for more than 35 years and ABIs for 30 years without any evidence of long-term decline in performance. Some of the original patients with these devices use them as much as 16 hours per day and performance and perceptual levels are stable.

Extensive animal studies (Agnew and McCreery, 1990; McCreery et al., 1990) have defined the limits of safe stimulation. Two factors contribute to neural damage from electrical stimulation: non-reversible ionic reaction products near the electrode-tissue interface, and excitotoxicity. Most reaction products that occur when charge is passed from an electrode are reversible if the charge is recovered by a reverse phase within a short time. Lilly et al. (1955) first proposed a brief biphasic charge-balanced waveform for limiting neural damage.

Neural damage can occur from excitotoxicity even if no damaging reaction products are generated near the electrode surface. In this case the neuron is driven to produce action potentials at a rate that cannot be sustained by the cell's metabolic machinery. With sustained stimulation the neuron's ionic balance is disrupted to the level that it is fatally damaged. Extensive chronic experiments (McCreery et al., 1990) have shown that such damage is determined both by the absolute level of charge and the charge density. A meta-analysis of this data resulted in a model of safe stimulation levels for electrical excitation of neurons (Shannon, 1992b). It appears that the primary factor determining toxicity of electrical stimulation is the charge density at the neuron. If the electrode is close to stimulable neurons, then the local charge density near the electrode surface is critical. Some electrode geometries can produce edge effects and "hot spots" where charge density is higher and it is in these areas where neurons are most likely to be damaged. If the neurons are more distant from the electrodes, these local concentrations of charge are dispersed by the distance and the relevant factor is simply the charge density at the neuron.

How is it possible to know the distance between the stimulating electrode and the neurons? A seminal paper by Ranck (1975) plotted the distance between the stimulating electrode and the neurons over hundreds of biophysical studies, including myelinated and unmyelinated neurons, in vivo and in vitro. Figure 6.9 replots the data from these studies. In general, a 200 µs/phase pulse of 1 mA can stimulate a neuron that is about 1 mm away. The consistency across studies was impressive, given the diversity of methods and preparations. We had an opportunity to confirm this result when we obtained the brain of an ABI patient who had died (Shannon et al., 1997). We were able to measure the actual distance between stimulating electrode and the cochlear nucleus in the brainstem. We also had years of measurements from this patient of the current levels necessary to produce auditory percepts. When we compared these results to the figure of Ranck the agreement was excellent. Our ABI patient had thresholds of 250-600 µA and the actual distance measured was 500 µm between electrode and brainstem. This consistency between a human implant and laboratory measures gives us confidence that we can estimate the distance between the stimulating electrode and the target neurons from the current levels needed to elicit a response.

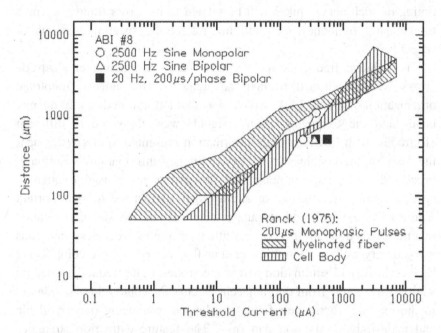

Figure 6.9. Composite plot of the meta-analysis of Ranck on the relation between stimulation amplitude and distance between electrode and neuron. Superimposed on Ranck's results are data from an ABI patient post-mortem. Note that the behavioral thresholds and the anatomical distances relate well to the animal experiments summarized by Ranck.

6.4 Signal Processing for Implants

The original single-channel implant simply placed a filtered version of the acoustic waveform on the electrodes. In some cases the acoustic waveform was compressed and used to modulate a high-frequency carrier for better coil-coupled transmission across the skin. Such a waveform is highly inappropriate for transmission of speech information because the raw acoustic waveform is not charge balanced and because the biological mechanisms of the deafened cochlea cannot extract frequency-specific information from an analog electrical waveform. All neurons near the electrode are stimulated whenever the electrical waveform delivers sufficient charge to trigger action potentials. The timing of such nerve spikes will be related to the gross timing of voice fundamental frequency, but will not reflect the spectral elements of speech.

To achieve frequency-specific stimulation, multichannel electrode arrays were developed to take advantage of the normal tonotopic organization of the cochlea. Sound was divided into multiple frequency bands and the frequency-specific signals were delivered to different electrodes, with low-frequency information presented to electrodes near the apex of the cochlea where low-frequency information is normally processed. The early multichannel processing either used frequency-specific analog waveforms, or attempted to extract the most important features from speech and stimulate with a simplified signal (so called feature extraction strategies). Neither of these processing methods worked very well. The multichannel analog strategies were complicated by electrical field summation across electrodes. The frequency-specific analog waveforms from two adjacent electrodes would add and subtract in the regions where their fields overlapped, producing uncontrollable and undesirable activation patterns. The feature extraction strategies were inconsistent in extracting speech cues, especially in noisy listening environments. When the background noise consisted of other voices the feature extraction strategies would select features from the background voices as well as the target voice. In contrast to single-channel analog implants, at least these multichannel strategies produced some limited open-set speech recognition (see second two bars in Fig. 6.1).

A breakthrough occurred in the 1990s when signal processing techniques were developed to present biphasic pulses that were interleaved in time across electrodes (Wilson et al., 1991). The use of non-simultaneous biphasic pulses eliminated the problem of electric field summation across electrodes. Brief biphasic pulses are sequentially presented to each electrode. The amplitude of each pulse represents the energy in that frequency band of speech at that moment in time. The overall rate of stimulation was originally about 250 pps/electrode, but newer hardware allows pulse rates of 1000 pps/electrode and higher.

The other breakthrough that occurred at the same time was to abandon feature extraction processing. When the hardware was limited in bandwidth it was felt that some reduction in information rate was necessary. Newer hardware has sufficient bandwidth that the raw information from each signal band is sent to the associated electrode with relatively little modification. The result has been a significant improvement in speech recognition (the 5th and 6th bars in Fig. 6.1). Research has demonstrated that the post-lingual human brain is better at extracting relevant information about speech than even the most reliable pre-processing strategy (a fact that has been widely appreciated in the automatic speech recognition community for many years). Humans are trained at speech pattern recognition over a lifetime, with more than 30 million words received just in the first 4 years of life (Hart and Risley, 1995). The pattern recognition ability of the average human brain for speech is amazing - we can extract the correct words from running speech of talkers with high or low pitch voices, heavy accents, spoken fast or slow, in high noise levels, and even heavily distorted by a bad communication channel. No machine or processing algorithm is even close to human performance. Cochlear implants experienced a dramatic improvement in performance when the processing algorithms simply presented the signals in tonotopic region of the cochlea and "got out of the way" and let the brain do the rest.

The next level of improvements in cochlear implant signal processing depend on achieving a better understanding of the trade-off between signal processing and allowing the over-trained brain pattern recognition system to recognize the patterns of speech. What information is not getting through to the patient in a cochlear implant? Is the limitation in the signal processing or in the damaged nervous system or is it simply an inescapable limitation of prosthetic stimulation? Let us look at the basic perceptual capabilities of cochlear implants and how they are affected by signal processing. In the next section we will review the basic perception of amplitude, timing, and frequency with a cochlear implant.

6.5 Perceptual Issues in Implant Design

6.5.1 *Amplitude cues*

All sensory systems incorporate some degree of amplitude compression at the periphery because the range of physical amplitudes far exceeds the range of neural firing. In hearing the normal ear can code sound levels over a range of 120 dB, which is a range in amplitudes of one million to one. Each auditory neuron can only code sound amplitudes over a range of about 30 dB. The cochlea normally provides a logarithmic compression of sound amplitudes to match the large range of sound amplitude to the smaller range of neural outputs. However, in electrical stimulation we must control the level of neural activity to mimic the normal range of perceptual loudness. If one acoustic sound is twice as loud as another then we need to code those two sounds into electrical amplitudes that will mimic this loudness ratio in the electrically stimulated ear. Studies have shown that loudness is an exponential function of the electric current level, whereas it is a power function of acoustic amplitude (Zeng and Shannon, 1992, 1994, 1999). Most commercial implant devices use a logarithmic compression of acoustic amplitude prior to conversion into electric current amplitude. While a logarithmic compression is not theoretically ideal, it is close enough mathematically to the ideal transformation that it is a reasonable compromise in a prosthetic device.

6.5.2 *Temporal cues*

Temporal cues in hearing are traditionally divided into three classes: envelope cues, periodicity cues, and fine structure (Rosen, 1992; Plomp, 1983). Envelope cues are low-frequency temporal fluctuations (<50 Hz) that are perceived as temporal fluctuations rather than as a distinct pitch. Periodicity cues are temporal fluctuations in the 50-500Hz range that produce a sensation of pitch that is related to the periodicity. Temporal fine structure cues are temporal fluctuations faster than 500 Hz. In the normal acoustic cochlea fine structure temporal information is conveyed by a complex combination of the cochlear place of activation and the temporal structure. Cochlear implants convey envelope cues quite well and CI listeners can generally detect periodicity cues up to 300-500 Hz. However, CI listeners cannot detect temporal fine structure cues. CI devices convey fine structure information by stimulating different electrodes in different cochlear locations. This allows a crude discrimination of pitch by utilizing the type of pitch information that is coded by cochlear location. However there is no indication that CI listeners can make use of temporal cues above 500 Hz strictly in the time domain and CI listeners do not appear to be able to combine timing and cochlear place information for complex pitch as occurs in acoustic hearing.

CI listeners appear to have relatively normal processing of global temporal cues. Global temporal processing is measured by several psychophysical techniques: gap detection measures the smallest detectable silent interval in an ongoing sound, forward masking measures the recovery from adaptation following a sound, and modulation detection measures the ability to detect fluctuations in an ongoing sound. On all of these measures implant listeners are similar in their capabilities to normal hearing, when compared at equivalent loudness levels (Shannon, 1989, 1990, 1992a). Implant listeners can detect gaps of 1-3 ms, have time constants of recovery of 60-100 ms following a stimulus, and can detect modulation of 1-3% up to modulation frequencies of 100-300 Hz. The implication is that these kinds of temporal processing utilize central processing mechanisms that are not adversely affected by deafness or by the lack of fine temporal structure delivered by a cochlear implant.

6.5.3 *Spectral cues: The number of spectral channels*

One of the most important factors in the success of cochlear implants is in the replication of spectral information presented to the correct tonotopic location along the cochlea. Many studies have shown that speech recognition performance improves as the number of spectral channels is increased (Dorman and Loizou, 1997; Dorman et al., 1997; Fishman et al., 1997; Friesen et al., 2001; Fu and Shannon, 1999;

Shannon et al., 2004). In cochlear implant listeners and in simulations of cochlear implants speech recognition improves dramatically as the number of spectral channels is increased from 1 to 8. Adding spectral channels beyond eight continues to improve performance in normal hearing but does not appear to improve performance in implants. It is not clear why implant performance seems to be limited in the number of effective spectral channels, but it is likely to be limited by interactions across electrodes. More spectral channels are needed for speech recognition in noise (Fu et al., 1998; Friesen et al., 2001; Fu and Nogaki, 2005) and for complex pitch and music (Smith et al., 2002; Shannon et al., 2004).

6.5.4 *Spectral cues: Warping and shifting the tonotopic map*

One of the potential problems in cochlear implants is that of presenting spectral information to the wrong tonotopic location in the cochlea. The normal cochlea in humans is 35 mm in length and frequency information is distributed approximately logarithmically along the cochlear length, with high frequencies near the base and low frequencies near the apex (Greenwood, 1990). However, cochlear implant electrode arrays are about 25 mm in length and so cover a region in the cochlea that would normally respond to acoustic frequencies of 500-5000 Hz. A cochlear implant signal processor typically takes acoustic information from 200-10,000 Hz and presents it to the electrodes. This type of processing distorts the normal tonotopic distribution of information: the frequency to cochlear place mapping in the implant is shifted and compressed relative to the normal acoustic mapping. Studies have shown that distortion in the tonotopic map results in a reduction in speech recognition (Shannon et al., 1998; Baskent and Shannon, 2003, 2004). Presumably, the central mechanisms for speech pattern recognition are developed over a lifetime of listening experience and there is a tight association between the correct tonotopic pattern in cochlear place with correct identification of the phoneme. It is not clear how flexible this association is, i.e. how long it might take to relearn the association of new speech patterns produced by the implant. There is some evidence that these patterns can be quickly relearned (Rosen et al., 1999; Fu et al.,

2005), but relearning may not be possible if the distortion is too great (Fu et al., 2002).

6.5.5 *Bilateral implants*

Localizing sounds in space is an important ability for locating the source of a sound and also for being able to recognize a single talker in a noisy environment like a restaurant or cocktail party. Normal acoustic listeners can follow conversations in a noisy room when the signal level is 10-20 dB less than the noise level. Implant listeners have generally only had a single implant and so are not able to use the binaural cues to locate sound sources and to understand speech in noisy conditions. Recently, many adults and children have received bilateral implants and the results are mixed (Litovky et al., 2004; Nopp et al., 2004; Schleich et al., 2004; Buss et al., 2008; Grantham et al., 2008). Some patients with bilateral implants can locate sound sources in space, although not as well as normal hearing listeners. Bilateral implants also allow some patients to understand speech in noisier conditions than with a single implant, but again the improvement is not as large as that observed for NH listeners. It appears that approximately one third of bilateral implant recipients can use the two implants better than either implant alone, one third benefit from improved performance by using the head shadow effect (the ear opposite a noise source will have a more favorable signal to noise ratio), and one third derive no additional benefit from two implants. Research into the causes of performance limitations and variations is ongoing.

6.5.6 *Combined acoustic and electric stimulation*

As CI performance improves the selection criteria have been relaxed to allow patients with more and more residual hearing. Some patients have a pattern of hearing loss in which they have good residual hearing at low acoustic frequencies (below 1000 Hz) and essentially no hearing at high frequencies. Cochlear implants are being used to supplement the residual hearing of such patients so that they use acoustic hearing and implant hearing in the same ear (Gantz et al., 2005, 2006; Vermeire et al., 2008). Although the residual hearing may not be sufficient to allow speech recognition by itself, the acoustic hearing often preserves fine spectral resolution and temporal resolution within the region of acoustic hearing. When this residual hearing is combined with electrical stimulation at higher frequency locations in the cochlea these patients are able to recognize speech at a high level, allowing telephone use in most. However, some patients have lost some or all of their residual hearing following implantation and others do no better than a full cochlear implant. It remains to be determined what the most appropriate approach is for such patients. Since hearing is usually present in the contralateral ear, preserving acoustic hearing in the implanted ear may not be necessary.

6.6 Future Directions in Device Design and Signal Processing

6.6.1 *Noise reduction pre-processing*

Speech recognition in real-world listening situations is often limited by noise, produced either by competing talkers or machines. Many companies making consumer electronics (cell phones, speech-to-text transcription, hearing aids) are actively working on techniques for improving the signal to noise ratio at the input to the device. Spectral enhancement methods have shown promise (Yang and Fu, 2005) as have active beamforming microphone arrays (Soede et al, 1993). Some of these methods show undesirable processing artifacts under some conditions, but have shown the potential to improve the real signal-to-noise ratio by about 3 dB.

6.6.2 *Virtual channels*

One factor that appears to limit the capabilities of cochlear implants is the limited number of spectral channels. Modern cochlea implants have 12-22 stimulating electrodes spaced along the tonotopic axis of the cochlea. However, studies have shown that implant patients are actually performing as if they were using only 8-10 channels (Fishman et al., 1997, Friesen et al., 2001) or even as few as 4 (Fu and Nogaki, 2005) when listening in noise. Although there are more stimulating electrodes the effective number of information channels is probably limited by the interaction of electrical fields from adjacent electrodes. If the distance between neurons and electrodes is large relative to the distance between electrodes, then the current fields from adjacent electrodes may be nearly indistinguishable at the point of stimulation. There have been several techniques proposed that would sharpen the stimulating electrical field by controlling the relative phase of stimulation across the electrode array in a manner similar to beamforming or phased array processing. There is now some evidence that such field sharpening can result in an increased number of distinct pitch sensations between adjacent electrodes that could be used as "virtual" channels of stimulation (Donaldson et al., 2006). The initial results of such schemes in clinical speech processors are encouraging.

6.6.3 *Photolithographic electrode arrays*

If the electrode array is in close proximity to the stimulable neurons then the performance of the device may be limited by the number of electrodes. All implant manufacturers are actively investigating modern photolithographic techniques for increasing the number of electrodes in a cochlear implant array. Electrode stimulating surfaces can be printed on a flexible polyimide substrate and overcoated with an insulating layer of parylene. Electrodes have also been designed with distributed stress gauges along the length so the position and force could be monitored during surgical insertion (Wang and Wise, 2008). The resulting unit could be inserted into the cochlea directly or mounted on a silicone carrier, much like present implant technology. However the high electrode counts, up to hundreds of stimulation sites would require sophisticated multiplexing telemetry to send and receive signals from outside the skin.

6.6.4 *Optimizing parameters*

As hearing aids and cochlear implants add more electrodes and evolve more complex signal processing algorithms, the number of parameters increases dramatically. For example, each stimulated electrode in a cochlear implant has electrical pulse parameters (pulse phase duration, inter-phase gap duration, stimulation rate, amplitude, temporal interleave with adjacent electrodes), perceptual parameters (threshold, maximum loudness level, loudness growth function), as well as parameters for the signal processing channel that feeds that electrode (spectral bandwidth, cutoff frequencies, filter slopes, amplitude compression etc.). As the number of electrodes increases from 16 to 120 the number of parameters becomes unmanageable. Some of these parameters can be fixed across electrodes, but some must be determined for each individual patient. Genetic algorithms have shown promise for achieving rapid optimization in this large parameter space (Wakefield et al, 2005; Baskent et al., 2007) and will likely be implemented in the near future to reduce the time required to fit a complex device to an individual patient.

6.6.5 *Totally implantable CI*

Research is progressing on a totally implantable cochlear implant device that would not require the use of an external processor, microphone, or transmitter coil. This obviously would have tremendous practical appeal in that it would not have any outwardly visible parts and it would allow activities like swimming. Periodic charging of the device would occur transcutaneously, using a charging module (Cohen, 2004). This technology would also require the implantation of a microphone (Maniglia et al., 1999). All major implant companies are actively developing the technologies that would allow totally implantable devices.

6.7 Summary and Conclusions

Cochlear implants and brainstem implants are highly successful sensory prostheses, exceeding all of our expectations. People who lose their hearing after acquiring language have an excellent chance at regaining a high degree of functional hearing from electronic implants. Advances in engineering technology are making the devices smaller, faster and have higher signal processing capability. The limitations in device improvements are probably not on the engineering side but in terms of matching the device design to the neurobiology of the damaged sensory system. As performance improves we learn more about the potential benefits and limitations of artificial hearing and more about auditory neuroscience. Each advance in neuroscience leads to engineering improvements in the next generation of devices. Although the level of performance with auditory prostheses is much higher that originally imagined, there is reason to think that we will see continued improvement in hearing quality from these devices in the future.

6.8 References

Agnew, W. F. and D. B. McCreery, Eds. (1990). *Neural Prostheses; Fundamental Studies*. Prentice Hall Biophysics and Bioengineering Series,Prentice-Hall, Englewood Cliffs, New Jersey.

Baser M. E., Evans, D. G., and Gutmann, D. H. (2003). Neurofibromatosis 2. *Curr. Opin. Neurol.*, 16, pp. 27-33.

Baskent, D. and Shannon, R. V. (2003). Speech recognition under conditions of frequency-place compression and expansion, *J. Acoust. Soc. Amer.*, 113, pp. 2064-2076.

Baskent D. E. and Shannon, R. V. (2004) Frequency-Place Compression and Expansion in Cochlear Implant Patients, *J. Acoust. Soc. Amer.*, 116, pp. 3130-3140.

Başkent, D., Eiler, C. L., and Edwards, B. (2007). Using genetic algorithms with subjective input from human subjects: implications for fitting hearing aids and cochlear implants. *Ear & Hearing,* 28(3), pp. 370-380.

Brackmann, D. E., Hitselberger, W. E., Nelson, R. A., Moore, J. K., Waring, M., Portillo, F., Shannon, R.V., and Telischi, F. (1993). Auditory Brainstem Implant. I: Issues in Surgical Implantation, *Otolaryngology, Head and Neck Surgery*, 108, pp. 624-634.

Buss, E., Pillsbury. H., Buchman, C., et al. (2008) Multicenter U.S. Bilateral Med-El Cochlear Implantation Study: Speech Perception over the First Year of Use, *Ear & Hearing,* 29, pp. 20-32.

Chouard C. H. (1980). The surgical rehabilitation of total deafness with the multichannel cochlear implant. Indications and results. *Audiology*, 19(2), pp. 137-145.

Clark, G. M., Tong,Y. C., and Patrick, J. F. (1990), *Cochlear prostheses*, Churchill Livingstone, Edinburgh, pp. 99-124.

Cohen, N. L. (2004). Cochlear implant candidacy and surgical considerations. *Audiol. Neurotol.*, Vol. 9, pp. 197-202.

Colletti. V and Shannon, R V. (2005). Open Set Speech Perception with Auditory Brainstem Implant? *The Laryngoscope,* 115, pp. 1974-1978.

Colletti, V., Shannon, R. V., Carner, M., Colletti, L., Sacchetto, L., Turazzi, S., Masotto, B. (2007). The first successful case of hearing produced by electrical stimulation of the human midbrain, *Otology and Neurotology*, 28, pp. 39-43.

Donaldson, G. S., Kreft, H. A., and Litvak, L. (2006). Place-pitch discrimination of single- versus dual-electrode stimuli by cochlear implant users, *J. Acoust. Soc. Amer.*, 118(2), pp. 623-626.

Dorman, M. F. and Loizou, P. C. (1997). Speech intelligibility as a function of the number of channels of stimulation for normal-hearing listeners and patients with cochlear implants, *Amer. J. Otol.*, 18(6 Suppl), pp. S113-S114.

Dorman, M. F., Loizou, P. C. and Rainey, D. (1997b). Speech intelligibility as a function of the number of channels of stimulation for signal processors using sine-wave and noise-band outputs, *J. Acoust. Soc. Amer.*, 102(4), pp. 2403-2411.

Eddington, D. K., Dobelle, W. H., Brackmann, D. E., Mladevosky, M. G., and Parkin, J. L. (1978). Auditory prosthesis research with multiple channel intracochlear stimulation in man, *Ann. Otol. Rhinol. Laryngol.*, 87, Suppl. 53, pp. 1-39.

Edgerton, B. J., House, W. F., and Hitselberger, W. (1982). Hearing by cochlear nucleus stimulation in humans, *Ann. Otol. Rhinol. Otolaryngol.*, 91 (Suppl.), pp. 117-124.

Eisen, M. D. (2003). Djourno, Eyries, and the First Implanted Electrical Neural Stimulator to Restore Hearing. *Otol. & Neurotol.*, 24, pp. 500-506.

Eisenberg, L. S., Maltan, A. A., Portillo, F., Mobley, J. P., and House, W. F. (1987). Electrical stimulation of the auditory brain stem structure in deafened adults, *J. Rehab. Res. Dev.*, 24, pp. 9-22.

Fishman K., Shannon R. V. and Slattery W. H. (1997). Speech recognition as a function of the number of electrodes used in the SPEAK cochlear implant speech processor. *Journal of Speech and Hearing Research*, 40, pp. 1201-1215.

Friesen, L., Shannon, R. V., Baskent, D., and Wang, X. (2001). Speech recognition in noise as a function of the number of spectral channels: comparison of acoustic hearing and cochlear implants, *J. Acoustical Society of America*, 110(2), 1150-1163.

Fu, Q.-J. and Shannon, R.V. (1999). Recognition of spectrally degraded and frequency-shifted vowels in acoustic and electric hearing, *Journal of the Acoustical Society of America*, 105(3), 1889-1900.

Fu, Q.-J., Shannon, R.V., and Wang, X. (1998). Effects of noise and spectral resolution on vowel and consonant recognition: Acoustic and electric hearing, *Journal of the Acoustical Society of America*, 104(6), pp. 3586-3596.

Fu, Q.-J., Shannon, R. V., and Galvin, J. (2002). Perceptual learning following changes in the frequency-to-electrode assignment with the Nucleus-22 cochlear implant, *J. Acoust. Soc. Amer.*, 112, pp. 1664-1674.

Fu, Q.-J., Galvin, J. J., III, Wang, X. and Nogaki, G. (2005). "Moderate auditory training can improve speech performance of adult cochlear implant users," *Acoustics Research Letters Online*, 6(3), pp. 106-111.

Fu, Q.-J. and Nogaki, G. (2005). "Noise Susceptibility of Cochlear Implant Users: The Role of Spectral Resolution and Smearing," *Journal of the Association for Research in Otolaryngology*, 6(1), pp. 19-27.

Gantz, B. J., Turner, C, Gfeller, K. E., and Lowder, M. W. (2005). Preservation of hearing in cochlear implant surgery: advantages of combined electrical and acoustical speech processing. *Laryngoscope*, 115(5), pp. 796-802.

Gantz, B. J, Turner, C. W., and Gefeller, K. E. (2006). Acoustic plus electric speech processing: Preliminary results of a multicenter clinical trial of the Iowa/Nucleus hybrid implant, *Audiol. Neurotol.*, 11, Suppl 1, pp. 63-68.

Grantham, W., Ashmead, D., Ricketts, T., Haynes, D. and Labadie, R. (2008) Interaural Time and Level Difference Thresholds for Acoustically Presented Signals in Post-Lingually Deafened Adults Fitted with Bilateral Cochlear Implants Using CIS+ Processing, *Ear & Hearing*, 29, pp. 33-44.

Greenwood, D.D. (1990). "A cochlear frequency-position function for several species - 29 years later", *J. Acoust. Soc. Am.*, 87, 2592-2605.

Hart, B. and Risley, T. R. (1995). *Meaningful Differences in the Everyday Experience of Young American Children*, Brookes Publishing, Baltimore.

Hochmair-Desoyer, I. J., Hochmair, E. S., Burian, K., and Stiglbrunner, H. K. (1983). Percepts from the Vienna cochlear prosthesis, in C.W. Parkins and S.W. Anderson (eds) Cochlear Prostheses: An International Symposium, *Annals of the N.Y. Academy of Sciences*, 405, pp. 295-306.

House, W. F., and Urban, J. (1973). Long term results of electrode implantation and electronic stimulation of the cochlea in man. *Ann. Otol. Rhinol. Laryngol.*, 82(4), pp. 504-517.

House, W. F., and Edgerton, B. J. (1982). A multiple-electrode cochlear implant. *Ann Otol. Rhinol. Laryngol., Suppl.*, 91(2 Pt 3), pp. 104-16.

Lenarz, M., Lim, H. H., Patrick, J. F., Anderson, D. J., and Lenarz, T. (2006). Electrophysiological validation of a human prototype auditory midbrain implant (AMI) in a guinea pig model, *JARO*, 7, 383-398.

Lilly, J. C., Hughes, J. R., Alvord, E. C., and Galkin, T. W. (1955). Brief, noninjurious electric waveform for stimulation of the brain. *Science*, 121, pp. 468-469.

Lim, H. H., and Anderson, D. J. (2006). Auditory cortical responses to electrical stimulation of the inferior colliculus: Implications for an auditory midbrain implant, *J. Neurophysiol.*, 96, pp. 975-988.

Lim, H. H., Lenarz, T., Joseph, G., Battmer, R. D., Samii, A., Samii, M., Patrick, J. F., and Lenarz, M. (2007). Electrical stimulation of the midbrain for hearing restoration: Insight into the functional organization of the human central auditory system. *J. Neurosci.*, 27, pp. 13541-13551.

Lim, H. H., Lenarz, T., Anderson, D. J., and Lenarz, M. (2008a). The auditory midbrain implant: Effects of electrode location, *Hearing Research*. 242, pp. 74–85.

Lim, H. H., Lenarz, T., Joseph, G., Battmer, R. D., Patrick, J. F., and Lenarz, M. (2008b). Effects of phase duration and pulse rate on loudness and pitch percepts in the first auditory midbrain implant patients: Comparison to cochlear implant and auditory brainstem implant results. *Neuroscience,* 154(1), pp. 370-380.

Litovsky, R. Y., Parkinson, A., Arcaroli, J., Peters, R., Lake, J., Johnstone, P., and Yu, G. (2004). Bilateral cochlear implants in adults and children. *Arch. Otolaryngol. Head Neck Surg.,* 130(5), pp. 648-655.

Maniglia, A. J., Abbass, H., Azar, T. et al. (1999). The middle ear bioelectronic microphone for a totally implantable cochlear hearing device for profound and total hearing loss. *Am. J. Otol.,* 20, pp. 602-611.

McCreery, D. B., Agnew, W. F., Yuen, T. G. H., and Bullara, L. (1990). Charge density and charge per phase as cofactors in neural injury induced by electrical stimulation, *IEEE Trans. BME,* BME-37, 996-1001.

McCreery, D. G., Shannon, R. V., Moore, J. K., Chatterjee, M., and Agnew, W. F. (1998). Accessing the tonotopic organization of the ventral cochlear nucleus by intranuclear microstimulation, *IEEE Trans. Rehabi. Engin.,* 6(4), pp. 391-399.

Merzenich, M. M., White, M., Vivion, M. C., Leake-Jones, P. A., and Walsh, S. (1979). Some considerations of multichannel electrical stimulation of the auditory nerve in the profoundly deaf; interfacing electrode arrays with the auditory nerve array. *Acta Otolaryngol.,* 87(3-4), pp. 196-203.

Michelson, R. P., Merzenich, M. M., Pettit, C. R., and Schindler, R. A. (1973). A cochlear prosthesis: further clinical observations; preliminary results of physiological studies. *Laryngoscope,* 83(7), pp. 1116-1122.

Moore, J. K. (1987). The human auditory brainstem: a comparative view, *Hear Res.,* 29: 1-32.

Nopp, P., Schleich, P., and D'Haese, P. (2004). Sound Localization in bilateral users of Med-EL COMBI 40/40+ cochlear implants, *Ear & Hearing,* 25, pp. 205-214.

Otto, S. A., Brackmann, D. E., Hitselberger, W. E., Shannon, R. V., and Kuchta, J. (2002). The multichannel auditory brainstem implant update: Performance in 60 patients, *Journal of Neurosurgery,* 96, pp. 1063-1071.

Otto, S. R, Shannon, R. V., Brackmann, D. E., Hitselberger, W. E., McCreery, D., Moore, J., and Wilkinson, E. (2008). Audiological Outcomes with the Penetrating Electrode Auditory Brainstem Implant, *Otology and Neurotology,* 29, pp. 1147-1154.

Plomp, R. (1983). The role of modulation in hearing, in *Hearing – Physiological Bases and Psychophysics,* R. Klinke and R. Hartmann, (Eds.), Springer-Verlag, Berlin, pp. 270-276

Ranck, J. (1975). Which elements are excited in electrical stimulation of mammalian central nervous system: A review, *Brain Res.,* 98, pp. 417-440.

Rosen, S. (1992). Temporal information in speech and its relevance for cochlear implants, in *Philos. Trans. Royal Soc. London Ser. B Biol. Sci.,* pp. 336, 367.

Rosen, S., Faulkner, A, and Wilkinson, L. (1999). Adaptation by normal listeners to upward spectral shifts of speech: Implications for cochlear implants, *J. Acoust. Soc. Amer.,* 106(6), pp. 3629-3636.

Schleich, P., Nopp, P., and D'Haese, P. (2004). Head shadow, squelch and summation effects in bilateral users of Med-EL COMBI 40/40+ cochlear implants, *Ear & Hearing*, 25, pp. 197-204.

Shannon, R. V. (1989). "Detection of gaps in sinusoids and pulse trains by patients with cochlear implants", *J. Acoust. Soc. Am.*, 85, pp. 2587-2592.

Shannon, R. V. (1990). Forward masking in patients with cochlear implants, *J. Acoust. Soc. Amer.*, 88, pp. 741-744.

Shannon, R.V. (1992a). Temporal modulation transfer functions in patients with cochlear implants, *J. Acoust. Soc. Amer.*, 91, pp. 1974-1982.

Shannon, R.V. (1992b). A model of safe levels for electrical stimulation, *IEEE Transactions on Biomedical Engineering*, 39(4), 424-426.

Shannon, R. V., Fayad, J., Moore, J. K., Lo, W., O'Leary, M., Otto, S., and Nelson, R. A. (1993). Auditory Brainstem Implant. II: Post-Surgical Issues and Performance, *Otolaryngology, Head and Neck Surgery*, 108, pp. 635-643.

Shannon, R. V., Moore, J., McCreery, D., and Portillo, F. (1997). Threshold-distance measures from electrical stimulation of human brainstem, *IEEE Trans. on Rehabilitation Engineering*, 5, pp. 1-5.

Shannon, R.V., Zeng, F.-G., and Wygonski, J. (1998). Speech recognition with altered spectral distribution of envelope cues, *J. Acoust. Soc. Amer.*, 104(4): 2467-2476.

Shannon, R.V., Fu, Q-J and Galvin, J. (2004). The number of spectral channels required for speech recognition depends on the difficulty of the listening situation, *Acta Oto-Laryngologica*, Suppl. 552: 50-54.

Simmons, F. B. (1966). Electrical stimulation of the auditory nerve in man, *Arch. Otolaryngol.*, 84, pp. 2-54.

Simmons, F. B., White, R. L., Walker, M. G., and Mathews, R. G. (1981). Pitch correlates of direct auditory nerve electrical stimulation. *Ann. Otol. Rhinol. Laryngol., Suppl.*, 90(2 Pt 3), pp. 15-8.

Smith, Z. M., Delgutte, B. and Oxenham, A. J. (2002) Chimaeric sounds reveal dichotomies in auditory perception, *Nature*, 416, pp. 87-90.

Soede, W., Bilsen, F. A., and Berkhout, A. J. (1993) Assessment of a directional microphone array for hearing-impaired listeners, *J. Acoust. Soc. Am.*, 94, pp. 799–808.

Spahr, A. J. and Dorman, M. F. (2006). Performance of subjects fit with the Advanced Bionics CII and Nucleus 3G cochlear implant devices, *Arch. Otolaryngol HNS*, 130, pp. 624-628.

Vermeire, K., Anderson, I., Flynn, M. and Van de Heyning, P. (2008) The Influence of Different Speech Processor and Hearing Aid Settings on Speech Perception Outcomes in Electric Acoustic Stimulation Patients, *Ear & Hearing*, 29, pp. 76-86.

Wakefield, G. H., van den Honert, C., Parkinson, W., and Lineaweaver, S. (2005). Genetic algorithms for adaptive psychophysical procedures: recipient-directed design of speech-processor MAPs. *Ear Hear.*, 26(4 Suppl), pp. 57S-72S.

Wang, V., and Wise, K. (2008). A Hybrid Electrode Array with Built-in Position Sensors for an Implantable MEMS-Based Cochlear Prosthesis." *IEEE/ASME Journal of Microelectromechanical Systems*, in press.

Wilson. B. S., Finley, C. C, Lawson, D. T., Wolford, R. D., Eddington, D. K., and Rabinowitz, W. M. (1991). New levels of speech recognition with cochlear implants, *Nature*, 352, pp. 236-238.

Yang, L.-P., and Fu, Q.-J. (2005). "Spectral subtraction based speech enhancement for cochlear implant patients in background noise," *J. Acoust. Soc. Am.* 117(3), pp. 1001-1005.

Zeng, F. G. and Shannon, R. V. (1992). Loudness balance between electric and acoustic stimulation, *Hearing Res.*, 60, pp. 231-235.

Zeng, F.-G. and Shannon, R. V. (1994). "Loudness coding mechanisms inferred from electric stimulation of the human auditory system", *Science*, 264, pp. 564-566.

Zeng, F.-G. and Shannon, R. V. (1999). Psychophysical laws revealed by electric hearing, *NeuroReport*, 10(9), pp. 1-5.

6.9 Review Questions

Q6.1   A cochlear implant restores perfect hearing. True or False.

Q6.2   People with a cochlear implant can understand speech in quiet but have difficulty in noisy rooms. True or False.

Q6.3   Cochlear implants and auditory brainstem implants provide similar levels of speech understanding. True or False.

Q6.4   Prosthetic electric stimulation of the auditory nervous system has been tried in humans with electrodes positioned in:

A. the cochlea

B. the cochlear nucleus in the brainstem

C. the inferior colliculus in the midbrain

D. the auditory cortex

E. all of the above

F. only A, B, and C

Q6.5   Because cochlear implants have a limited bandwidth it is necessary to extract only the most important features of speech and present a simplified version of the speech signal to the implant. True or False.

Q6.6   Cochlear implants are only for the totally deaf. Anyone with even the slightest amount of residual acoustic hearing should not get an implant. True or False.

Q6.7   Single channel implants present the full bandwidth acoustic signal in electric form to the electrode. Thus single channel implants can provide speech recognition performance that is as good as that of a multichannel implant. True or False.

IV

HEART

Chapter 7

Vascular Mechanics in Artificial and Human Arteries

Michael D. Whitt, Ph.D.[1] and Gary M. Drzewiecki, Ph.D.[2]

[1] Miami Dade College, Department of Engineering
Miami, FL 33132
PH: 305-237-7532; FX: 305-237-7900; EM: mwhitt@mdc.edu

[2] Rutgers University, Dept. of Biomedical Engineering
617 Bowser Road, Piscataway, NJ 08854
PH: 732-445-3727; FX: 732-445-3753; EM: drzewiec@rci.rutgers.edu

7.1 Introduction

The arterial system in its role of cardiovascular resistance system has a different function and importance than the venous system which acts as the capacitance system of the circulatory system. Although the venous system contains approximately 2/3 of the total volume of the entire circulatory system, the arterial system ensures that the heart is able to provide adequate flow to all tissues providing adequate nutrients and oxygen while also providing adequate removal of carbon dioxide and other toxins.

The vascular mechanics of arteries play a significant role in the speed of the pressure and flow waveforms traveling through the arterial system in addition to the amount of work that the ventricles must supply to the blood. As patients age, the magnitude of pulse pressure increases and systolic hypertension occurs as a result of increasing vascular stiffness (Franklin et al., 2001).

Aging and diseased states such as aneurysm, arteriosclerosis, and artheromatosis can have an effect on the elastic properties of the artery. Arteriosclerosis and artheromatosis are often grouped under the term artherosclerosis. The two diseases are differentiated as arteriosclerosis is a generalized thickening and stiffening of the arterial media related primarily to hypertension while artheromatosis is an imflammatory arterial occlusive disorder related primarily to endothelial dysfunction and excessive deposition of oxidized lipids (Izzo et al., 2001). In some cases these diseases are treated via interventional methods such as balloon angioplasty, atherectomy, or stenting tools in the case of arterial blockages. However, in specific cases of arterial blockage grafts are performed. Autografts are performed where the mammary artery or subclavian vein is used for coronary artery bypass grafts (CABG). These vessels are chosen for their superior mechanical properties. In other cases allografts are performed to replace the vessel that is not meeting the mechanical and structural requirements.

The remainder of vascular graft procedures is performed with synthetic materials made up of materials that closely simulate the mechanical and structural properties of the human artery. However, the mechanical properties of these vascular graft materials exhibit differences from human arteries as a result of their being passive vessels.

These mechanical differences in human arteries can be quantified by comparative analysis of pressure-area (P-A) curves of the synthetic vascular graft materials and human arteries which provides a method where the mechanical properties can be graphically observed. This P-A curve can be obtained via invasive methods such as IVUS or noninvasive methods such as through the use of an instrument referred to as a Calibrated Cuff Plethysmograph which will be discussed in this chapter.

7.2 Basic Vascular Mechanics and the Pressure-Area Curve

The human artery is a viscoelastic tube that can have a varying change in lumen area at a constant pressure change. These changes in mechanical properties can be measured via observation of the velocity of pressure and flow waves along these vessels (Callaghan et al., 1986). This value is quantified by looking at the Moens-Korteweg equation (Eq. 7.1):

$$c_0 = \sqrt{(Eh/2R\rho)} \qquad (7.1)$$

Where c_0 is the velocity of the pressure wave, E is the Young's Modulus in the circumferential direction, h is the wall thickness, R is Radius of the tube, and ρ is the density of fluid.

The mechanical properties of the artery can also be estimated through observation of its characteristic pressure-flow relationship where the pressure drop measured over the length of the tube is described as a function of flow and the quantity external pressure minus downstream pressure (Brower et al., 1973). The incremental elastic modulus, E_{inc}, defined as the ratio of the force required to produce the elongation to the actual elongation or length change does have an effect on compliance and distensibility of the human artery. However, it is important to recognize that compliance, defined as a volume change for any given pressure change, will be larger in larger arteries while distensibility, defined as compliance per unit volume provides a normalized measurement.

Graphical representations of crossectional area and compliance as the measured variable versus transmural pressure as the independent variable provide a method of observation to compare the mechanical properties of a single human artery under control or vasodilator and vasoconstrictor effects. Addtionally, comparisons to the human artery can be graphically observed against vascular grafts. The active portion of the human artery and its physiology differentiates itself from synthetic grafts and plays a significant role in the differing mechanical properties between human artery and synthetic vascular grafts.

The anatomical zones of the artery are the following:

- Intima – bounded by endothelium and the internal elastic membrane (IEM). The IEM is primarily made up of elastic fibers while the endothelium acts as a semipermeable membrane between the blood vessel wall and the luminal wall.

- Media – bounded by the IEM and the external elastic membrane (EEM). Smooth muscle, collagen, and elastin are present here. The elastic fibers are oriented more concentric in thoracic arteries than in coronary arteries where the orientation is more random.
- Adventitia- bounded by the EEM and the tissues surrounding the blood vessel. The adventitia is innervated and primarily made up of randomly arranged collagen and elastin.

The tissue proteins collagen and elastin play an important role in the mechanics of the artery. Various researchers have found that at lower stresses the elastin present in the artery supports the greatest part of the load (Roach et al., 1959). Low strain elastic modulus and elastin composition directly correlate. However a poor correlation exists between high strain elastic modulus and collagen content (Kalsner, 1982). The majority of the collagen exists in the adventitia although collagen also exists in the media.

Experimental results showed that the stress-strain characteristics of the artery did not change within the physiological range (0-250 mm Hg) following the removal of approximately 50% of the arterial wall collagen from the adventitia. The conclusion was made that medial collagen had the more significant effect on arterial mechanical properties in the physiological pressure range.

The material characteristics of the artery are viscoelastic and anisotropic. Dynamic elastic modulus values are greater than the static elastic modulus values. The anisotropic properties are due to the collagen in the arteries being primarily oriented circumferentially and axially. Within the physiological diameter range, elastic modulus value is greatest circumferentially. Radial and axial values are smaller and approximately equal.

The crossbridge formation taking place between the contractile proteins, actin and myosin, provide the force generated from smooth muscle activation. Increased smooth muscle activation leads to decreased lumen diameter, increased pressure, increased static and dynamic modulus and decreased stresses within the tissue (Cox, 1979). As with collagen orientation and modulus, smooth muscle has its greatest effect circumferentially.

The collagen/elastin ratio in coronary arteries is highest. The arterial elastic modulus is made up of contributions from the passive elements (mainly collagen and elastin) and active elements (smooth muscle activation). Coronary arteries have shown a lesser maximum force development than arteries from other parts of the body. The decreased force development is due to decreased actomyosin content. There is a direct correlation between % cell fraction actomyosin and maximum force development.

In general, muscles with larger actin/myosin ratios have greater force generating capacity. This is due to the increased number of crossbridges formed per thick filament. For example, patients with high blood pressure generally have higher actin/myosin ratios. Research done with rat carotid and tail arteries have shown that the maximum active stress response decreases with age (Cox, 1983). This is believed to be due to the decrease in the contractile proteins; actin and myosin.

As previously mentioned, the passive elements of the artery are primarily collagen and elastin. The endothelial cells are where the synthesis takes place. There are different types of collagen and elastin which are synthesized. The differing types of collagen and elastin have differing mechanical properties. Type III collagen dominates at birth and decreases with aging. Amounts of Type I collagen also varies with diameter of the blood vessel (Kalsner, 1982). However, collagen synthesis can take place throughout life.

Collagen and elastin molecules both contain intermolecular crosslinks which have a large impact on the elastic modulus. The degree of crosslinking between these molecules increases with aging. Therefore, elastic modulus increases and has been found to increase linearly with age (Gonza et al., 1974). The relationships were found to be (Eqs. 7.2 and 7.3):

- $E_p = 90.0 + 16[\text{Age}]$ for the ascending aorta and, $\qquad$ (7.2)

- $E_p = 105.0 + 2.6[\text{Age}]$ for the right pulmonary artery $\qquad$ (7.3)

Elastin, a hydrophobic molecule, is the primary material in the IEM and EEM in smaller arteries. It is found in the medial elastic laminae in larger arteries. The number of elastic fibers present is set during the early development of the vessel wall. Elastin is not synthesized from this point. Lysis only occurs with aging.

As elastin lyses, the distance between elastin lamellae increases. This increased void space fills with collagen, proteoglycans, lipids, calcium, and salts. Also lipids accumulation inside the elastic fibrils leads to increased fibrillar lysis thus decreasing the elasticity of the fibrils. The remaining elastin (after lysing) undergoes increasing binding of nonelastin protein-polysaccharide to elastin chains as well as an increased number of interchain crosslinks with aging. This also contributes to the increased stiffness with age.

The observation of elastin lysis increasing with age is explained by smooth muscle cells migrating toward the intima with aging. These cells during migration resynthesize various molecules. Collagen and elastin fibers are included in this list. Cellular molecule synthesis was shown to decrease with aging and artherosclerotic plaque formation. Also elastolytic protease (causing elastin lysis) has been shown to increase exponentially with both aging and % of arteriosclerosis (Hornebeck et al., 1978)

Covalently crosslinked elastin (CE) decreases with aging in the aorta. The decrease of CE is believed to be a factor in the aging of the artery and artherosclerosis. A correlation was found to exist between increased elastin lysis and decreased CE.

Elastin lamellae in the thoracic aorta have the following increases with age (O'Rourke, et al., 1987):

- Increased diameter
- Increased wall thickness
- Increased interlamellar spacing
- Decreased elastin fibre density
- Increased medial thickness
- Increased tension per lamellar unit causing stiffness through causing each lamellae to become taut at lower stresses. As a result collagen fibers are recruited earlier and each lamellar unit must support a greater load.

Collagen and elastin support the load placed on the artery together. Elastin provides the support in the regions of lower stress while collagen provides the support in the higher stress regions. As collagen is recruited at the higher stresses, arterial stiffness increases as aortic volume distensibility (D) decreases with increased pressure (Eq. 7.4 – Distensibility Equation).

$$D = \frac{100}{V} X \frac{dV}{dP} \qquad (7.4)$$

Collagen has a greater stiffness than elastin. Measured values from differing animal arteries place the elastin fibers in 10^6 dyn/cm^2 range while collagen is in the 10^9 dyn/cm^2 range (Cox, 1977). Differences have been measured between human brachial arterial properties of a young group (<35) and an old group (>60) and significant differences in pressure modulus and compliance are observed (Mozersky et al., 1973). Many studies support the increase in arterial modulus with age (Table 7.1).

Table 7.1. Change in Pressure Modulus/Compliance with Age (Source: Mozersky, et al. 1973).

Measurement	Young (<35 Years Old)	Old (>60 Years Old)
E_p(dyn/cm^2)	2.64	6.28
%dV/V	6.0%	3.3%

The collagen/elastin ratio also increases with age. This leads to increased stress at any given strain. The ratio of collagen to elastin is high at birth before the elastin synthesis of the early years of life (Newman et al., 1978). It was seen that aortic strain at a given stress decreases with the collagen/elastin ratio increase with age.

The modulus of a collagen/elastin composite with loading parallel to the fiber direction (Voight model) can be expressed through an isostrain model equation (assuming strain is equal in both phases):

$$E_{total} = W_e E_e + f_c W_c E_c \qquad (7.5)$$

where:

- E_{total} = the Young's Modulus of the composite
- W_e = weight fractional content of elastin
- E_e = Young's Modulus for elastin
- f_c = fraction of collagen fibers supporting the wall load at any given transmural pressure
- W_c = weight fractional content of collagen
- E_c = Young's Modulus for collagen

With increasing aging, circumferential and tangential tension increase. However at any given pressure more tension is seen circumferentially than tangentially. Circumferential tension (T_c) is defined as:

$$T_c = PR \qquad (7.6)$$

where P = intraluminal pressure and R = vessel internal radius. This is also commonly referred to as the law of LaPlace.

Longitudinal tension (T_L) is defined as:

$$T_L = \frac{PR}{2} \qquad (7.7)$$

Arteries are anisotropic where the mechanical properties are not the same in all three dimensions. An isotropic cylindrical tube would be more distensible circumferentially at any given pressure per the relationships in Eqs. 7.6 and 7.7. However, a human artery is more distensible longitudinally as a result of its anisotropic properties. The distensibility is greater in the thoracic region and suggests a greater elastin content in this region or a difference in the helical organization of the elastic elements in the differing regions. Previous research supports that the arterial wall media resists loading in the transverse direction. The intima and media resist loading in the longitudinal direction (Roy, 1980).

Observations of volume distensibility changes with age show that within physiological blood pressure range distensibility decreases with age. The previous observations can be explained through the earlier mentioned synthesis/catabolism of elastin and collagen. The reason that distensibility decreases with age is due to the catabolism of elastin with increasing age. As elastin catabolizes there is a lesser resistance to the lower stress/strain loads. Also, the collagen helices become fully extended at lower stress/strain values with age. Therefore, distensibility decreases with age. Additionally, volume distensibility and compliance are maximum values at mean arterial pressure as seen in oscillometry where Mean Arterial Pressure is found at maximum volume distensibility and compliance (Drzewiecki, et al., 1994).

Pulse wave velocity (c_0), used in the diagnosis of artherosclerosis, is the linear velocity that a pulse wave generated by a systole propogates along an artery. The Moens-Korteweg equation shows that c_0 increases with both arterial wall modulus and wall thickness. Both of these factors increase with age leading to increased pulse velocity with age. Additionally, the arterial elastin content increases with radius and collagen content does not (Milch, 1965). However, the general radius of the artery increases with age. This alone would cause a decrease in pulse velocity with age. The increase in pulse velocity with age is a result of the product of modulus and wall thickness being greater than the increase in radius with age. Pulse wave velocity has been found to increase linearly with age as seen in (Eqs. 7.8 – ascending aorta) and (Eq. 7.9 – right pulmonary artery) (Gonza, et al., 1974):

$$c_0 = 3.0 + 0.10 \text{ (age)} \tag{7.8}$$

$$c_0 = 2.2 + 0.02 \text{ (age)} \tag{7.9}$$

Intimal sclerosis and degeneration of the elastic lamellae that make up the internal elastic membrane (IEM) increase with age. These factors also favor an increase in the Young's Modulus leading to increased pulse velocity. Observations have shown that calcification in the media always takes place in aging arteries prior to the intimal changes (Lansing, 1955). This occurs simultaneously with the decrease in elastin with aging where hydroxyapatite is seen to be the main contributor to vascular deposit (Carlstroem et al., 1953).

Additional studies have shown that after approximately 25 years of age, aortic distensibility decreases (Yater and Birkeland,1929-30). Eighty percent of this decrease is attributed to tissue elasticity/smooth muscle function and 20% is attributed to fibrosis.

Polysaccharides present in the arterial wall decrease with advancing age. They interact with the arterial proteins, and bind water and cations. The strong attraction for water allows the polysaccharides to act as a plasticizing agent therefore decreasing the modulus. The decrease in polysaccharides with aging contributes to the increasing arterial stiffness.

The increase in stiffness with stress relationship can be graphically and mathematically expressed from the mathematical form as seen in (Eq. 7.10 – age group 29 to 85 years) (Mirsky et al., 1976):

$$E = k\rho + c \qquad (7.10)$$

where c = value of stiffness at 0 stress, ρ= stress, and k = stiffness constant (i.e. slope of stiffness-strain relation in linear area). The slope of these relationships represents a stiffness constant that has been observed to increase with age from 29-75 years of age with no significant increase from 75-85 years of age.

The viscoelastic properties of arteries change with age where the phase lag between force and length is greater in young arteries than in older arteries. However, there is no difference in the collagen/elastin ratio with increasing age (Yin et al., 1983). Hydroxyproline, an amino acid $C_5H_9NO_3$ that occurs naturally as a constituent of collagen, is used in the identification of collagen. The stiffness differential between old and young arteries is greater when smooth muscle is activated. However, the differential still exists with 100% smooth muscle inactivation although to a lesser degree.

Experiments have successfully measured the P-A relationship of human arteries using IVUS. However, the experiments only provide measurements in the region that is above 0 mm Hg Transmural Pressure where the data for the collapse region of the vessel is not obtainable (Kinlay et al., 1995; Bank et al., 1995). The P-A relationship that occurs in human arteries provides a methodology to observe the arterial vascular mechanics changes that occur with age. Relative changes can be measured where subject to subject comparisons can be made using initial area as a baseline and obtaining normalized data similar to a distensibility value obtained for two different subjects.

7.3 Vascular Graft Mechanics

7.3.1 *Review of literature*

Vascular grafts are classified into two major categories. Large diameter grafts (>10 mm) primarily made up of Dacron (80%) and PTFE (20%) are primarily used for aortic and iliac artery reconstruction. The small caliber grafts (<10 mm) are primarily used for CABG, lower-extremity bypass procedures, and hemodialysis access. The patency rates for the synthetic graft material are better for the aortic and iliac artery reconstruction than for when small caliber grafts are used. Saphenous vein grafts and internal mammary grafts both have greater patency rates than the small caliber vascular grafts with the internal mammary artery providing the superior patency rates.

Dacron (polyethylene terphthlate) and PTFE (polytetrafluoroethylene) maintain their tensile strength for years after being implanted. However other materials such as Nylon (polyamide), Ivalon, and Orlon decrease in tensile strength after months of being implanted. Woven Dacron grafts are nonporous with no stretch while knitted Dacron grafts have variable stretch and are porous. As previously mentioned, the patency rates for the use of these grafts is better for large vessel grafts (Ku et al., 2000).

Neointimal hyperplasia, which occurs in the anastomotic area, is the prime reason of failure of small caliber grafts. The low compliance rates leading to compliance mismatch plays a role as well. The neointimal hyperplasia could be caused by platelet deposition with local release of platelet derived growth factor (PDGF), other growth factor stimulation of smooth muscle cell (SMC) proliferation (e.g., transforming growth factor (TGF), fibroblast growth factor (FGF)), monocyte recruitment, complement activation, leukocyte deposition, chronic inflammation, and mechanical stimuli such as stress and shear abnormalities (Greisler, 1991). Additionally, the optimal sizing of a graft is important to provide a wall shear rate that will increase the long term patency of the synthetic grafts (Binns et al., 1989).

7.3.2 *Measurements and previous data*

The mechanics of the vascular graft differs from that of the human artery. X-ray imaging has been performed where a stiffness parameter (β) and diameter compliance were calculated. A stiffness parameter has been determined from Eq. 7.11:

$$Ln\ (P/P_s) = \beta(D/D_s - 1) \qquad (7.11)$$

where P is the pressure and D is the diameter at P, and P_s and D_s are the standard intraluminal pressure and the internal diameter at the standard pressure. As β increases the vessel becomes more rigid.

Diameter compliance (C_d) was calculated from the formula in Eq. 7.12:

$$C_d = \Delta D/(D \times \Delta P) \qquad (7.12)$$

where D is the internal diameter of the vessel and ΔD is the diameter change associated with a ΔP change at standard pressure. C_d provides a normalized measurement of compliance similar to distensibility.

Although the anostomotic region was seen to have a greater stiffness than the arterial region, the artery was more compliant. The ePTFE graft measured was significantly more stiff and less compliant than both (Sonoda et al., 2002).

Table 7.2. Stiffness and Diameter Compliance Values for Artery, Graft and Anastomosis (Hayashi et al., 1985).

	β Value	C_d (%/mm Hg x 10^{-2})
Artery	10.6	6.8
ePTFE	164	0.51
Anastomosis	14.4	5.5

The pressure area curve for the PTFE graft shows no change as it is all one material while the human artery shifts the stress from elastin to collagen with the intraluminal pressure change (Figure 7.1).

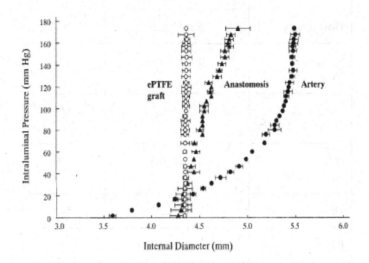

Figure 7.1. P-A Relationships between Artery, Anastomosis, and ePTFE Graft (Hayashi et al., 1980).

The compliance mismatch is not the only possible factor influencing wall shear rate that is a cause of anastomosis. Impedance phase angle (IPA), the phase angle between pressure and flow wave is a factor causing anastamosis (Annis et al., 1987, 1984). Compliance mismatch remains the primary factor having a significant effect on low patency rates (Salacinsk et al., 1978).

As seen in Table 7.3, the mechanical property differences between the human artery and synthetic graft materials have a significant effect on patency ratès. As newer material grafts are developed, the importance of measuring the compliance will be key to the success of patency ratẹ increases. Development of P-A curves will be an important measurement towards this goal.

Table 7.3. Relationship between Compliance and Patency Rates (Dardik et al., 1978; Veith et al., 1986).

Graft Type	Compliance (% mm Hg x 10^2)	Patency %
Host Artery	5.9 +/- 0.5	-
Saphenous Vein	4.4 +/- 0.8	75
Umbilical Vein	3.7 +/- 0.5	60
Bovine heterograft	2.6 +/- 0.3	59
Dacron	1.9 +/- 0.3	50
PTFE	1.6 +/- 0.2	40

7.4 Human Artery Mechanics

7.4.1 *In vivo measurements*

The brachial artery is the common site for noninvasive blood pressure measurement. During routine measurement, an occlusive cuff is applied to the arm over the brachial artery and inflated over a range of pressure extending from 0 to near 150 mm Hg. This effectively alters the pressure that the brachial artery is subjected to by changing the transmural pressure. As the cuff pressure falls from high values to zero, the vessel, in turn, undergoes complete collapse of its lumen, partial collapse, and then an increase in lumen size. This leads to mixture of vessel collapse mechanics and vessel elastic wall distension mechanics, depending on the transmural pressure. As a consequence, the relationship between the brachial lumen area and transmural pressure is curvilinear.

Ths pressure-lumen area (P-A) relationship ultimately permits occlusive blood pressure determination to be feasible. The role that the P-A curve plays in affecting the accuracy of blood pressure measurement is not certain (Coats et al., 1992). Moreover, an accurate model of the P-A curve of the collapsible brachial artery is not available for humans.

The most common methods of blood pressure determination today are the method of Korotkoff and the oscillometric method. It has been shown that the Korotkoff sound arises as a consequence of the strong influence of the P-A relationship on pressure and flow dynamics under the cuff (Drzewiecki et al., 1987, 1989). Alternatively, the oscillometric method employs small oscillations in the cuff pressure to determine blood pressure. These oscillations have been empirically determined to maximize in amplitude when the cuff pressure equals the mean arterial pressure (Geddes et al., 1983; Ramsey, 1979). Theoretical analyses of the cuff pressure oscillations have been derived from the brachial P-A relationship (Drzewiecki, 1995; Drzewiecki et al., 1994).

There are relatively few noninvasive methods available for measuring the P-A relationship Kelly et al. (1989) and Van der Hoeven et al. (1973) have employed pulse wave velocity to indirectly find compliance from pulse propagation obtained using an upstream and downstream pulse sensor. Alternatively, plethysmography has been employed to find the arterial volume pulse. The volume pulse amplitude is then divided by the pulse pressure amplitude to find compliance. These approaches, though, only provide a single value of compliance at the subject's normal blood pressure and the change in lumen area. Arterial compliance in the arm has also been evaluated as a function of the instantaneous pressure by means of vascular ultrasound (Simon et al., 1983). This technique also permits the real time tracking of vessel diameter. The simultaneous measurement of intra-arterial pressure then permits the evaluation of lumen area versus pressure. This method, though, is limited to the range of the subject's pulse pressure. Recently, intravascular ultrasound of the brachial artery has been employed under an occlusive cuff (Bank et al., 1996). The instantaneous measurements of arterial diameter are obtained, and the P-A curve is generated. However, values are not obtained over the range of vessel collapse and the method is invasive.

Other researchers have attempted to combine plethysmography with the occlusive arm cuff as an alternative noninvasive approach (Shankar et al., 1991; Shimazu et al., 1989). Electrical impedance plethysmography has been popular, since it permits calibration of volume records. These approaches are noninvasive, repeatable, and implemented as simply as routine blood pressure measurement.

Duplex ultrasonography is one noninvasive method where change in arterial area can be measured by obtaining an arterial area diameter measurement at a given EKG cycle point. Multiple transcutaneous measurements can be made taking arterial diameter measurements at the same EKG cycle point. This method provides a relative change in arterial diameter when performed at multiple times. This technique is currently one of the standards used for performing testing where changes in vascular mechanics need to be measured.

Additionally, duplex ultrasonography provides a method to obtain an arterial compliance measurement. However, duplex ultrasonography provides all measurements assuming that the measured diameter is taken from a perfectly circular artery. This compliance measurement only can be done at the equivalent of 0 mm Hg cuff pressure and requires the accurate edge detection and quantitative maearuement of a trained sonographer.

Thermodilution is another method that is considered a standard for the noninvasive measure of relative vascular mechanical changes over time. This provides an estimate of the change in the vascular mechanics as related to a temperature change measurement distal of the point of measure that is a function of the change in flow.

Tonometry provides a noninvasive measure of arterial vascular mechanics. One of the keys for obtaining accurate arterial compliance values is the proper transducer placement over the artery. However, arterial compliance measurements vary depending on tonometer pressure. Additionally, compliance and flow measurements obtained are not calibrated but only provide estimates.

In studies conducted where the electrical impedance technique is compared with other standard methods of measuring stroke volume and cardiac output, correlation coefficients were determined as a function of patient condition. The correlation coefficient in subjects without valve problems or heart failure and with a stable circulatory system is 0.8 to 0.9. In patients with a failing circulatory system and valvular or other cardiovascular problems, the correlation coefficient may be less than 0.6 (Patterson, 1989).

There are various methods currently in existence to obtain vascular mechanics data that are accepted as standards of measure. Each of these standards of measure has its own individual strengths and weaknesses. One fact is that none of these current standards provides a calibrated P-A curve over the entire transmural pressure region from full collapse to fully dilated.

7.4.2 *The passive vessel*

The interaction between collagen, elastin, and smooth muscle provides the mechanical properties of the human artery. It has been proposed that the smooth muscle in the arterial wall is in series with collagen and that both are in parallel with elastin (Burton, 1954; Nichols et al., 1990). The P-A curve can be analyzed in both the distension region as measured with IVUS as well as the collapse region (Drzewiecki et al., 1997). These two regions make a transition at a point that was denoted by the buckling area, A_b, and buckling pressure, P_b. The buckling point was identified from the data as the point at which compliance is a maximum and assumes a constant axial tension.

Beginning with distension, the extension ratio, λ, was defined as the ratio of lumen area, A, with reference to the buckling area, A_b. This ratio measures distension for values greater than one, since, by definition, it will be less than unity once the vessel begins to collapse. It was limited to values above one for distension by using the hyperbolic relation

$$\lambda = [1 + (\frac{A}{A_b})^C]^{1/C} \tag{7.13}$$

The value of c is a constant that is not critical in value and has been set at a value of 40 in a previous study (Drzewiecki et. al. 1997). It should be sufficiently large to force the extension ratio rapidly to one when $A < A_b$. For the range of collapse, bending stresses occur that lead to the development of a negative valued collapse pressure, P_c. The inverse extension ratio was defined to represent the range of vessel bending as:

$$\lambda^{-1} = [1 + (\frac{A_b}{A})^c]^{1/c} \tag{7.14}$$

The value of c was chosen to be the same as in Eq. 7.13. The use of Eqn. 7.13 and 7.14 also permits a smooth transition between the collapse and distention ranges depending on the choice of c. The arterial pressure was then determined by summing the pressures caused by vessel collapse, buckling, and distention, respectively:

$$P = -E((\lambda^{-1})^n - 1) + P_b + a(e^{b(\lambda-1)} - 1) \tag{7.15}$$

where a and b are the arterial elastance constants for distention, E is the vessel elastance during collapse, and n is a constant that determines the rate of change of pressure with respect to change in area during collapse.

Equation 7.15 requires the determination of parameters a,b, E, n, A_b, and P_b. A_b and P_b were measured directly from the data. They were determined as the point on the P-A curve that corresponds with maximum compliance. Their values were inserted into Eq. 7.15 for the specific subject, leaving the remaining constants to be found using nonlinear least squares regression (Marquadt-Levenberg algorithm). Parameter dependencies were reduced by substituting a/b for a and E/n for E and then performing the nonlinear regression for a/b and E/n. The value of a was then determined by multiplying the regression result for a/b by b, and similarly, E/n by n. It should be noted that when lumen area is zero, the first term of Eq. 7.15 goes to infinity. Hence, this point was not included in the data set for nonlinear regression. Lastly, the value of n was constrained to positive values only. This forces the first term of Eq. 7.15 to maintain a hyperbolic form, as required by collapse mechanics. The above method has successfully yielded rapid and unique convergence for all parameters using actual subject data sets.

7.4.3 *The active vessel: flow mediated dilation*

7.4.3.1 *Introduction*

The arterial pressure-lumen area (P-A) curve provides potential clinical benefit in various areas of cardiovascular disease such as congestive heart failure, hypertension, and coronary and peripheral arterial disease in addition to providing monitoring benefits for patients undergoing anesthesia. The P-A curve could supply valuable information not currently provided by ultrasonography and potentially eliminate subjective error currently found in ultrasound diameter measurements. These benefits are provided through the quantification of smooth muscle activity.

An instrument referred to as a calibrated cuff plethysmograph (CCP) was used to obtain a P-A curve (Figure 7.2) while performing oscillometric blood pressure measurement. The P-A curve is generated by performing numerical integration of the arterial compliance versus transmural pressure curve (Figure 7.3) using the trapezoidal rule (Larson et al., 1982). The scale of transmural pressure for each individual subject's P-A curve and arterial compliance curves are equivalent. Each arterial compliance curve and subsequent P-A curve includes transmural pressures ranging from arterial wall collapse to above venous pressure. Transmural pressure is defined as:

$$\text{Transmural Pressure} = \text{Intralumen Mean Arterial Pressure}$$
$$- \text{External Pressure Applied}$$

$$(7.16)$$

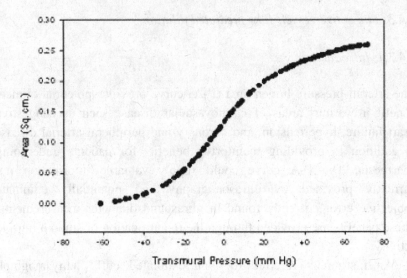

Figure 7.2. CCP Output: Arterial Pressure-Area Curve.

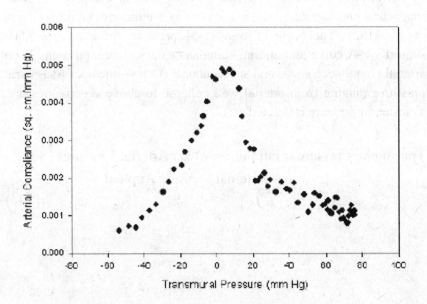

Figure 7.3. CCP Output: Arterial Compliance Curve.

CCP Benefit

The CCP is able to provide an arterial compliance vs. transmural pressure curve and pressure-area curve while performing a standard oscillometric blood pressure measurement. As a result, earlier diagnosis of diseases can be made through the use of this practical tool.

Transmural pressure is used as the independent variable providing a standard reference point for all patients' P-A and arterial compliance curves. As previously mentioned, the clinical data obtained from the CCP has value in varied arenas. For example, congestive heart failure has been associated with increased sympathetic activity measured as decreased arterial compliance (Grassi et al., 1995). Hyperemic reaction that results in reduced arterial compliance and area decrease may be an indicator of coronary artery disease (Lekakis et al., 1998). Hypertension patients can be treated with calcium channel blockers, alpha blockers, or beta blockers. General physiological effects of these treatments include decreased heart rate and workload as a result of decreased strength of myocardial contraction, and peripheral and coronary vasodilation (Schauf et al., 1990). The magnitude effect that each drug has on vasodilation and strength of myocardial contraction is not quantified. As a result, treatment of hypertensive patients is often an iterative process at best.

Additionally, activity of nicotinic antagonists providing skeletal and smooth muscle relaxation for patients undergoing anesthesia can be quantified by measuring the vasodilatory effects via a percent increase in peripheral arterial lumen area. In cases where curare-like compounds are used as an anesthetic to accomplish skeletal and smooth muscle relaxation without the inhibition of the brainstem visceral control system caused by higher levels of a general anesthetic, quantification of smooth muscle activity is valuable.

In all of the above cases, the quantitative hemodynamic information obtained from CCP potentially provides a better understanding of the physiological mechanisms involved in classifying congestive heart failure, patient response to anesthesia, clinical benefits and response of hypertension drug treatments as well as providing useful information for patient care decision in the diagnosis and treatment of coronary and peripheral artery disease.

The objective of the studies performed was to provide comparative measurements of brachial artery lumen area using Doppler ultrasonography and CCP. Additionally, the error from both techniques was observed. Measured responses to hyperemic stimuli were observed for similarity between the two methods. In all experiments, the Doppler ultrasound measurement was taken as the control measurement.

7.4.3.2 *Materials and methods*

CCP Fundamentals and Calculations

The CCP consists of a pressure transducer, amplifier, diaphragm pump, inline flowmeter, motor speed control, power supply, blood pressure cuff, tubing, and stopcock and needle valves (Fig. 7.4). The technique combines the concepts of plethysmography and oscillometry.

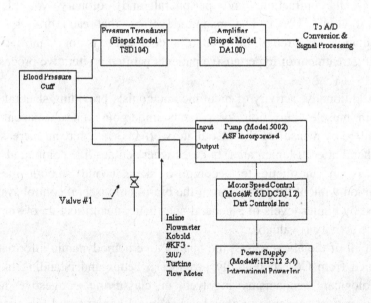

Figure 7.4. Schematic of Calibrated Cuff Plethysmograph.

CCP calibration and repeatability were demonstrated in previous experiments (Whitt et al., 1997, 1998). The experiments discussed here include transcutaneous ultrasound and CCP experiments performed on eight healthy subjects. Brachial artery lumen measurements from the ultrasound technique were used as the control measurement to evaluate the accuracy of the CCP.

Oscillometry is defined as the use of an instrument for measuring changes in pulsations in the arteries especially of the extremities (Merriam-Webster, 1993). Oscillometric data provides systolic, diastolic, and mean arterial pressure values (Geddes et. al, 1983). Mean arterial pressure can be found where the pressure oscillations are at a maximum. Systolic blood pressure is found at 55% of the maximum amplitude while diastolic blood pressure is found at 85% of the maximum amplitude (Drzewiecki et al., 1994).

Plethysmography is defined as the use of an instrument for determining and registering variations in the size of an organ or limb and in the amount of blood passing through it (Merriam-Webster, 1993). An ideal gage for the measurement of limb volumetric changes has a linear relationship between the actual volume change and measured independent variable used to predict the volumetric change (Whitney, 1953). The CCP uses change in cuff pressure as the measured independent variable. Segmental plethysmography is the specific technique through which the oscillometric volume pulses are obtained by the CCP. The ideal segmental plethysmograph system would be linear where a given change in cuff pressure would result in an equal volume change over the entire cuff pressure range (Winsor, 1957; Hyman et al., 1960). However, the CCP does not provide a resultant relationship where the cuff pressure change is directly proportional to the vascular volume change over the entire range of cuff pressures. This phenomenon is caused by a nonlinear pressure volume (P-V) relationship in cuff compliance caused by the effect of Boyle's Law and tightness of the cuff on the limb (Drzewiecki et al., 1993).

Cuff compliance is defined as:

Cuff Compliance = [Change in cuff volume (ml)]/[Change in cuff pressure (mm Hg)]   (7.17)

Segmental plethysmography provides accurate measurements of limb volumetric displacements at all pressures where cuff compliance can be determined. Obtaining a value for cuff compliance allows for accurate measurement of limb volumetric displacements through the following relationship:

$$dV_{artery} = dV_{cuff} = (dV/dP)_{cuff} \times dP_{cuff} \qquad (7.18)$$

The relationship $dV_{artery} = dV_{cuff}$ is only true if the pressure applied to the artery under the cuff is uniform throughout the entire cuff length. If however, the pressure applied to the artery under the cuff is not uniform, this relationship does not hold. As a result, the actual cuff length is not equal to the effective cuff length (L_{cuff}) (Alexander et al., 1977).

The effective cuff length (L_{cuff}) can then be defined as:

Effective Cuff Length = [Fraction of artery under the actual cuff length subjected to cuff pressure] x [Actual Cuff Length]

$$(7.19)$$

L_{cuff} values can be determined for each subject or a group of experiments by observing the ratio of brachial artery lumen measurements of ultrasound experiments versus CCP experiments.

The CCP data acquisition is made up of standard oscillometric and flowmeter data that are simultaneously obtained. (Fig. 7.5) This information is used to determine the cuff compliance curve, arterial compliance curve, and P-A curve. The signal recorded at the cuff consists of a pump pressure pulse resulting from each stroke of an external pump operating between 25-35 Hertz. (Figure 7.6) and the subject's arterial pressure pulses (Fig. 7.7) which is developed by band pass filtering the data between 0.5 – 5.0 Hz.

Observation of a Fast Fourier Transform (FFT) of the overall cuff signal resulting from both waveforms (Figure 7.8) permits verification that the energy from each signal is discrete.

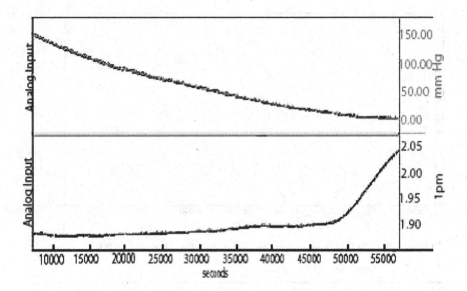

Figure 7.5. CCP Data Acquisition: Oscillometric Data (Top) and Flowmeter Data (Bottom).

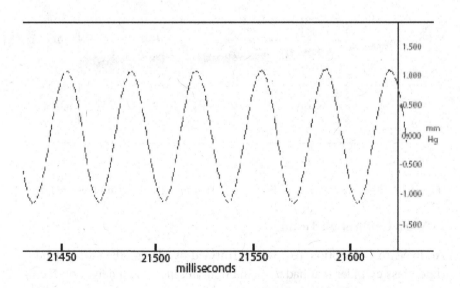

Figure 7.6. CCP Data Acquisition: Pump Calibration Pulse - Band Pass Filter (25-35 Hertz).

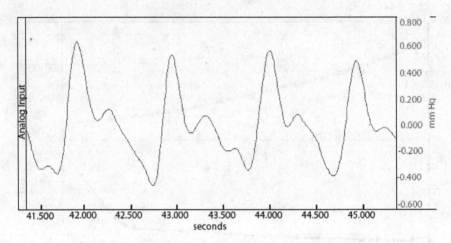

Figure 7.7. CCP Data Acquisition: Arterial Pulse - Band Pass Filter (0.5 - 5.0 Hertz).

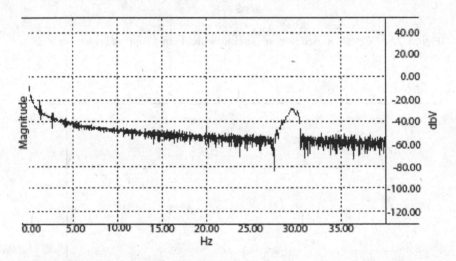

Figure 7.8. CCP Data Acquisition: Fast Fourier Transform (FFT) of Cuff Pressure Data.

In Vitro Calibration Testing

An In Vitro Calibration Test was performed by placing the cuff around a rigid glass cylinder that had a 30cm circumference and a height of 20cm. An Intravenous (IV) bag filled with 100 cc of water manufactured by Harmac Medical Products, Inc. was placed between the cylinder and the cuff.

The experimental model for the In Vitro Calibration Test was performed for each set of independent variable conditions shown in the Design of Experiments where the dependent variable was % Error. The two independent factors observed were cuff pressure and pump frequency. Cuff pressure was observed from over five levels ranging from 40 mm Hg to 160 mm Hg and pump frequency was observed at two distinct levels ranging from 27 Hertz to 37 Hertz. At least one replicate was performed at most conditions. The dependent variable, % Error, for all experiments of the In Vitro Calibration test is defined as:

% Error = [Plethysmograph Measured Volume Change– Actual Volume Change(2.0 ml)] ÷ [Actual Volume Change(2.0 ml)]

$$(7.20)$$

Following setup, data acquisition was initiated. All data acquisition was performed at 500 samples per second. The IV bag was filled with water removing all air and dead space. The stopcock attached to the bag was placed in the closed position. The desired pump frequency and cuff pressure were then set. A syringe was filled with 2.0 ml of water. The syringe was connected to the stopcock valve. The valve was opened and the 2.0 ml of water was injected into the IV bag. Cuff pressure change was recorded.

Patient Information

All human subject CCP testing was performed at the University of Maryland; Baltimore, MD. Comparitive testing was performed using Doppler ultrasonography as the control measurement. All data acquisition was performed at 500 samples/second using eight subjects. The eight subjects for the CCP and ultrasound experiments included five healthy women and three healthy men ranging in age from 23 to 57 years of age (Table 7.4). Independent oscillometric blood pressure measurements were performed on all subjects using both an automated oscillometer and the CCP.

Table 7.4. Patient Information.

PATIENT #	SEX	AGE	HEIGHT(IN)	WEIGHT (LBS)
1	M	57	71	147
2	F	37	69	160
3	F	23	66	128
4	M	33	75	170
5	M	28	70	138
6	F	45	62	144
7	F	42	67	156
8	F	42	64	159

CCP Experimental Procedure

Test setup began for each experiment by a blood pressure cuff being placed around the subject's left upper arm while the subject was in a resting position with the subject's back parallel to the floor. While the cuff was around the subject's upper arm, a manual bulb was used to fill the blood pressure cuff to 200 mm Hg. For the five minute hyperemia experiments, the cuff pressure was held for five minutes at approximately 200 mm Hg prior to data acquisition. Cuff pressure and flowmeter data are obtained while allowing the cuff pressure to slowly descend from 200 mm Hg to 0 mm Hg. Data analysis was performed to obtain the arterial compliance and arterial lumen area values for each subject at all arterial transmural pressures.

Ultrasound Experimental Procedure

All ultrasound imaging measurements were taken using each subject's left brachial artery for diameter measurements. The equipment used was a 5-11 MHz bandwidth broadband transducer on an Advanced Technology Laboratory Apogec 8004 Ultrasound Machine. The system specifications were 640 x 480 pixels with no lateral distortion. All studies were done in a temperature controlled room at 22C with the subject in a resting position with their back parallel to the floor. Electrocardiogram data was continuously obtained. Blood pressure and heart rate data were recorded from the right arm every five minutes with an automatic sphygmomanometer. The subject's left arm was comfortably immobilized in an extended position to allow constant access to the brachial artery for imaging. All measurements were performed by a highly skilled sonographer. The brachial artery of the left arm was imaged at a location 3-7 cm above the antecubital fossa. The artery was located by use of ultrasound attenuators taped to the subject's left arm. Images were obtained in the longitudinal view with great care to maximize vessel diameter and provide optimal blood vessel wall definition. The image depth was set at 4 cm and gain settings were adjusted to best delineate the arterial wall. The images were then magnified by a resolution box function (Fig. 7.9). Additionally, Doppler flow velocity measurements were recorded although they were not analyzed. All measurements were taken by two independent observers using the same image. The measurements of the two observers are averaged to obtain the overall final brachial artery diameter value. All sessions were recorded on videotape for subsequent off line analysis.

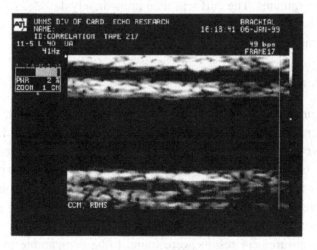

Figure 7.9. Ultrasound Image: Brachial Artery Following Magnification.

Experimental Schedule

All experiments were performed in a single day session. The CCP experiments were performed prior to the ultrasound experiments. Between each experiment a ten minute rest break was given to the subject to allow for recovery of the arterial smooth muscle. First, the noninvasive CCP technique was performed under normal conditions for data acquisition.

Following the data acquisition collection under normal conditions, a five minute hyperemia experiment was performed using the CCP. This experiment followed the same procedure as the normal condition experiment with the exception of data acquisition taking place following the cuff pressure being held at approximately 200 mm Hg around the subject's left upper arm for five minutes. This effectively restricts blood flow and creates a five minute reactive hyperemia experiment.

Following CCP data acquisition, ultrasonography was performed. Measurements were taken under normal and five minute hyperemic conditions. First, the left brachial artery was measured under normal conditions. Immediately following this measurement, the blood pressure cuff was placed around the left arm of the subject and inflated to 200 mm Hg for five minutes. The cuff was then immediately deflated to 0 mm Hg and another ultrasound measurement of the left brachial artery was taken after one minute.

7.4.3.3 *Results*

ANOVA analysis of the in vitro calibration testing corroborates that the independent variables, cuff pressure ($P = .594$) and pumping frequency ($P = .088$), did not significantly affect the %Error in measured volume from the CCP technique. Mean percentage error for all experiments performed was 1.5%. Mean square error is 2.9%. CCP demonstrated a high degree of accuracy in measuring the volume change of the IV bag.

The independent oscillometer systolic, diastolic, and mean arterial pressure measurement results were found to be comparable to the CCP results (Table 7.5). CCP brachial artery measurements for each subject under normal conditions were reproducible. Brachial artery area measurements at approximately +60 mm Hg transmural pressure were used for all recorded CCP area measurements where comparisons are made to Doppler ultrasonography.

Table 7.5. Automatic Oscillometeric (O) and CCP Blood Pressure Measurements (mm Hg).

Patient #	O Systolic BP	CCP Systolic BP	O Diastolic BP	CCP Diastolic BP	O Mean Arterial Pressure	CCP Mean Arterial Pressure
1	158	165	85	90	114	110
2	118	123	67	71	86	84
3	110	111	66	79	83	86
4	119	110	72	80	90	88
5	116	115	71	75	87	85
6	132	140	84	95	105	113
7	121	115	73	75	92	88
8	108	120	65	78	80	90
Mean	122.75	124.88	72.88	80.38	92.13	93
SD	16.00	18.80	7.74	8.11	11.61	11.60

Systolic, diastolic, and mean arterial blood pressure were observed for all subjects of more than 40 years of age and less than 40 years of age. All oscillometric and CCP blood pressure values were higher and had a greater standard deviation for all subjects of more than 40 years of age.

Following CCP data acquisition and observation of the arterial compliance curve under normal conditions, arterial compliance was observed to increase in the five minute hyperemia CCP experiments (Figure 7.10) and corresponds to an increase in brachial artery area (Fig. 7.11). The arterial compliance versus transmural pressure relationship is nonlinear (Roach et al., 1959; Drzewiecki et al., 1997) where arterial compliance has its greatest sensitivity at positive transmural pressures. The increase in arterial compliance was most evident at the transmural pressure of +60 mm Hg where the smooth muscle in series with collagen dominates the arterial mechanics (Bank et al., 1996; Perregaux et al., 1999). The observed CCP arterial area diameter increase at +60 mm Hg transmural pressure was contrasted against the arterial diameter increase observed from the normal and five minute hyperemia experiments performed with ultrasound. CCP indicated a brachial artery lumen area increase of 15.8% +/- 11.7% while ultrasound indicated an increase of 10.3% +/- 7.4% following the five minute hyperemia experiments.

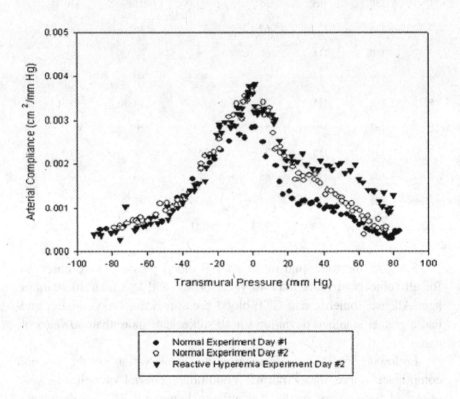

Figure 7.10. CCP Results: Normal vs. Five Minute Hyperemic Arterial Compliance Curves.

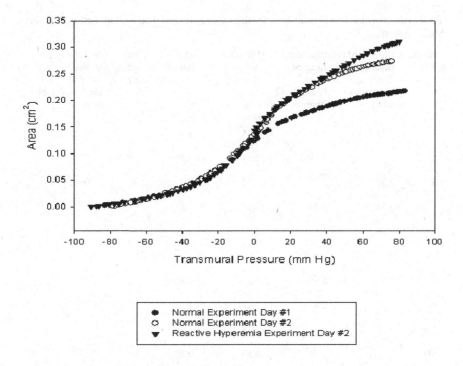

Figure 7.11. CCP Results: Normal vs. Five Minute Hyperemic.

Pressure-Area Curves

Normal experiment brachial artery diameter averaged 44.5% +/- 20.1% larger for CCP measurements than Doppler ultrasound (Table 7.6).

Table 7.6. Normal Condition: Cuff Plethysmography and Ultrasound Brachial Artery Measurements.

Patient #	Ultrasound Brachial Artery Diameter #1 (mm)	Ultrasound Brachial Artery Diameter #2 (mm)	Ultrasound Avg. Brachial Artery Diameter (mm)	Plethysmography Area Converted to Diameter (mm)	% Difference between ultrasound and plethysmography diameter
1	2.78	3.31	3.05	3.9	27.9
2	2.69	3.19	2.94	3.55	20.7
3	2.32	2.72	2.52	3.0	19.0
4	3.71	4.45	4.08	5.5	34.8
5	2.39	2.78	2.59	3.9	50.6
6	2.42	2.96	2.69	3.9	45.0
7	2.5	2.96	2.73	4.1	50.2
8	2.25	2.6	2.43	4.1	68.7
Mean			2.88	3.99	39.6
SD			0.53	0.71	17.11

Observation of the five minute hyperemia condition experiments from the same eight patients showed that the CCP diameter was 47.7% greater than the ultrasound diameter with a standard deviation of 15.1%.

A correction factor of 0.69 could be applied to all CCP diameter measurements. This would provide a common baseline for all diameter measurements between ultrasound and CCP experiments. Additional experimentation will be required to fully understand the proper use of the correction factor with the CCP. Currently, the differential measurements between CCP and ultrasound measured diameters can not be fully expressed as a mathematical relationship with a high degree of confidence.

While using the correction factor, the relationship between all normal condition experiments contrasting ultrasound and CCP is described by the mathematical relationship:[CCP Measured Diameter (mm)]=0.76 [Ultrasound Measured Diameter (mm)] + 0.63. The linear relationship can be described at greater than 95% Confidence (P =.01 and r^2 = .65). Additionally, the relationship between all hyperemia condition experiments contrasting ultrasound and CCP is described by the mathematical relationship: [CCP Measured Diameter (mm)] =0.75[Ultrasound Measured Diameter (mm)] + 0.90. As observed in the normal condition experiments, the linear relationship can be described at greater than 95% Confidence (P= .02 and r^2 = .67) (Fig. 7.12).

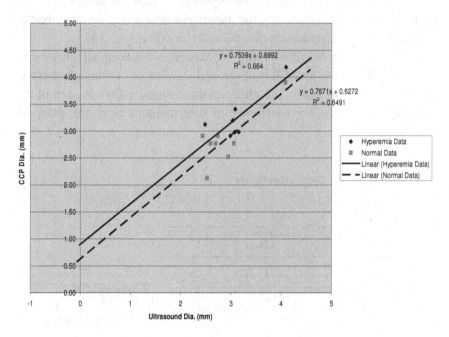

Figure 7.12. Mathematical Relationships: CCP Measured Diameters versus Ultrasound Measured Diameter (Correction Factor Applied).

However, it is believed that the use of the correction factor is unnecessary. The slopes of the two graphs are approximately parallel (1.7% difference). The y-intercept has a differential of 43.4% between the normal condition measurements and five minute hyperemia experiments.

Without taking the correction factor into account, the relationship between all normal condition experiments contrasting ultrasound and CCP is described by the mathematical relationship [CCP Measured Diameter (mm)]=1.08[Ultrasound Measured Diameter (mm)] + 0.88. The linear relationship can be described at greater than 95% Confidence (P =.01 and r^2 = .65). Additionally, the relationship between all hyperemia condition experiments contrasting ultrasound and CCP is described by the mathematical relationship: [CCP Measured Diameter (mm)] =1.07[Ultrasound Measured Diameter (mm)] + 1.26. As observed in the normal condition experiments, the linear relationship can be described at greater than 95% Confidence (P= .02 and r^2= .67) (Fig. 7.13).

There is a direct relationship in existence between all ultrasound measured diameters and CCP developed diameters. Although there is subjective error present in the ultrasound measured values as seen in the individual measures, the coefficient of determination is greater than .64 in all cases.

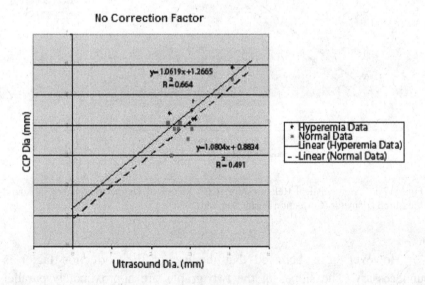

Figure 7.13. Mathematical Relationships: CCP Measured Diameters versus Ultrasound Measured Diameter (No Correction Factor Applied).

CCP Benefit

The CCP provides measurements that are calibrated for each patient. As a result, there is not subjective error and a high degree of confidence in the measurements obtained.

7.5 Discussion

The in vitro experiment hypothesis results support that cuff pressure and pump frequency have no significant effect on CCP measured volume. Additionally, the accuracy of these measurements had minimal error. Cuff compliance did vary as expected in all experiments performed (Fig. 7.14).

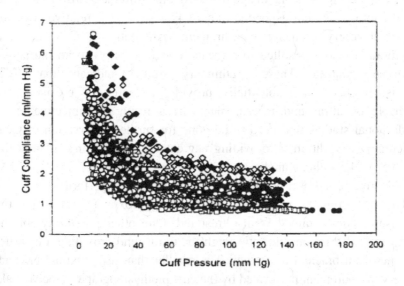

Figure 7.14. CCP Results: Cuff Compliance for All Experiments.

Additionally, in vivo testing of seven of the eight healthy subjects reveals that reactive hyperemia conditions result in increased brachial artery compliance and area measurements. These results are supported by both CCP and ultrasound experiment results. The magnitude of brachial artery ultrasound measurements in our experiments were compared with previous similar studies performed (Perregaux et al., 1999; Corretti et al., 1995) and found to be in the same range.

Initially, the difference in diameter measurement between CCP and ultrasound was believed to be the result of CCP signal incorporation of different vessels than the ultrasound experiments. The CCP volume signal recording is all inclusive measuring all arteries under the cuff including the deep brachial artery, radial collateral artery, and middle brachial artery in addition to the brachial artery. Although the diameters of all ultrasound measurements were smaller magnitudes than all CCP measurements, the order of magnitude from smallest measurement to largest measurement was similar between CCP and ultrasound.

Observation of the ultrasound results showed that two independent observers using the same image obtained a measurement difference of up to 0.7 mm which corresponded to a 18.47% +/- 2.16% relative error for brachial artery diameter measurement. Alternatively, CCP in vitro calibration testing resulted in a mean % error of 1.5% from the actual volume changes. These preliminary studies indicate that CCP measurements could potentially provide a degree of precision not capable of ultrasound measurements as a result of subjective error. Additional studies will need to be done for further observation of CCP accuracy in addition to providing a greater understanding of how the CCP signal should be analyzed.

Normal condition brachial artery measurements performed with the CCP were found to be consistently an approximate 1.4 times the measurements obtained from ultrasound. One other possibility for the existence of this constant ratio might be ultrasound providing a measure of the distal brachial artery which is smaller than the proximal brachial artery measurement performed by the cuff plethysmograph (Ciocca et al., 1995). Additionally, previous studies have provided evidence that a transition point exists along the length of the brachial artery indicating a transition between elastic and muscular artery behavior (Bjarnegard et al., 2003, 2004). These regions have demonstrated different distensibility responses to sympathetic activation.

All CCP lumen area measurements were taken at a transmural pressure of +60mm Hg. This is believed to be a source of error introduced into all CCP lumen area measurements. Values taken at +60mm Hg transmural pressure are valuable for comparison data. However, in future CCP experiments where discrete values of brachial artery lumen area are required higher transmural pressure values should be used. Additionally, the transmural pressure used to obtain the brachial artery area for each subject should be maximized to provide maximal lumen area measurement above venous pressure.

The mean CCP measured percent change in arterial diameter following five minute hyperemia conditions was found to be only slightly greater than the percent change found in the ultrasound experiments (15.8% vs. 10.25%). The ultrasound results generally corresponded with previous experiments where the percentage increase in brachial arterial diameter following five minute hyperemia experiments was measured at 12.6% +/- 5.7% (Bank et al., 1995).

The correction factor of 0.69 was applied to each diameter calculated by the CCP. This correction factor takes into account that the cuff may not provide a uniform collapse of the artery it is acting upon. As a result, the correction factor should provide an effective cuff length which would need to be determined for any cuff used. Review of the regression equation provided by the normal and hyperemic data did not show confidence in the y-intercept representing the differential measurement between CCP and ultrasound with or without the correction factor. Additional studies will be required to understand the proper use of the correction factor in providing discrete measurements of arterial lumen diameter.

The CCP discussed in this chapter is in its initial form. Presently, the CCP is most valuable in providing relative changes using CCP readings as a baseline. Additional testing and modifications will be required to provide discrete measurements of brachial artery diameter with a high degree of confidence in addition to a commercial product capable of providing the benefits of early diagnosis and treatment benefits for various cardiovascular diseases.

7.6 Acknowledgements

Rutgers University Department of Biomedical Engineering, Susanne and Mark Kelley for their editing, Kathy Magliato, M.D., for her time and efforts in reviewing this manuscript, and Vladimir McKenzie (undergraduate) and Monica Rodriguez (graduate student) for their research efforts.

7.7 References

Alexander, H., Cohen, M., and Steinfield, L. (1977). "Criteria in the choice of an occluding cuff for the indirect measurement of blood pressure," *Med. and Biol. Eng. and Comput.* 15:2-10.

Annis, D., Fisher, A.C., How, T.V. (1987). "A compliant small-diameter arterial prosthesis," In Williams DF, editor. Blood compatibility, Volume 11, Boca Raton, FL: CRC Press; pp.63-78.

Annis, D., Fisher, A.C., How, T.V. (1984). "A compliant small-diameter arterial prosthesis," In: Planck H, Egbers G, Syre, editors. Polyurethanes in biomedical engineering. New York: Elsevier Science Publishers; pp.279-285.

Bank, A.J., Wilson, R.F., Kubo, S.F., Holte, J.E., Dresing, T.J., and Wang, H. (1995). "Direct Effects of Smooth Muscle Relaxation and Contraction on In Vivo Human Brachial Artery Elastic Properties" *Circulation Research.* 77(5):1008-16.

Bank, A.J., Wang, H., Holte, J.E., Mullen, K., Shammas, R., and Kubo, S.H. (1996). "Contribution of collagen, elastin, and smooth muscle to in vivo human brachial artery wall stress and elastic modulus" *Circulation.* 94(12):3263-70.

Binns, R.L., Du, D.N., Stewart, M.T., Ansley, J.P., and Coyle, K.A. (1989). "Optimal graft diameter: Effect of wall shear stress on vascular healing" *J. Vasc Surg.* 10:326.

Bjarnegard, N., Ahlgren, A.R., Sandgren, T., Sonesson, B. and Lanne, T. (2003). "Age affects proximal brachial artery stiffness; Differential behavior within the length of the brachial artery," *Ultrasound in Medicine and Biology.* 29(8):1115-1121, Aug.

Bjarnegard, N., Ahlgren, A.R., Sonesson, B., and Lanne, T. (2004). "The effect of sympathetic stimulation on proximal brachial artery mechanics in humans – differential behaviour within the length of the brachial artery?," *Acta Physiologica Scandinavica.* 182(1):21-27, Sept.

Brower, R.W. and Noordergraff, A.N. (1973). "Pressure-Flow Characteristics of Collapsible Tubes: A Reconciliations of Seemingly Contradictory Results," *Annals of Biomedical Engineering.* 1, 333-355.

Burton, A.C. (1954). "Relation to structure to function of the tissues of the walls of blood vessels," *Physiol. Rev.* 34:619-642.

Callaghan, F.J., Geddes, L., Babbs, C.F., and Bourland, J.D. (1986). "Relationship between pulse-wave velocity and arterial elasticity," *Med. Biol. Engng. Comput.,* 24:248-254.

Carlstroem, D., Engfelt, B., Engstroem, A., and Ringertz, N. (1953). "Studies on the chemical composition of normal and abnormal blood vessel walls," I. Chemical nature of vascular calcified deposits. *Lab. Invest.* 2:325.

Ciocca, R.G., Madison, D.L., Wilkerson, D.K. and Graham, A.M. (1995) "Fibromuscular Dysplasia of the Brachial Artery – An Endovascular Approach," *American Surgeon.* 61(2):161-164, Feb.

Coats, A.J.S., and Clark, S.J. (1992). "Validation of ambulatory monitors in special populations", *Am. J. Hypertension.* 5:664-665.

Corretti, M., Plotnick, G. and Vogel, R. (1995). "Technical aspects of evaluating brachial artery vasodilation using high-frequency ultrasound," *American Journal of Physiology.* 268(4 Pt 2): H1397-1404.

Cox, R.H. (1979). "Regional, Species, and Age Related Variations in the Mechanical Properties of Arteries," *Biorheology,* 16:85-94.

Cox, R.H., (1983). "Age-Related Changes on Arterial Wall Mechanics and Composition of NIA Fischer Rats," *Mechanisms of Aging and Development,* 23:21-36.

Cox, R.H. (1977). "Effects of age on the mechanical properties of rat carotid artery," Am. J. Physio. 233(2):H256-H263.

Dardik, H., Ibrahim, I.M., and Dardik, I. (1978). "Evaluation of glutaraldehyde tanned human umbilical cord vein as a vascular prosthesis for bypass to the popliteal, tibial and peroneal arteries.", Surgery B3(5): 577-88, May.

Drzewiecki, G., Hood, R., and Apple, H. (1994). "Theory of the Oscillometric Maximum and the Systolic and Diastolic Detection Ratio," *Annals of Biomedical Engineering.* 22:88-96.

Drzewiecki, G.M., Melbin, J., and Noordergraaf, A. (1987). "The noninvasive measurement of blood pressure and the origin of the Korotkoff sound." In: *Handbook of Bioengineering,* edited by S. Chien and R. Skalak. New York: McGraw-Hill.

Drzewiecki, G.M., Melbin, J., and Noordergraaf, A. (1989). "The Korotkoff Sound," *Ann. Biomed. Eng.* 17:325-359.

Drzewiecki G. (1995). "Noninvasive assessment of arterial blood pressure and mechanics" In: *The Biomedical Engineering Handbook,* edited by J. Bronzino. Boca Raton, FL: CRC Press, pp.2367-2374.

Drzewiecki, G., Field, S., Moubarak, I., and Li, J. K-J. (1997). "Vessel growth and collapsible pressure-area relationship," *Am. J. Physiol.* 273:H2030-H2043.

Drzewiecki, G., Karam, E., and Bansal, V. (1993). "Mechanics of an occlusive arm cuff and its application as a volume sensor," *IEEE Trans. Biomed. Eng.* 40:704.

Franklin, S.S., Khan, S.A., Wong, N.D., Larson, M.G., and Levy, D. (2001). "Is Pulse Pressure Useful in Predicting Risk for Coronary Heart Disease? The Framingham Study," *Circulation* 100(4):354-360.

Geddes, L., Voelz, M., Combs, C., and Reiner, D. (1983). "Characterization of the oscillometric method for measuring indirect blood pressure" *Am. Biomedical Eng.* 10:271-280.

Gonza, E.R., Marble, A.E., Shaw, A., and Holland, E.G. (1974). "Age-related changes in the mechanics of the aorta and pulmonary artery of man," *Journal of Applied Physiology.* 36(4):407-411.

Grassi, G., Giannattasio, C., Failla, M., Pesenti, A., Peretti, G., Marioni, E., Fraschini, N., Vailati, S., Mancia, G. (1995). "Sympathetic Modulation of Radial Artery Compliance in Congestive Heart Failure," *Hypertension.* 26:348-354.

Greisler, H.P. (1991). *New Biologic and Synthetic Vascular Prosthesis,* Austin, TX, RG Landes.

Hayashi K. and Nakamura T. (1985). "Material test for the evaluation of mechanical properties of biomaterials." *J. Biomed. Mater. Res.*19:133-144.

Hayashi K., Handa H., Nagasawa, S., Okumura A., and Moritake K (1980). "Stiffness and elastic behavior of human intracranial and extracranial arteries." J. Biomech. 13:175-184.

Hornebeck, W., Adnet, J.J., and Robert, L. (1978). "Age Dependent Variation of Elastin and Elastase in Aorta and Human Breast Cancers," *Exp Geront.* 13:293-298.

Hyman, C. and Winsor, T. (1960). "The Application of the Segmental Plethysmograph to the Measurement of Blood Flow Through the Limbs of Human Beings," *American Journal of Cardiology.* 6:667-671, Sept. 1960.

Izzo, J.L. and Shykoff, B.E., "Arterial Stiffness: Clinical Relevance, Measurement, and Treatment," *Rev. Cardiovasc. Med.,*2(1):29-40,2001.

Kalsner S. (1982). "The Coronary Artery", New York: Oxford University Press.

Kelley, R., Daley, J., Avolio, A., and O'Rourke, M. (1989). "Arterial dilation and reduced wave reflection-Benefit of dilevalol in hypertension," *Hypertension.* 14:14-21.

Kinlay, S., Creager, M.A., Fukumoto, M., Hikita, H., Fang, J.C., Selwyn, A.P., Ganz, P. (2001). "Endothelium-Derived Nitric Oxide Regulates Arterial Elasticity in Human Arteries in Vivo," *Hypertension.* 38:1049-1053.

Ku, D.N., Allen, R.C. (2000). *Vascular Grafts. In: The Biomedical Engineering Handbook:* Second Edition. Ed. Joseph D. Bronzino, Boca Raton: CRC Press LLC.

Lansing, A.L. (1955). "Experimental Studies on Arteriosclerosis," *Symposium on Arteriosclerosis. Publication 338,* Washington DC, National Academy of Sciences, National Research Council, p. 50-60.

Larson, R.E., Hostetler, R.P. (1982). "Numerical Integration," In: Calculus: With Analytical Geometry. New York: DC Heath and Company, pp.491-500.

Lekakis, J., Papamichael, C., Vemmos, G., Voustas, A., Stamelopoulos, and Moutopoulos, S. (1998). "Peripheral vascular endothelial dysfunction in patients with angina pectoris and normal coronary angiograms," *Journal of the American College of Cardiology.* 31(3):541-6.

Merriam-Webster's Medical Desk Dictionary: (1993) Springfield, MA: Merriam-Webster Inc.

Milch, R.A. (1965). "Matrix Properties of the Aging Arterial Wall." *Monographs in the Surgical Sciences.* 2(4):261-341.

Mirsky, I. and Jantz, R.F. (1976). "The Effect of Age on the Wall Stiffness of the Human Thoracic Aorta: A Large Deformation 'Anisotropic' Elastic Analysis," *J Theory Biol.* 59:467-484.

Mozersky, D.J., Sumner, D.S., Hokanson, D.E. and Strandness, D.E. (1973). "Transucutaneous Measurement of Arterial Wall Properties As a Potential Method of Estimating Aging," *Journal of the American Geriatics Society.* 21:18-20.

Newman, D.L. and Lallemend, R.C. (1978). "The Effect of Age on the Distensibility of the Abdominal Aorta of Man" *Surgery, Gynecology,and Obstetrics,* 147:211-214.

Nichols,W.W., O'Rourke, M.F. (1990). "Therapeutic interventions," In: Nichols WW, O'Rourke MF, eds. McDonald's Blood Flow in Arteries. London, England: Edward Arnold: p.421-437.

O'Rourke, M.F., Avolio, A.P., Lauren, P.D., and Yong, J. (1987). "Age-Related Changes of Elastin Lamellae in the Human Thoracic Aorta," *JACC.* 9(2),53A.

Patterson, R.P. (1989). "Fundamentals of impedance plethysmography," *IEEE Eng. Med. Biol. Magazine,* 8:35.

Perregaux, D., Chauduri, A., Moharty, P., Bukari, L., Wilson, M., Sung, B., Dandona, P. (1999). "Effect of gender differences and estrogen replacement therapy on vascular reactivity," *Metabolism: Clinical and Experimental.* 48(2):227-32.

Ramsey III, M. (1979). "Noninvasive blood pressure determination of mean blood pressure," *Med. Biol. Eng. Comput.* 17:11-18.

Roach, M.R. and Burton, A.C. (1959). "The reason for the shape of the distensibility curves of arteries," *Canad J Biochem,* 37,557.

Roy, C.S. (1980). "The elastic properties of the arterial wall," *J. Physiol.(Lond).* 3:125-162.

Salacinski, H.J., Goldner, S., Giudiceandrea, A., Hamilton, G., and Seifalian, A.M. (2001). "The Mechanical Behavior of Vascular Grafts: A Review," *Journal of Biomaterials Applications.* 15:241-278.

Schauf, C., Moffett, D., and Moffett, S. (1990). "Somatic and Autonomic Motor Systems," In: Human Physiology: Foundations and Frontiers. St. Louis: Times Mirror/Mosby College Publishing, pp.254-283.

Shankar, R., and Webster, J.G. (1991). "Noninvasive measurement of compliance of human leg arteries.," *IEEE Trans. Biomed. Eng.* 38:62-67.

Shimazu, H., Kawarada, A., Ito, H., and Yamakoshi. K. (1989). "Electric impedance cuff for the indirect measurement of blood pressure and volume elastic modulus in human limb and finger arteries," *Med J Biol Eng Comput* 27:477-483.

Simon, A.C., Laurent, S., Levenson, A., Bouthier, J.E., and Safar, M.E. (1983). "Estimation of forearm arterial compliance in normal and hypertensive men from simultaneous pressure and flow measurements in the brachial artery, using a pulsed Doppler device and a first-order arterial model during diastole," *Cardiovasc. Res.* 17:331-338.

Sonoda, H., Urayama, S.I., Takamizawa, K., Nakayama, Y., Uyama, C., Yasui, H., and Matsuda, T. (2002). "Compliant design of artificial graft: compliance determination by new digital X-ray imaging system-based method," *J Biomed Mater Res.* 60:191-195.

Van der hoeven, G.M.A., de Monchy, D., and Beneken, J.E.W. (1973). "Studies on innocent praecordial vibratory murmers in children; I. Systolic time intervals and pulse wave transmission lines in normal children," *Br. Heart J.* 35:669.

Veith, F.J., Gupta, S.K., Ascer, E., White-Flores, S., Samson, R.H., Scher, L.A., Towne, J.B., Bernhard, V.M., Bonier, P., Flinn, W.R., Astelford, P., Yao, J.S.T., and Bergan, J.J. (1986). "Six-year prospective multicenter randomized comparison of autologous saphenous vein and expanded polytetraflouroethylene graft in infrainguinal arterial reconstruction," *J Vasc Surg.* 3:104-114.

Whitney, R. (1953). "The measurement of volume changes in human limbs," *J Physio. Lond.* 121, 1-27.

Whitt, M. and Drzewiecki, G. (1997). "Repeatability of Brachial Artery Area Measurement," *Annals of Biomedical Engineering.* 25 (Supplement 1) : S12.

Whitt, M. and Drzewiecki, G. (1998). "Repeatability of Noninvasive Brachial Artery Area Measurement in Humans," *AAMI '98 Final Program and Abstracts*: 66.

Winsor, J. (1957). "The segmental plethysmograph. A description of the instrument." *Angiology.* 8,87.

Yater, W.M., and Birkeland, I.W. (1929-30). "Elasticity (extensibility) of the aorta of human beings," *Amer. Heart J.* 5:781.

Yin, F.C.P., Spurgeon, H.A., and Kallman, C.H. (1983). "Age-Associated Alterations in Viscoelastic Properties of Canine Aortic Strips," *Circulation Research.* 53(4):464-472.

7.8 Glossary of Terms

Arteriosclerosis – a chronic disease in which thickening, hardening, and loss of elasticity of the arterial walls result in impaired blood circulation. It develops with aging, and in hypertension, diabetes, hyperlipidemia, and other conditions.

Autograft – tissue transplanted from one part of the body to another in the same individual.

Allograft – the transplant of an organ or tissue from one individual to another of the same species with a different genotype.

Distensibility – the capability of being distended or stretched under pressure.

Transmural Pressure – the pressure difference between the pressure inside and the pressure outside a walled structure.

Collagen – the fibrous protein constituent of bone, cartilage, tendon, and other connective tissues including that of the walls of arteries and veins.

Elastin – a protein that coils and recoils like a spring within the elastic fibers of connective tissue and accounts for the elasticity of structures such as skin, blood vessels, heart, lungs, intestines, tendons, and ligaments.

Oscillometry – measurement of oscillations of any kind. In medicine, it is used in studying cardiovascular and respiratory physiology.

Plethysmography – a test used to measure changes in blood flow or air volume in different parts of the body.

Hyperemia – a condition in which blood congests in a particular area of the body.

7.9 Review Questions

Q7.1   The elastic properties of an artery is not affected by:
   A. atheramotosis
   B. aging
   C. diameter

Q7.2   Coronary artery grafts is not performed by using:
   A. arteries
   B. veins
   C. nylon stents

Q7.3   What independent factor has the greatest significant effect on graft patency rates?

Q7.4   The arterial pressure-area curve summarizes the effect of the following except:
   A. vessel diameter
   B. elastin
   C. collagen
   D. blood pressure flow

Q7.5 Endothelial function is evident in:

A. normal vascular physiology

B. dacron graft

C. inflammatory disorder

Q7.6 The velocity of pulse pressure is not dependent on:

A. elastic stiffness

B. wall stiffness

C. mass density of blood

D. radius

E. length

Q7.7 Arterial distensibility normalizes compliance by volume. True or False.

Chapter 8

Hemodynamic Monitoring: Invasive, Noninvasive, and Wireless Applications

John K-J. Li, Ph.D.[1] and Hongjun Zhang, Ph.D.[1]

[1] Dept. of Biomedical Engineering, Rutgers University
599 Taylor Road, Piscataway, NJ 08854
PH: 732-445-4500, ext. 6305; FX: 732-445-3753; EM: johnkjli@rci.rutgers.edu;
EM: hongjun@rci.rutgers.edu

8.1 Introduction

For centuries, monitoring of cardiovascular function has intrigued physicians, scientists and innovators alike. It has become a necessity in modern day diagnose of the state of the circulation in patients suffering from cardiovascular and related diseases. With the advancement of modern technology, "Bionics of the Circulation" has indeed come of age. Some of the inventions have seen their ways through improved monitoring of blood pressure and flow, geometric and elastic properties, others through cardiac pacing and defibrillation and still others through temporary and implantable cardiac assist devices.

In this chapter, we will focus on classic and modern invasive and noninvasive hemodynamic monitoring and cardiac assist devices and introduce wireless technology for cardiovascular applications.

8.2 Blood Pressure Measurements

8.2.1 *Invasive blood pressure measurement*

8.2.1.1 *The needle-pressure transducer combination*

The combination of a fluid-filled catheter and a pressure transducer continues to be the most commonly used measurement system for in-vivo recording of pulsatile blood pressure waveforms. This blood pressure recording system can be applied to cardiac chambers, major arteries and veins, as well as smaller (~1 mm) vessels of the circulation. This is because of the long, well-established and improved catheterization techniques in combination with angiographic imaging modalities in clinical catheterization laboratories. The catheter system has the added advantage of the ease of injecting radio-opaque dyes for visualization of the vasculature, assessing the severity of blockage, as well as administering therapeutic drugs. Balloon catheter for angioplasty applications and micro-pore catheter for intravascular local drug delivery have also become popular. Multi-lumen, multi-functional catheters afford thermodilution for cardiac output measurement, as well as either atrial or ventricular pacing capabilities through electrodes mounted on the catheter. These technological advances have promoted the popularity of interventional cardiology.

From a historical perspective, Forssmann and Cournand, who shared the 1956 Nobel prize in Medicine with Richards, were the original inventors who first recorded blood pressure waveforms in peripheral arteries and cardiac chambers. The catheter has the flexibility and maneuverability that allows accessibility to different parts of the circulation. There are instances, where a combination of a hyperdermic needle and a pressure transducer suffices, particularly when the blood vessel is superficial or under intra-operative conditions. Brachial, radial or femoral arteries are common superficial sites for pressure measurements with needle-transducer systems. Left ventricular chamber pressure measurement with direct apex insertion of a needle is also common under open chest conditions.

The performance of a needle-pressure transducer system can be evaluated through basic mechanical and electrical modeling. The simplest representation of the system is a spring-mass system of natural frequency:

$$f_n = \frac{1}{2\pi}\sqrt{\frac{\pi r^2}{\rho l} \cdot \frac{dp}{dV}} \tag{8.1}$$

where r is the internal lumen radius of the needle, l is the length of the needle and ρ is the fluid density. Typically the needle and pressure transducer dome are filled with heparinized saline, providing the necessary fluid coupling. Blood pressure pulsation is transmitted via fluid coupling resulting in the movement of the pressure transducer diaphragm. The greater the amount of fluid, the greater is the fluid movement or inertia. Thus, the inertia is represented by

$$L = \frac{\rho l}{\pi r^2} \tag{8.2}$$

The compliance of the pressure transducer is determined by the movement of the stainless steel diaphragm within the fluid-filled transducer dome. Compliance which is defined as volume displacement per unit distending pressure, is the inverse of stiffness:

$$C = \frac{dV}{dp} \tag{8.3}$$

$$Compliance = \frac{1}{dp/dV} = \frac{1}{stiffness} \tag{8.4}$$

Equation 8.1 can be re-written as:

$$f_n = \frac{1}{2\pi}\sqrt{\frac{1}{LC}} \tag{8.5}$$

When the needle is narrow, the Poiseuille resistance, R, becomes important in the determination of the frequency response.

Blood pressure waveform is periodic and can be represented by a Fourier series as the sum of a mean pressure and a number of sine waves of fundamental frequency f (heart rate/sec) and harmonics, nf (n = 1,2, ..., N):

$$p(t) = \overline{p} + \sum_{n=1}^{N} p_n \sin(n\omega t + \phi_n) \qquad \omega = 2\pi f \qquad (8.6)$$

which, when substituted into the second order differential equation describing the fluid motion, results in the amplitude ratio for the nth harmonic:

$$\frac{P_{mn}}{P_{on}} = \sqrt{\frac{1}{1 - (n\omega)^2 LC + (n\omega RC)^2}} \qquad (8.7)$$

The corresponding phase angle is:

$$\phi_n = \tan^{-1} \frac{n\omega RC}{1 - n\omega LC} \qquad (8.8)$$

where P_{mn} = measured pressure for the nth harmonic and P_{on} = actual pressure of the nth harmonic component. For a distortion-free blood pressure measurement system, or one with a flat frequency response, it is necessary that the amplitude ratio P_{mn}/P_{on} =1.0, or there is no difference between the measured pressure and the actual pressure. Under this condition, the phase angle ϕ_n = 0, i.e., there is no phase shift between the two. For the pressure measurement system to record the arterial blood pressure waveform faithfully, it must have sufficient dynamic frequency response (Li et al., 1976).

8.2.1.2 *The catheter-pressure transducer combination*

For a catheter-pressure transducer system, frequently an underdamped system, compliance as well as geometric factors are important. Figure 8.1 provides a lumped approximation of the system and the previous linear second-order representation is sufficient for evaluating the dynamic frequency response of the system.

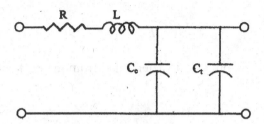

Figure 8.1. Lumped model representation of the catheter-pressure transducer system. R= Poiseuille resistance of the fluid in the catheter. C = compliance combination of the catheter and the manometer (C=Cc+Ct; Cc=compliance of the catheter and Ct= compliance of the transducer). L = inertia of fluid.

Either a sinusoidal pressure generator or a step-response "pop-test" (Fig. 8.2) is the common method for evaluating the dynamic frequency response of the catheter system. Clinically and experimentally used catheter-transducer combinations are usually underdamped, resulting in oscillations in amplitude (Fig. 8.2).

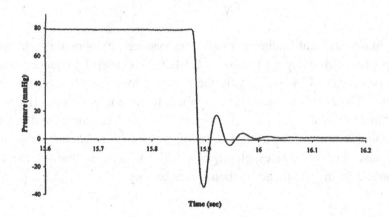

Figure 8.2. The pop-test (step response) for the dynamic testing of transducer system performance, f = 1/T = resonant frequency. The catheter transducer system is seen to be an underdamped system.

The damped natural resonance frequency, f_d , is obtained as the inverse of the period (T) of oscillation:

$$f_d = \frac{1}{T} \tag{8.9}$$

The exponential damping, α_e is determined from the peak amplitudes A_1 and A_2 ,

$$\frac{A_1}{A_2} = e^{-\alpha_e t} \tag{8.10}$$

Express in terms of amplitude ratio, A_p ,

$$A_p = \ln \frac{A_2}{A_1} \tag{8.11}$$

The relative damping factor, α_d , is obtained from the following expression:

$$\alpha_d = \frac{A_p}{\sqrt{4\pi^2 + A_p^2}} \tag{8.12}$$

Many clinical catheter-transducer systems exhibit underdamped responses with damping factors of 0.1-0.3. The useful frequency range can be estimated by multiplying the resonant frequency by the damping factor. The flat frequency response refers to an amplitude ratio (Eq. 8.7) within ±5% of unity, or 1. The higher resonant frequencies and greater damping factors (up to critical damping) offer better dynamic frequency response. For derivatives of pressure (dP/dt), such as that for the left ventricle, higher frequency response is necessary.

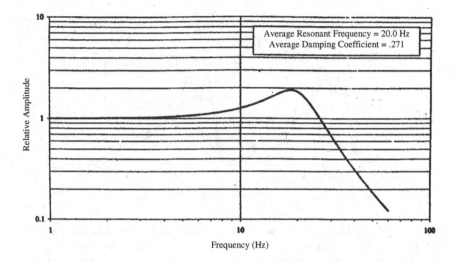

Figure 8.3. Dynamic frequency response shown as the relative amplitude ratio vs. frequency. The resonance frequency in this example is 20 Hz.

Li and Noordergraaf (1977) have analyzed responses of differential manometer systems. For these systems, the individual frequency responses, as well as static and dynamic imbalances are important factors to be considered. Catheter-tip pressure transducers (Fig. 8.4) offer superior frequency response, sufficient even for cardiac sound recording. They, however, suffer from fragility, temperature-sensitivity, and the need to be calibrated against known manometric systems. The efficacy of catheterization in the diagnostic setting has been discussed by Li and Kostis (1984).

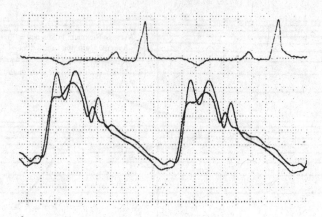

Figure 8.4. Aortic blood pressure waveform measured with an underdamped catheter-pressure transducer system and a high-fidelity catheter-tip pressure transducer. Overshoot and oscillations are clearly seen in the fluid-filled underdamped catheter-pressure transducer system.

8.2.2 *Noninvasive blood pressure measurements*

8.2.2.1 *Auscultatory measurement of blood pressure*

The auscultatory Korotkoff sound cuff method remains the most popular form of noninvasive blood pressure measurement in the clinical setting. This method however, lacks accuracy when compared to invasive catheter technique. Errors of 5-10 mmHg error are common. This technique, however, is simple to employ and has surprisingly high repeatability. It allows both systolic and diastolic pressures to be determined. The width and length of the cuff are important considerations in the application of the auscultatory method. Typically, a width to circumference ratio of 0.4 is used.

The first vascular sounds that emerge is generally referred to as phase 1, define Ps. When either the vascular sounds become muffled (phase IV) or disappear completely (phase V), the diastolic pressure (Pd) is obtained. There remains debate as to whether phase IV or V is a better indicator of diastolic pressure. Figure 8.5 illustrates the Korotkoff vascular sounds recorded in a brachial artery. When vascular reactivity is altered with hand-grip, the spectral content is shifted, such that the Korotkoff sound intensity is increased, together with a higher observed blood pressure (Fig. 8.5; Matonick and Li, 1999). Numerous theories have been proposed as to the generation of the Korotkoff sounds. Their origins have been a controversial subject of research. Some have suggested that they are pressure-related rather than flow-related (Drzewiecki et al., 1987).

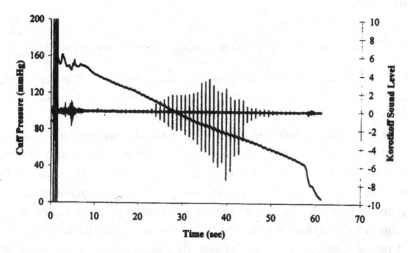

Figure 8.5. Korotkoff vascular sounds recorded in a brachial artery.

8.2.2.2 *Blood pressure measurement with the oscillometric method*

Alternative to the use of the stethoscope is the oscillometric method. Marey in 1885 found that cuff pressure oscillated over a considerable range of mean cuff pressures. He suggested that the oscillation is maximal when the arterial wall is not stressed circumferentially. Removal of this circumferential stress, provides a basis for noninvasive tonometry. This is "vascular unloading", as Marey termed it. The tension within the wall of the artery under such circumstance is zero when the transmural pressure is zero. The maximal oscillation was found to correspond to mean arterial pressure. The oscillometric method continued to gain popularity, although this technique is rather accurate for systolic and mean blood pressure detection, its accuracy is much less so for diastolic pressure measurement.

Geddes (1984) has provided a detailed analysis and comparison of the cuff technique and oscillometry. Maximum oscillation in cuff pressure corresponds to mean blood pressure as shown. Thus, in addition to systolic and diastolic pressures, mean blood pressure can be obtained. The radial pulse distal to brachial artery measurement site is also shown.

8.2.2.3 *Noninvasive blood pressure monitoring with tonometer*

There are several methods for noninvasive recording of blood pressure waveforms, including the volume pulse method, the pressure pulse method, the cantilever and optical deflection methods.

In the volume pulse method (Fig. 8.6), the successful recording hinges on the relationship between intravascular pressure distension and radial displacement. The pressure pulse method (Fig. 8.6), such as the tonometer, is dependent on the interplays of contact stress, the deformation stress and arterial pressure. Arterial pressure is actually a fraction of the contact stress. Drzewiecki et al. (1983) have shown that in arterial tonometery, with arterial flattening, shear stress becomes negligible compared with the normal stress in the arterial wall and skin, and uniform contact stress is developed over the transducer-skin interface. This is the ideal state for pulse recording with tonometry. Arterial tonometry for measuring blood pressure is based on the principle that when a pressurized blood vessel is partially collapsed by an external object, the circumferential stresses in the vessel wall are removed and the internal and external pressures are equal. Since tonometers are basically force transducers, they are useful only when applied to superficial arteries with solid bone backing.

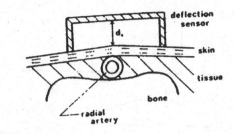

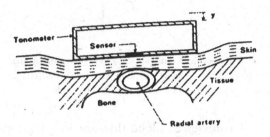

Figure 8.6. Illustration of the volume pulse method (top) and the pressure pulse method (bottom). Notice the difference in the sensor placement.

8.3 Blood Flow Measurements

8.3.1 *Electromagnetic flowmeter*

In-vivo accurate measurement of blood flow lagged behind that of pressure for decades. The electromagnetic flowmeter is based on Faraday's law of induction:

$$e = v \times B - J / \sigma_c \qquad (8.13)$$

where the induced electric field is E, in a conductor moving with a velocity v in a magnetic field intensity *B*. *J* is the current density and σ_c is the conductivity (of blood). Figure 8.7 illustrates the principle. Bevir's (1971) virtual current theory, however, presents a more practical analysis.

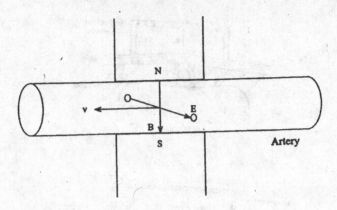

Figure 8.7. Illustration of the electromagnetic blood flow measurement principles. The moving conductor (blood with velocity, v) in a magnetic field (B) induces an electric motive force and the potential (E) is picked up by the electrodes.

Wyatt (1984) has reviewed blood flow and velocity measurement by electromagnetic induction. The cannular flowmeters with uniform field and point electrodes have the defect of a high degree of dependence on velocity distribution when they are not symmetric. The perivascular flowmeters have two defects: in addition to their sensitivity to velocity distribution, they are also sensitive to wall conductivity effects. The former can be reduced by using insulated- or multiple-electrodes which improves the signal-to-noise ratio. Mills' (1966) catheter-tip flowmeter has the advantage that it is unaffected by the vessel wall. Boccalon et al. (1978) has devised a noninvasive electromagnetic flowmeter which provides useful clinical applications.

8.3.2 *Ultrasound Doppler velocimeters*

Ultrasonic methods of measuring blood flow velocity are based on either the transmission or the reflection of ultrasound. Ultrasound propagation velocity through biological tissue is about 1560 m/s. Its associated wavelength can be easily calculated from

$$\lambda = \frac{c}{f} \qquad (8.14)$$

Typical diagnostic ultrasound utilizes frequencies in the range of 1 MHz to 15 MHz. Thus, the corresponding wavelengths are 0.78 mm and 0.156 mm, respectively.

The transit-time ultrasound measurement of blood velocity utilizes two crystal transducers placed at two different locations, serving as transmitter and receiver. With known ultrasound velocity, c, and the transit time $\Delta t = t_1 - t_2$, we have:

$$\Delta t = \frac{2vD}{c^2 \cos \theta} \tag{8.15}$$

where $D/\cos\theta$ is the distance between the transceiver and θ is the angle between the axial blood velocity and the transceiver.

A more common approach is the ultrasound Doppler technique, based on the back scattering of ultrasound by red blood cells. Turbulence, therefore, increases the scattering. Two commonly used types are continuous wave Doppler (CWD) and pulsed wave Doppler (PWD). In the CW mode, the Doppler shifted frequency, f_d, of the back scattered ultrasound is:

$$f_d = \frac{2v \cos \theta}{c} \cdot f_0 \tag{8.16}$$

where v is the blood velocity, θ is the angle between the ultrasound beam and the centerline, and f_o is the transmitted ultrasound frequency. In the PW mode, a velocity profile across the vessel can be obtained. Signal from cells scatters in a range at a depth of:

$$z = \frac{ct_d}{2} \tag{8.17}$$

By pulsing the ultrasound beam, one can obtain range resolution along the beam. Generally, a short burst of ultrasound is transmitted with a repetition frequency f. The backscattered signal is received and sampled after a time delay t_d.

Velocity profiles can also be obtained by the use of thermal-convection velocity sensors, such as hot-wire anemometers. Thermistors have been popular thermal velocity probes mounting on either a catheter or a needle. These sensors have been applied to clinical settings (Roberts, 1972).

In general, Doppler measured blood flow velocity compares well with that obtained by electromagnetic method.

8.3.3 *Indicator dilution methods and thermodilution*

Quantification of blood flow, even in the microcirculation by the introduction of indicators to the circulatory system has been exercised for quite some time. Dye dilution has been used for many decades. The indicator dilution method for measurement of blood flow has been well described (Geddes, 1984) in which an indicator of known mass is injected upstream. With the velocity of blood flow, the indicator is diluted and its concentration is detected and sampled downstream. The amount of flow, Q, is calculated from the following relation:

$$Q = \frac{m}{C_c \times t}$$
(8.18)

where m is the mass of the injectate, C_c is the concentration, and t is time.

The Stewart-Hamilton principle states that if a known concentration of indicator is introduced into a flow stream and its temporal concentration is measured at a downstream site, then the volume flow can be calculated. The Stuart-Hamilton principle relates the flow (Q) to the mass (m) of indicator injected and the concentration (c(t)) of the indicator measured downstream at time t:

$$Q = \frac{m}{\int_0^\infty c(t)dt}$$
(8.19)

Thus, if the area under the concentration vs. time curve is found, flow can be easily obtained. For measurement of blood flow in a single vessel, the above formulation works well. When applied to measuring cardiac output, however, the continuous pumping of the heart introduces the problem of recirculation. To overcome this, an exponential extrapolation of the concentration-time curve's descending limb is imposed such that an approximation of the integral with the area under the curve is achieved.

Indicators that have commonly been used include Evans blue dye, Indocyanine green and some radioactive isotopes, such as Albumin Iodide131. The advantage of the non-toxicity and affordability of repeated determinations within a short time span makes cold solutions excellent choices as indicators. This was demonstrated by Fronek and Ganz (1960) in the measurement of flow in single vessels and cardiac output by local thermodilution. The advent of thermodilution has made cold saline and dextrose popular indicators.

In thermodilution, normal saline or isotonic dextrose (5%) in water is used as the injectate, either at 0°C or at room temperature. The most popular site of injection is the right atrium and the sampling site is the pulmonary artery. By this choice of the sites, the effect of recirculation is minimized. In this approach, a flow-directed balloon-tipped catheter can be introduced into a vein and upon inflation of the balloon, the catheter is guided with the flow into the right atrium, the right ventricle or the pulmonary artery. The thermodilution catheter typically has a thermistor near the tip of the catheter to monitor sampling site temperature. The faster the flow, the greater the temperature increase.

Ganz et al. (1971) demonstrated this method (Fig. 8.8) by injecting a 10 ml of cold (0.5-5°C) isotonic dextrose solution into the superior vena cava of a patient with normal circulation. The injectate was delivered in 1-2 seconds. The area under the thermal curve was found by planimetry which is now substituted with an analog integrator or with a digital computer.

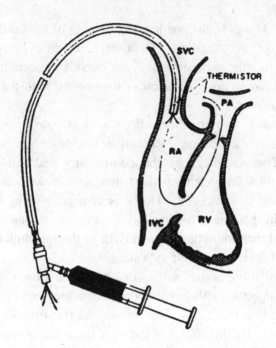

Figure 8.8. Thermodilution method in man. The injection catheter is in the superior vena cava (SVC). The thermistor for measurement of indicator temperature is inside the injection catheter 1 to 2 cm from the tip. The thermistor for measurement of blood temperature is in a main branch of the pulmonary artery (PA). RA and RV are right atrium and right ventricle, respectively.

For the thermodilution technique (Li, 2000), the standard cardiac output (CO) determination in-vivo is normally calculated from the following formula:

$$CO = \frac{V_i(T_b - T_i)S_iC_i 60}{S_bC_b \int \Delta T_b(t)dt} F_c \qquad (8.20)$$

where

V_i = volume of the injectate in ml

T_b, T_i = temperature of the blood and injectate, respectively

S_b, S_i = specific gravity of the blood and injectate, respectively

C_b, C_i = specific heat of blood and injectate, respectively

The ratio of $(S_iC_i)/(S_bC_b)$ is 1.08 when 5% dextrose in water is used as an indicator. This ratio is 1.10 when normal saline is used.

The indicator heat loss along the catheter between the site of injection and the delivery site is accounted for by a correction factor, F_c:

$$F_c = \frac{T_b - T_{id}}{T_b - T_i} \tag{8.21}$$

where T_{id} is the temperature of the injectate through the catheter at the delivery site. F_c has been reported to be between 0.8 and 0.9.

8.4 Measurement of Cardiac and Vascular Dimensions

Measurements of geometric dimensions of blood vessels, such as length, diameter and wall thickness, are of considerable importance in quantifying dynamic behavior. Strain gages are popular for length measurements. Mercury-in-silastic rubber, constantan, silicon, and germanium transducers are examples. They are based either on dimensional change or resistivity change. Change in resistance (ΔR) is derived from:

$$R = \frac{\rho_r l}{A} \tag{8.22}$$

where A is the cross-sectional area and l is the length of the strain gage wire. The fractional change in resistance is given by:

$$\frac{\Delta R}{R} = (1 + 2\sigma)\frac{\Delta l}{l} + \frac{\Delta \rho_r}{\rho_r} \tag{8.23}$$

where σ is the Poisson ratio (ratio of radial strain to longitudinal strain). The first term on the right-hand side is due to dimensional effect, the second term to piezo-resistive effect. Strain gage transducers can be applied to measure length as well as pressure. In both cases, the resultant change in resistance is detected by a Wheatstone bridge circuitry.

Superior resolution with high gage factors can be obtained with semiconductors.

High-resolution dimension measurement can also be obtained with ultrasonic dimension gages. The disadvantage is more complex circuitry. The method requires a pair of piezoelectric transducers (1-15 MHz) either sutured or glued on to the opposite sides of a vessel for pulsatile diameter measurement or for wall thickness measurement. It is operated in the PW mode at f =I KHz. Dimensional measurement, such as vessel diameter, cardiac chamber long and short axes and cardiac muscle segment length can be readily made with the ultrasonic dimension gages. The small size of piezoelectric crystal ultrasonic dimension transducers allows their implantation for chronic and conscious animal studies. Dynamic measurements of large vessel diameter and wall thickness can be simultaneously recorded with ultrasound operating in M-mode. However, its limitation lies in boundary identification and resolution. Similar problem is encountered with angiographic recording. Magnetic resonance imaging affords high resolution, but the disadvantage of the inability to provide real time recording. Recent advance in intravascular ultrasound (IVUS) provides structural detail, as well as dimension measurements.

8.5 Multi-sensor Hemodynamic Monitoring

For a more comprehensive diagnostic analysis of cardiovascular diseases, single sensor is often inadequate. Multiple sensors with capability of simultaneous monitoring of ECG, blood pressure and blood flow are often deployed. Multi-sensor pressure-velocity catheters are available. With the advent of inexpensive data acquisition systems, multi-channel recoding is commonplace.

Figure 8.9 illustrates high-fidelity blood pressure recordings measured at multiple arterial sites, such as the ascending aorta, abdominal aorta, iliac artery and the femoral artery. Simultaneously electromagnetic flow probe registered aortic flow is also shown. Aortic flow is commonly measured for the ease of direct calculations of stroke volume, hence cardiac output when heart rate is known from the ECG.

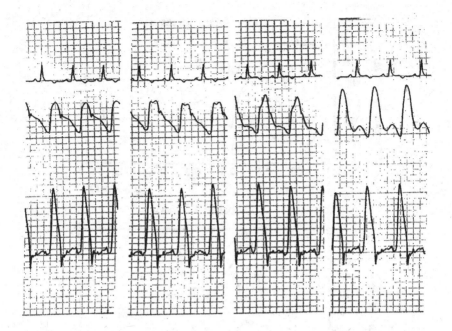

Figure 8.9. Simultaneously recorded electrocardiogram (top panel), blood pressure (middle panel) and ascending aortic flow (bottom panel) waveforms. Pressure waveforms in the ascending aorta (first left), descending thoracic aorta (second left), the abdominal aorta (second right) and the iliac artery (first right) are shown.

Further hemodynamic analysis with recorded aortic pressure and flow waveforms are possible. For instance, Figure 8.10 illustrates the resolved forward and reflected components of the measured waveforms. Notice that increased reflected pressure wave tends to decrease flow, since reflected pressure and flow waves are 180 degree out of phase. Increased wave reflection has been shown to augment systolic pressure and thus increase the afterload to ventricular ejection. Significantly increased wave reflection beyond normal is also found to be a main contributing factor to isolated systolic hypertension (ISH) in the elderly (Li et al., 2007). In the case of ISH, although systolic pressure is increased beyond 160 mmHg, diastolic pressure can remain normal. ISH is attributed to a significantly reduced arterial compliance in combination with a moderate increase in peripheral resistance.

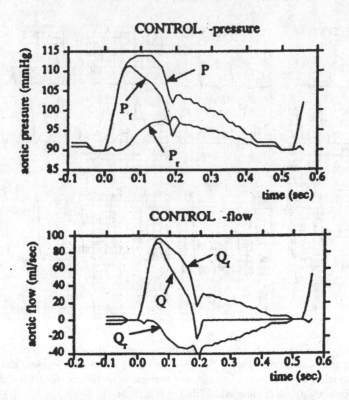

Figure 8.10. Ascending aortic pressure (top) and flow (bottom) waveforms resolved into their respective forward (P_f, Q_f) or antegrade, and reflected (P_r, Q_r) or retrograde components. Notice that wave reflection exerts opposite effects on pressure and flow waveforms, as seen from Q_r and P_r. Courtesy of Dr. Ying Zhu (affiliation: c/o Dr. Li}.

Figure 8.11 is yet another example in which pressure, flow and geometric dimension, in this case, the cardiac muscle segment, are recorded simultaneously for analysis of cardiac hemodnamics or myocardial function. The temporal relations of the onset of cardiac muscle shortening, the developed aorto-ventricular pressure gradient and the eventual ventricular ejection are critical aspect of monitoring cardiac hemodynamics.

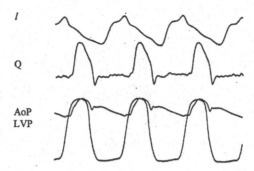

Figure 8.11. Simultaneously measured cardiac muscle segment length (top trace), left ventricular pressure (LVP), aortic pressure (AoP) and aortic flow (Q) are shown. Ejection begins when LVP exceeds AoP and ends with aortic valve closure. Cardiac muscle shortening from end-diastole to end-systole is clearly shown.

8.6 Concluding Remarks: Noninvasive and Wireless Hemodynamic Monitoring

With the advent of advanced sensor technology and wireless capabilities, the next generation of hemodynamic monitoring is taking place rapidly. Noninvasive monitoring has come of age for screening, diagnosis and therapeutic treatment efficacy evaluation.

Figure 8.12 illustrates how rapid and reliable simultaneous recordings of ECG, radial pressure pulse and radial artery blood flow velocity can be obtained in a human subject.

Biotelemetry has been around for some time, but its use has been limited to implantable sensors for ECG and hemodynamic monitoring. With the popularity and rapid advancement of wireless technology, and its combination with noninvasive wearable sensors (e.g. Zhang and Li, 2008), the next generation of hemodynamic monitoring in the hospital, clinic, home and remote settings will be the primarily beneficiary. To this end, we are making good progressive to contribute to such a goal. Figure 8.13 demonstrates such an example in wireless remote monitoring of arterial blood velocity with noninvasive Doppler ultrasound.

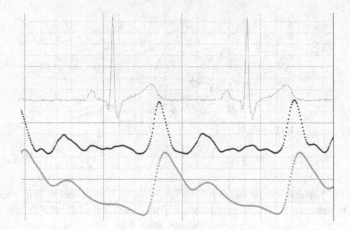

Figure 8.12. Simultaneous recordings of ECG (upper trace), radial artery Doppler ultrasound velocity (middle trace), and radial artery tonometer pressure (lower trace). Temporal relations can be clearly seen.

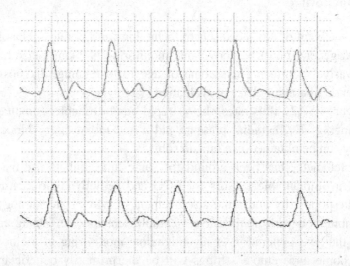

Figure 8.13. Wirelessly transmitted (top trace) and received (bottom trace) arterial Doppler ultrasound blood velocity. Upper: Transmitted signal. Lower: Received signal. Time scale: 0.167s per division.

8.7 References

Bevir, M. (1971). Sensitivity of electromagnetic velocity probes. *Phys. Med. Biol.* 16, pp. 229-232.

Boccalon, H., Candelon, B., Puel, P., Enjalbert, A., and Doll, H. (1978). Assessment of pulsatile blood flow by a noninvasive electromagnetic device. In *Noninvasive Cardiovascular Diagnosis,* E.B. Dietlifich, ed., Univ. Park Press, Baltimore, pp. 231-240.

Drzewiecki, G. M., Melbin, J., and Noordergraaf, A. (1987). Noninvasive blood pressure recording and the genesis of Korotkoff sound. Chap.8, *Handbook of Bioengineering,* R. Skalak and S. Chien, eds. New York: McGraw-Hill.

Drzewiecki, G. M., Melbin, J., and Noordergraaf, A. (1983). Arterial tonometry: review and analysis. *J. Biomech.* 16, pp. 141-152.

Fronek, A. and Ganz, V. (1960). Measurement of flow in single vessels including cardiac output by local thermodilution. *Circ. Res.* 8, pg. 175.

Ganz, W., Donoso, R., Marcus, H. S., Forrester, J. S., and Swan, H. J. (1971). A new technique for measurement of cardiac output by thermodiluation. *Am. J. Cardiol.* 27, pp. 392-396.

Geddes, L. A. *Cardiovascular Devices and Their Applications.* Wiley, New York, 1984.

Li, J. K-J. *The Arterial Circulation: Physical Principles and Clinical Applications. Human Press, Totowa, New Jersey, 2000.*

Li, J. K-J. and Kostis, J. B. (1984). Aspects determining accurate diagnosis and efficacy of catheterization. *Proc. Ist Int. Congr. Med. Instrument.* pp. A07-A08.

Li, J. K-J. and Noordergraaf, A. (1977). Evaluation of needle-manometer and needle differential-manometer systems in the measurement of pressure differences. *Proc. 3rd NE Bioeng. Conf.* 5, pp. 275-277.

Li, J. K-J., Van Brummelen, A. G. W., and Noordergraaf, A. (1976). Fluid-filled blood pressure measurement systems. *J. Appl. Physiol.* 40, pp. 839-843.

Li, J. K-J., Zhu, Y., O'Hara, D., and Khaw, K.. (2007). Allometric Hemodynamic Analysis of Isolated Systolic Hypertension and Aging. *Cardiovasc. Eng.* 7, pp. 135-139.

Matonick, J. P., and Li, J. K-J. (1999). Noninvasive monitoring of blood pressure during hand-grip stress induced vascular reactivity. *Proc. 34th. Assoc. Adv. Med. Instrum.* pp. 81-82.

Mills, C. J. (1966). A catheter-tip electromagnetic flow probe. *Phys. Med. Biol.* 11, pp. 323-324.

Roberts V. C. (1972). *Blood Flow Measurements.* Williams and Wilkins, Baltimore.

Wyatt D. G. (1984). Blood flow and blood velocity measurement in vivo by electromagnetic induction. *Med. Biol. Eng. Comput.* 22, pp. 193-211.

Zhang H. and Li, J. K-J. (2008). Noninvasive monitoring of transient cardiac changes with impedance cardiography. *Cardiovasc. Eng.* 8, pp. 225-231.

8.8 Review Questions (Find the most correct answer)

Q8.1 A Rutgers senior was seen running to cast his election vote on Tuesday. If his heart rate at the time was 98 beats/min and stroke volume is 70 ml per beat, his cardiac output must be:

A. 5 L/min

B. 70 ml/sec

C. 7 L/min

D. 686 ml/min

Q8.2 An ultrasound Doppler probe was used to measure blood flow velocity in a femoral (thigh) artery. Given that ultrasound transducer frequency of 5 Mhz, ultrasound velocity in blood of 1550 m/s, blood velocity of 30 cm/s and $\theta=60°$, the Doppler-shifted frequency is about

A. 1 KHz

B. 2 MHz

C. 2 KHz

D. 100KHz

Q8.3 An M-mode ultrasound is used track pulsatile diameter change and a pressure transducer to track pulse pressure change of a patient's carotid artery. For a pulse pressure of 50 mmHg and diameter change of 3%, the elastic modulus of the subject's artery is about (in units of $x10^6/dyns/cm^2$, where 1mmHg = 1332 dynes/cm^2)

A. 6.6

B. 1.5

C. 50.0

D. 2.0

Q8.4 In laminar Poiseuille flow, which of the following is the most important in determining the amount of resistance, hence flow through a vessel:

A. vessel length

B. vessel diameter

C. viscosity

D. pressure gradient

Q8.5 Thermodilution technique is used to measure
   A. blood pressure
   B. blood flow
   C. impedance
   D. cardiac output

Q8.6 Normal ejection fraction is about
   A. 0.95
   B. 0.70
   C. 0.40
   D. 0.25

Q8.7 Resonant frequency of a fluid-filled blood pressure measurement system is most critically dependent on
   A. catheter lumen diameter
   B. catheter length
   C. viscosity
   D. pressure transducer

Q8.8 The following combination provides the best frequency response for blood pressure measurement when compared with that through the atrial or ventricular muscles:
   A. a compliant catheter and a compliance transducer
   B. a compliant catheter and a stiff transducer
   C. a stiff catheter and a stiff transducer
   D. a stiff catheter and a compliant transducer

Q8.9 Blood pressure waveform can be measured noninvasively with a
   A. sphygmomanometer
   B. catheter
   C. pressure transducer
   D. tonometer

Q8.10 In isolated systolic hypertension,
   A. reflected pressure is significantly increased.
   B. retrograde flow is increased.
   C. systolic and diastolic pressures are both increased.
   D. flow is significantly decreased.

V

TISSUE ENGINEERING AND GENE THERAPY

Chapter 9

Tissue Engineering of the Heart

Michael O. Zembala, M.D., Ph.D.[1], Ricardo A. Bello, M.D., Ph.D.[1], and Robert E. Michler, M.D.[1]

[1] Dept. of Cardiothoracic Surgery, Montefiore Medical Center, Albert Einstein College of Medicine, New York, NY 10467
PH: 718-920-2100; FX: 718-231-7113; EM: rmichler@montefiore.org

9.1 Introduction – The Rationale for Cardiac Regenerative Therapy

Despite many breakthroughs in cardiovascular medicine, the complications of myocardial infarction, particularly congestive heart failure, remain among the most prominent health problems worldwide. Congestive heart failure (CHF), defined as progressive inability of the heart to contract, afflicts today an estimated 5 million people in United States alone (Thom et al., 2006). It has become the most common admitting diagnosis for patients over the age of 65 years and also, one of the most expensive. It is associated not only with a decreased quality of life, but also with significant morbidity and mortality. Improvements in the medical, surgical and minimally invasive, percutaneous treatment of acute coronary syndromes (ACS) have led to an increasing number of patients surviving with myocardial infarction and advanced coronary artery disease.

These improvements, combined with other advances in health and technology, have now allowed the average US life expectancy to rise to 77 years. While mortality in ACS is decreasing, the morbidity is increasing as more people survive the ACS to develop, with time, CHF or other major forms of left ventricular dysfunction. Myocardial infarction associated with an acute coronary syndrome results in abrupt left ventricular (LV) dysynergy and leads to global systolic dysfunction. To compensate for the loss of the contractile apparatus, neurohumoral mechanisms are rapidly activated. However, sustained neurohumoral activation provokes late remodeling of the remote non-infarcted myocardium, characterized by an abnormal and progressively increasing LV volume/mass ratio, that leads to further left ventricular dysfunction. Therefore CHF is a progressive disorder, a vicious cycle caused in part by the persistent non-functioning scar that perpetuates abnormal loading conditions and neurohumoral activation.

Regardless of advances in pharmacological therapies, cardiology and cardiovascular surgery, an additional 400,000 patients are newly diagnosed with CHF each year. Moreover, the age-adjusted mortality rate for CHF exceeds that of breast cancer and AIDS combined. Recent data suggests that CHF carries a mortality rate of at least 40% within 2 years of diagnosis, but for those patients with the most advanced stages of CHF (New York Heart Association class IV) the one-year mortality rate exceeds 50%. Only 35% of patients with clinically evident heart failure are still alive 5 years after their initial diagnosis (Murdoch et al., 1998). In addition to its poor prognosis, the treatment of CHF is associated with very high and continuingly escalating costs. Not only is CHF the most expensive diagnosis currently covered by the US government, it is estimated that the total medical costs (inpatient and outpatient) associated with the treatment of CHF exceed $50 billion per year (O'Connell et al., 1994).

Heart transplantation is considered to be the gold standard for the treatment of advanced, end-stage CHF. Cardiac transplantation has unrivaled late survival with over 50% of patients surviving 10 years (Terrovitis et al., 2006). Quality of life after cardiac transplantation improves greatly, as does exercise capacity and freedom from rehospitalizations. Unfortunately, the number of donors has reached a plateau over the past few years, at a time when the number of potential recipients has continued to grow. This critical discrepancy mandates that patients be strictly evaluated for candidacy for transplantation. Although organ shortage remains the most significant limiting factor of the heart transplantation, it is definitely not the only one. Heart transplant recipients face a rigorous scheme of immunosupression that is associated with many adverse reactions and, in some cases, contributes to kidney failure, lymphoproliferative diseases and skin cancer. (Gao et al., 2003).

Over the past years several surgical alternatives to heart transplantation have been considered, but none have gained wide spread acceptance (Goldstein et al., 2006). Surgical ventricular reconstruction (SVR), along with left ventricular assist device (LVAD) implantation, are among the most successful alternative surgical approaches to treatment of CHF.

In patients with ischemic cardiomyopathy and a substantial amount of dysfunctional but viable myocardium, improvement of left ventricular ejection fraction is determined by the extent of left ventricular remodeling. Patients with a high end-systolic volume due to left ventricular remodeling will not benefit from surgical revascularization despite the increased mass of viable myocardium. SVR aims at reducing and reshaping the left ventricle, thus restoring its native architecture (Di Donato et al., 2004). Restoration of the conical shape enables the heart to contract more efficiently, providing a better supply of oxygen and nutrients to previously hypoperfused organs and tissues. With promising early results, SVR has become a valuable alternative for many patients previously referred to, and waiting for, heart transplantation. A large, international, randomized clinical trial named STICH (Surgical Treatment for Ischemic Heart Failure) is currently being conducted under auspices of the NHLBI to evaluate the long term impact of the SVR on left ventricular function. SVR is compared with medical therapy alone, and with coronary revascularization in patients with severely damaged LV (Menicanti et al., 2004).

While SVR is thought to restore and retain LV shape and function, it carries a substantial risk of failure in patients with end-stage CHF. For those patients, mechanical circulatory support remains an important alternative. Ventricular assist devices, or VADs, are blood pumps used to support the failing heart in critically ill patients with end-stage CHF (Goldstein et al., 1998). Whether placed intracorporeally or paracorporeally, these pumps take over the function of the damaged left (and/or right) ventricle and restore more normal hemodynamics and end-organ perfusion. Left ventricular assist devices have been used in three clinical situations: (1) as a bridge to transplantation in patients who are listed for transplantation but decompensate before a suitable donor heart becomes available, (2) as a bridge to recovery in patients who are expected to recover left ventricular function (e.g. fulminant myocarditis), or (3) as a permanent alternative to transplantation in patients who are not considered to be candidates for transplantation. LVAD implantation, however, carries a substantial peri- and postoperative risk of failure. The most common early complications are peri- and postoperative bleeding and right heart failure (Goldstein et al., 2003; Ochiai et al., 2002). Wound infection and pump reliability are considered to be the most important late complications of LVAD support.

Still, several patient subsets remain without viable medical, percutaneous or surgical treatment options. These include not only patients with end-stage CHF, disqualified for transplantation and SVR, but also patients with angiographically proven coronary disease: diffuse small-vessel disease, in-stent restenosis (ISR), chronic total occlusions and degenerated vein grafts. It has been estimated that over 100,000 patients may be in this "no-option" group in the US each year (Lenzen et al., 2005).

Functional restoration of the damaged heart presents a formidable challenge, and developing strategies for treatment and prevention of post-infarct heart failure remains of utmost priority. The past decade witnessed a growing attention in regenerative therapy of the failing heart. Concepts that coronary collaterals could be grown under the influence of growth factors, and cardiomyocytes regenerated by omnipotent stem cells, changed the direction of cardiovascular research. Pioneering work, concentrated on augmenting myocardial perfusion by developing blood vessels, brought more questions than answers. It became evident that angiogenesis is a complex and still poorly understood process, requiring specific conditions and number of different growth factors and cells (Asahara et al., 1995). Similarly, the notion that stem cells are present in an adult, fully-differentiated organism created the opportunity of using these cells to regenerate damaged tissues and organs. This chapter focuses on efforts to regenerate the heart by cell transplantation.

Different stem cells will be described, together with their experimental and clinical application.

9.2 Sources of Stem Cells

The possibility of using cell-based therapies is tempting, as more promising experimental and clinical data are published each year. We have witnessed enormous advances in cardiovascular research aimed at restoring or even rebuilding, damaged myocardium. Many well established and almost indisputable paradigms have been displaced by a recent wave of remarkable discoveries. Traditionally, the heart has been viewed as a terminally differentiated organ. This important theory of the past 50 years (MacLellan et al., 2000) has been recently abolished due to the extraordinary findings of Anversa and collaborators (Beltrami et al., 2003).

Stem cells are defined by their ability to renew themselves and to differentiate into a wide array of specialized cell types. Such cells can be grouped in a number of ways: anatomically, functionally, or by cell surface markers, transcription factors and expressed proteins. The clearest division is between stem cells isolated from the embryo (therefore named Embryonic Stem Cells or ESCs) and stem cells discovered in adult, somatic and differentiated tissue (known as non-embryonic, or Adult Stem Cells).

The prospect of cardiac regeneration by stem cells is intriguing, novel, and complex. Recent research has provided evidence that both embryonic and adult stem cells may be useful in strategies that aim to both prevent and treat heart disease. However, their ability to regenerate cardiac tissue varies. The following sections of this chapter will focus on the multitude of cells, their advantages and disadvantages, and also on experimental and clinical applications and results.

9.2.1 *Embryonic stem cells*

Embryonic stem cells (ESC), as descendants of totipotent cells, are pluripotent and therefore possess ability to differentiate into cells derived from the three germ layers: ectoderm, endoderm and mesoderm. Embryonic stem cells are derived from a 3-5 day old embryo from the inner cell mass of a blastocyst, which contains approximately 30 of these highly undifferentiated cells. Because of this pluripotency, they hold the greatest potential to cure the broadest range of diseases and injuries, ranging from cardiovascular diseases to neurological disorders (such as Alzheimer's and Parkinson's diseases).

First isolated from murine blastocysts by Evans, Kaufman and Martin in 1981, ESC have been shown to grow for an indefinite period *in vitro* while maintaining the potential to differentiate into derivatives of all three embryonic germ layers. In 1998, Thompson derived the first successful ESC line, opening the field of stem cell research. Since then, ESC have been demonstrated to be capable of generating functional cardiac, neuronal and pancreatic cells. Rolletschek and collaborators (Rolletschek et al., 2004) were able to show that during ESC cell differentiation, tissue-specific genes, proteins, as well as functional properties, are expressed in a developmentally regulated manner recapitulating processes of early embryonic development. In another experiment, Boheler and colleagues proved that ESC are able to differentiate into cardiomyocytes representing all specialized cell types of the heart, such as atrial-like, ventricular-like, sinus nodal-like, and Purkinje-like cells (Boheler et al., 2002). These cardiomyocytes exhibit not only cell morphology similar to that of adult cardiac cells, but also have similar physiology; cultured ESC beat spontaneously, and when clustered, synchronously. Moreover, expression of several cardiac-specific genes and transcription factors such as GATA4 and Nkx2.5 were discovered in human ESC-derived cardiac-like cells. These cardiac-like cells were also found to express several proteins including atrial natriuretic peptide (ANP), troponin I and T (cTnI, cTnT) as well as being responsive to pharmacologic stimuli, demonstrating the presence of fully functional adrenergic and cholinergic receptors.

In vivo experiments shortly followed success of bench top discoveries. Min and collaborators (Min et al., 2002) injected ESC into a severely damaged, ischemic heart in an experimental model of myocardial infarction in a rat. As a result, cardiac function in the ESC-treated animals improved significantly just six weeks after cell transplantation. The area of infarcted myocardium was reduced, as well as the severity of left ventricular hypertrophy, resulting in improved hemodynamics. ESC engraftment was confirmed by labeling the cells with green fluorescent protein prior to injection. Four years later, Min once again approached the problem of ESC transplantation, but in a slightly different way. Based upon studies on intravenous administration and cell homing, he proposed a study of systemic injection of ESC in a previously mastered model of myocardial ischemia. The findings were truly astonishing as the ESC's homed into the area of ischemic injury. Thus, while the ESC's potential to migrate and differentiate into adult cardiac tissue were shown, knowledge of cells' ultimate fate and destination remained elusive. In another study Nelson and collaborators (Nelson et al., 2006) used ESC to evaluate cardiac regeneration in a mouse model of myocardial infarction in which the left anterior descending (LAD) and the first proximal branch of the left circumflex (LCx) arteries were permanently ligated. Myocardial infarction was followed 1 hour later by injection of a relatively low number (5×10^5) of pluripotent cells. While geometry and thus hemodynamics of the left ventricle improved, over 20% of examined animals developed teratomas in the pericardial space. Similar findings published by others raise serious safety concerns about use of ESC in human patients.

Regardless of the enormous regenerative potential, ESC are surrounded by numerous questions and controversies. Firstly, human ESC cannot be obtained in sufficient quantities because of widely discussed medical ethical issues. Secondly, current isolation and culture techniques allow cells to be differentiated into somatic cell populations that may yield impure products with possible tumorogenic and immunogenic potential. Therefore, to date, no clinical studies have been initiated.

9.2.2 *Adult, non-embryonic stem cells*

Stem cells are found in a variety of tissues and organs in a mature, fully developed organism. Adult stem cells, unlike ESC, have less self-renewal ability and the array of cells that can be created through their transdifferentiation is narrower. Despite these limitations a variety of stem and progenitor cell populations are being explored as potential therapeutic solutions. Since these cells reside in the bone marrow, blood, skeletal muscle, fatty tissue and the heart, harvesting them can be a relatively simple and safe procedure. For heart regeneration, the most intensively studied cells include skeletal myoblasts, bone marrow stem cells (including mesenchymal stem cells) and cardiac stem cells.

9.2.2.1 Skeletal myoblasts

The regenerative capacity of skeletal muscle it is now well established, as the first satellite cells and their properties were discovered by Mauro in 1961 (Mauro, 1961). It is now known that each mature skeletal muscle fiber contains a small number of undifferentiated and inactive satellite cells or myoblasts. Skeletal myoblasts (SM) remain in quiescent state until the muscle fiber is damaged, but act rapidly when injury does occur. They then proliferate and fuse with each other and with the injured cell providing continuity of the entire fiber. The ability of SM to proliferate and differentiate into muscle fibers, regenerating injured and replacing lost muscle cells, suggests that these cells may be a valuable source for cardiac repair.

SM availability, greater potential to withstand ischemia, and a relatively simple harvesting procedure create almost the perfect portrait of a suitable candidate for cellular transplantation. On the other hand, skeletal muscle cells are not capable of constant or repetitive contractions and their ability to adapt within myocardium is questionable.

Myoblasts survival and engraftment have been proven in various experimental models of heart injury (Ghostine et al., 2002). However, the transplanted SM cells were unable to transdifferentiate into functional cardiomyocytes. Instead, multinucleated myotubes were formed, electromechanically uncoupled from local cardiac muscle cells. Moreover these myotubes did not express any of the recognizable cardiac protein markers, such as alpha-myosin –heavy –chain (α-MHC) or troponin I. The most substantial problem was that implanted myoblasts appeared to remain electromechanically isolated from the host myocardium.

The functional unit that integrates and synchronizes cardiac myocyte contraction is the intercalated disc (Perriard et al., 2003). This structure is composed of intercellular adhesion molecules, mostly N-cadherin, and structures called gap junctions. These channels permit exchange of small metabolites between the cytoplasm of adjacent cardiac myocytes and provide a low resistance electrical pathway between cardiac muscle fibers. The dominant gap junction protein in cardiac myocytes is connexin-43 (Cx43). Loss of either N-cadherin or Cx43 has profound implications for myocyte morphology, and loss of N-cadherin itself can result in a dilated cardiac phenotype. Isolated skeletal myoblasts, in co-culture with neonatal cardiac myocytes *in vitro*, express cardiac specific proteins (GATA4, Nkx2.5 and ANP) together with N-cadherin and Cx43 at the junctions with neighboring cells (Formigli et al., 2005). In addition, approximately 10% of myotubes contract synchronously with surrounding cardiac myocytes (Reinecke et al., 2000). Taken together, these experiments demonstrate that skeletal myotubes and cardiomyocytes can indeed achieve electromechanical coupling given optimal conditions.

This same level of integration is not observed *in vivo*. Intracellular recordings of grafted myoblasts in infarcted rat myocardium showed that the contractile activity of newly formed myotubes is hyper-excitable and fully independent of neighboring cardiac myocytes (Leobon et al., 2003). These studies are supported by biochemical analysis of the engrafted cells. The majority of reports indicate absence of N-cadherin and Cx43 expression in the engrafted, differentiated myoblasts at all times examined up to 3 months after implantation (Reinecke et al., 2000) despite high expression of both proteins in undifferentiated skeletal myoblasts. A number of potential reasons may explain the discord between the *in vitro* and *in vivo* findings. One explanation is that myotubes *in vitro* are relatively immature and might retain a small yet functional population of junctional proteins. The expression of these proteins is completely abolished in engrafted myotubes as the differentiation is more complete in the myocardial environment (Reinecke et al., 2000). Another factor may be that skeletal muscle grafts are often separated from the host myocardium by intervening scar tissue

(Reinecke et al., 2000). This would compromise the ability of implanted skeletal myoblasts to develop significant cell-cell contacts with the surrounding cardiac myocytes, a key criteria identified by the co-culture studies for transdifferentiation. However, since injection of skeletal myoblasts into uninjured myocardium results in the same phenotype, this is at best an incomplete explanation. Another contributing factor is that the constant motion of the ventricular wall might exert unfavorable stretch/strain forces on the grafted cells preventing stable contacts from being formed. Whatever the reason, this phenomenon has lead multiple studies to recognize arrhythmogenesis as a major complication of myoblast transplantation.

Another basic biochemical difference between the cell types is dihydropyridine receptor (DHPR) expression (Garcia et al., 1994). Dihydropyridine receptors determine the mechanism of excitation-contraction coupling in myocytes. In cardiac muscle, DHPRs function as fast calcium channels that allow an influx of extracellular calcium that then triggers the release of sarcoplasmic calcium stores. Conversely, skeletal muscle DHPRs function as slow calcium channels and voltage sensors that directly control the release of calcium from the sarcoplasmic reticulum. The greatly different electrical properties of the skeletal isoform are inconsistent with the contractile properties of cardiac myocytes and might also add to the genesis of arrhythmias observed upon treatment with skeletal myoblasts.

Despite these substantial differences, a number of experimental studies have demonstrated that myoblast transplantation limits the deterioration of infarcted ventricle and improves its systolic and diastolic function. Skeletal myoblast transplantation in cardiomyopathic hamsters showed a significant 24% increase in fractional area change compared to a 6% decrease in controls after 4 weeks. Furthermore, cells were able to attenuate ventricular remodeling with no significant change in the development of myocardial fibrosis (Ohno et al., 2003). In the hypertensive rats, the treated group showed a significant alleviation of LV dilation and contractile dysfunction with a 9% decrease in LV end-diastolic dimension and fractional shortening of 38.5±1.5% vs. 32.1±1.4% six weeks after implantation. Moreover, up-regulation of the renin-angiotensin and endothelin systems during the transition to heart failure was attenuated by myoblast transplantation. Collectively, these studies show that cellular cardiomyoplasty is an effective therapy to prevent deterioration of ventricular morphology and cardiac function in both ischemic and non-ischemic models of cardiomyopathy.

A positive effect on ventricular remodeling seems to be the most significant and most commonly reported benefit of SM transplantation (McConnell et al., 2005). Lack of synchrony with beating cardiomyocytes *in vivo* is by far the most limiting factor of SM, as it substantially increases the risk of severe and life-threatening arrhythmias in the clinical setting (Mocini et al., 2005).

9.2.2.2 *Bone marrow cells (BMC)*

Bone marrow consists of bone marrow cells (BMC) and the extracellular substance harboring cytokines and growth factors (Antman et al., 2004). Within BMCs two cell populations can be distinguished: differentiated cells, such as osteoblasts and osteoclasts, and small but very diverse group of undifferentiated cells. The former group of bone marrow or bone-marrow derived mononuclear stem cells contains hematopoietic (HSC) and non-hematopoietic or mesenchymal stem cells (MSC) that have the potential for self-renewal and differentiation or plasticity.

Hematopoietic stem cells give rise to all hematopoietic lineages. They are characterized by specific cell markers, whose constellation varies among species. In humans HSC are positive for antigens CD34, CD45, CD117 (c-kit), Thy-1.1, but are lineage (Lin) and CD38 negative (Kawashima et al., 1996). Although hematopoietic stem cells are primarily involved in hematogenesis (Furness et al., 2006) HSC were surprisingly found to transdifferentiate into other phenotypes such as skeletal muscle (Ferrari et al., 1998), neurons (Mezey et al., 2000), hepatocytes (Lagasse et al., 2001), endothelial cells (Jackson et al., 2001), and cardiomyocytes (Orlic et al., 2001), both *in vivo* and *in vitro*. Moreover, hematopoietic stem cells include hemangioblasts and endothelial progenitor cells, both well recognized for their role in angiogenesis (Kocher et al., 2001).

This enormous plasticity of HSC encouraged Orlic and collaborators to undertake a challenging experimental study on myocardial repair after acute myocardial infarction. HSC injected directly into infarcted heart resulted in decreased left ventricular diameter and improved contractility just nine days after injection (Orlic et al., 2001). Detailed evaluation revealed transdifferentiation of these Lin(-), c-kit(+) cells into functional cardiomyocytes. Although the repair of the infarcted heart occurred only in 12 out of 30 animals, the promising study results invigorated the field of cardiovascular medicine. The very first clinical trial was started just one year later (Strauer et al., 2002). With time, strong evidence has accumulated opposing the beneficial role of HSC in cardiac regeneration. Several groups reported failure to duplicate Orlic's findings (Balsam et al., 2004), despite the use of sophisticated protocols and methodology. HSC failed to activate cardiac genes and restore damaged myocardium by formation of new cardiomyocytes as they were able to differentiate into hematopoietic cells only (Balsam et al., 2004). New theories emerged, viewing HSC as cells able to generate cardiac muscle cells at a very low frequency where new cardiomyocytes are being formed, not via transdifferentiation of the HSC but rather through cell fusion (Alvarez-Dolado et al., 2003). Kajstura et al added new fuel to HSC controversy, supporting the thesis of possible cardiac regeneration with bone marrow derived lin(-), c-kit(+) cells. In a meticulously conducted study, Kajstura et al demonstrated the cells' engraftment and positive impact on acutely damaged myocardium in mice. However, the authors noted a large diversity of cells out of which 63% were negative for lymphocytes, monocytes and granulocytes and only 48% were positive for markers of hematopoietic cell lineages. Thus, a mixture of enriched c-kit(+) bone marrow cells was used in this study.

For the past 5 years discussion has arisen on the plasticity of HSC. Theories favoring hematopoietic stem cells differentiation have been heavily questioned, suggesting cell fusion as more likely explanation of their action. Moreover, imperfections in cell characterization resulting in impurity of administered cells cast a shadow on HSCs potential.

In addition to HSC, bone marrow contains a population of non-hematopoietic stem cells. These multipotent cells were initially recognized for their ability to form colonies of fibroblasts *in vitro* and named Colony Forming Unit – Fibroblasts (CFU-F) (Castro-Malaspina et al., 1980). Subsequently, these cells were found to differentiate into cells of mesenchymal origin and are known today as mesenchymal stem cells (MSC) or mesenchymal progenitor stem cells. MSC are identified by surface proteins including CD29, CD44, CD17, CD90, CD106, CD120a and CD124 (Pittenger et al., 1999). They are however CD45(-)/CD34(-) and do not express hematopoietic lineage markers. Furthermore, they are limited in their lineage developmental potential. MSC represent a very small fraction of bone marrow stem cells, ranging from 0.001 to 0.01%. of the total population. This translates into approximately 2–5 MSC per 1 x 10^6 mononuclear cells (Castro-Malaspina et al., 1980; Pittenger et al., 1999).

Bone marrow is not the only host of MSC, several other tissues and organs have been discovered to harbor MSC. These include liver, testis, prostate, skeletal muscle and fatty tissue. It is a subject of dispute, however, whether MSC truly reside in remote niches, as more evidence is gathered on stem cells homing and trafficking (Kraitchman et al., 2005).

The earliest proof that MSC were able to differentiate into cardiomyocytes was published by Shinji Makino and collaborators (Makino et al., 1999). The Japanese scientists were capable of isolating a cardiomyogenic cell line from murine bone marrow stromal cells. Cultured cells were then treated with cytidine analogue 5-azacytidine, known for its potential to activate genes responsible for differentiation. Cells gradually increased in size and lengthened in one direction, connecting to each other with myotube-like structures. Such clusters began to beat synchronously just 3 weeks later, simultaneously expressing cardiomyocyte-specific markers (Nkx2.5/Csx, GATA4, TEF-1) (Makino et al., 1999). Clustered myotube-like structures were also found to be susceptible to adrenergic and cholinergic stimuli (Hakuno et al., 2002). It seems, however, that MSC require a direct cell-to-cell contact and distinct mediators to induce cell differentiation into specific lineage, as co-culturing MSC with cardiomyocytes results in differentiation of stem cells into cells presenting cardiac phenotype, distinguished by the expression of structural and contractile proteins and production of specific peptides, such as troponin T (Fukuhara et al., 2003).

Experimental studies following the success of *in vitro* discoveries have proven the feasibility and efficacy of MSC transplantation in the setting of myocardial ischemia. Various experimental models have been used to prove whether MSC truly engraft and improve regional and global left ventricular performance.

Toma and collaborators (Toma et al., 2002) were the first to demonstrate that human MSC can differentiate into cardiomyocytes when injected into murine myocardium. At the same time MSC were proven to possess low immunogenecity, thus allowing for cellular xenotransplantation. Mangi et al (Mangi et al., 2003) injected genetically modified autologous MSC into the ischemic rat myocardium. Transplanted cells inhibited the process of cardiac remodeling by reducing inflammation, collagen deposition and cardiomyocyte hypertrophy. Moreover Mangi noticed over 80% regeneration of lost myocardial volume, and completely normalized systolic and diastolic cardiac function in MSC treated animals. Similarly Tang and collaborators (Tang et al., 2006) found left ventricular function improving after MSC injection. Interestingly, Tang designated the combined effect of myogenesis and angiogenesis as a main reason of MSC-mediated myocardial regeneration, as he observed increased myocardial vessel density alongside newly formed myocardial cells.

Nevertheless, the number of stem cells harbored in bone marrow is insufficient for organ or tissue repair. Aspiration of bone marrow, isolation and *in vitro* expansion of specific cell population is required in order to achieve quantities sufficient for successful therapy.

Evidence has been accumulated on the existence of multipotent cells within the bone marrow, which are able to differentiate into cardiomyocytes and significantly contribute to myocardial repair. As of today, the identity of such intensively sought cell remains elusive.

9.2.2.3 *Endothelial progenitor cells*

In 1997 Asahara and collaborators (Asahara et al., 1997) discovered that human peripheral blood contained a pool of cells capable of differentiation to endothelial cells *in vitro*. Further investigation revealed that these bone-marrow derived cells possessed properties of stem cells, such as self-renewal, clonogenecity and, of course, differentiation capacity. Cells were found to express common hematopoietic stem cell markers – CD34 and CD133 in addition to vascular endothelial growth factor receptor 2 (Buhring et al., 1999) (VEGFR2 or kinase-domain-related – KDR), but since their differentiation potential was limited to one lineage, they were named as Endothelial Progenitor Cells (EPC). Subsequent studies have suggested existence of at least 2 sub-populations of EPC – so called "Early EPC" or Circulating Angiogenic Cells (CAC) and "Late EPC" which are exceedingly rare in peripheral blood (1 cell in 20ml of blood) (Hur et al., 2004). CAC are thought to produce proangiogenic cytokines and factors while EPC differentiate into endothelial cells. Just recently EPC were found to possess the ability to acquire a myocyte phenotype when in close proximity to such. *In vivo* studies revealed that EPC contribute not only to vasculogenesis but also myogenesis, through transdifferentiation, not cell fusion (Murasawa et al., 2005). Regardless of the sub-molecular differences, EPC were found to circulate in peripheral blood of both healthy and diseased individuals. Their pool significantly increases in various cardiovascular disorders such as coronary artery disease. Although currently disputable, several theories have emerged on the EPC source, mobilization and role. The first theory perceives inflammatory cytokines as homing beacons for EPC that mobilize a quiescent, bone-marrow harbored pool of progenitor cells. A second hypothesis assumes EPC reside within the vascular endothelium, and are released into the blood when damage (shear stress or ischemia) occurs. While the exact role of EPC in cardiovascular physiology remains unidentified, numbers of studies indicate their protective role in cardiovascular homeostasis. Transplantation of EPC has been shown to promote neovascularization and improve function in various experimental models of myocardial ischemia. Transdifferentiation to endothelial cells, smooth muscle cells and cardiomyocytes has been characterized by immunohistochemistry. Encouraging results of these experimental studies have led to human clinical studies of ESC transplantation; these studies are described in more detail later in this chapter.

9.2.2.4 *Cardiac stem cells*

Cells capable of self-renewal and bearing the potential of plasticity have recently been proven to reside in the myocardium (Beltrami et al., 2003). These specific Cardiac Stem Cells (CSC) are multipotent and clonogenic, giving rise to cardiomyocytes, smooth muscle cells and endothelial cells both *in vivo* and *in vitro* (Dawn et al., 2005). CSC are characterized by presence of the surface stem cells antigens c-kit, Sca-1 and MDR1, but they do not express the transcription factors or surface proteins of cardiomyocytes and endothelial cells (Beltrami et al., 2003). CSCs, together with supporting cells and early lineage committed cells (LCC) cluster in so-called niches, where they divide and partially differentiate. LCC are one step further in differentiation process, as they express markers typical for cardiomyocytes and vascular smooth muscle cells along with typical stem cell markers. Stem cell niches are distributed throughout the heart with the apex and atrial tissue being the most occupied locations. These specific compartments offer CSC an appropriate microenvironment, hosting growth factors, cytokines and other molecules.

The role of CSC in myocardial physiology is now under investigation. It is believed that CSC and LCC participate in the normal turnover of cardiac cells, by forming new myocytes and capillaries (Urbanek et al., 2003). Although limited in number, as there is 1 CSC per 8000-20,000 myocytes, the cells are powerful enough to generate nearly 3×10^6 cardiomyocytes a day in the fully functional and healthy heart. Considering the equal number of cells decreasing each day due to apoptosis/necrosis, we are led to a conclusion that myocardium replaces its entire cell population every ~5 years (Anversa et al., 2006).

Despite its regenerative potential, the heart appears defenseless against the consequences of acute or chronic ischemia. Reasons may be twofold: the ischemic insult affects the CSC and LCC as well, as they die together with the cardiomyocytes and endothelial cells. Secondly, the number of c-kit(+) cells within the myocardium decreases with age, therefore their gross regenerative potential decreases. It seems however that it is not the number of cells that matters most, but their inability to translocate and home to an area of injury (Urbanek et al., 2005). In turn, CSC contribute to myocardial thickening and remodeling by intense proliferation and differentiation in non-ischemic regions.

In 2003 Beltrami (Beltrami et al., 2003) published a groundbreaking paper describing the direct injection of cardiac stem cells into the border zone of an experimentally induced myocardial infarction. Cellular transplantation resulted in improved left ventricular performance after just 20 days of observation. Interestingly, 10 days after the injection, small and immature muscle cells, capillaries and arteries composed the reconstituted tissue. 10 days later the number of cells remained unchanged, but their volume and size doubled, leading to conclusion that cell proliferation prevails during the first phase, and is followed by cell hypertrophy. It is also worth noticing that left ventricular function improved after 20 but not 10 days indicating insufficient strength of newly developed tissue.

Beltrami's findings were confirmed by Axel Linke and collaborators (Linke et al., 2005), who also examined if resident cardiac stem cells could be activated and attracted by two potent growth factors, IGF (insulin-like growth factor) and HGF (hepatocyte growth factor), in a setting of myocardial injury. In fact, previously performed studies revealed that the CSC of the murine heart possesses the HGF c-Met receptor (HGFR) and the IGF-1-IGF-1 receptor systems. HGF and IGF had been successfully used as proangiogenic factors in both experimental and clinical settings to treat peripheral vessel disease (Morishita et al., 2004). In Linke's experiment, both factors activated and recruited resident CSC, which in turn migrated into the ischemic tissue, restoring blood supply and myocardial contractility. It is worth mentioning that in humans HGF levels were found not to correlate with evidence of ischemia, but with angiographically visible collateralization of the vessel.

Basing upon the abovementioned discoveries, Dawn and collaborators (Dawn et al., 2005) sought for a more clinically oriented approach to stem cell injection. The hypothesis was that CSC could migrate via the vessel wall into the myocardium, when injected into the coronary circulation. This was tested in a model of myocardial infarction followed by reperfusion, closely mimicking the most commonly seen clinical scenario, as patients with acute myocardial infarction often undergo spontaneous or iatrogenic reperfusion prior to hospital admission. In such settings CSC were found to successfully cross the vessel wall and enter the interstitium of the heart. Moreover, injected and labeled CSC were able to regenerate ischemic myocardium by forming not only cardiomyocytes but also coronary vessels.

Following this path towards clinical application, a group of scientists guided by Eduardo Marban (Smith et al., 2007) successfully isolated, expanded and characterized human cardiac stem cells obtained by percutaneous endomyocardial biopsy. Percutaneous right ventricular biopsy is a relatively simple and safe procedure, and can ultimately be used as a method of harvesting CSC for cellular therapy. Marban's revolutionary work provided evidence that CSC can be safely obtained using this minimally invasive technique, and despite the very limited amount of harvested tissue, can be grown *in vitro*, providing a large population of cells in a relatively short time.

Cardiac stem/progenitor cells will soon enter the clinical arena (Fig. 9.1). These undifferentiated, multipotent and clonogenic cells form cardiomyocytes and elements of coronary vessels. Their limited commitment makes them an interesting alternative in cellular transplantation. A recently published study by Smith and colleagues (Smith et al., 2007) described the feasibility and safety of isolation and expansion of adult cardiac stem cells from endomyocardial biopsy specimens. Endomyocardial biopsy is a minimally invasive procedure performed by insertion of a bioptome into the right ventricle via the internal jugular vein under fluoroscopic guidance. Small pieces of myocardium are then grasped, biopsied, and processed for stem cell isolation. The patient is usually discharged from the hospital later that same day and return to their normal activities the following day.

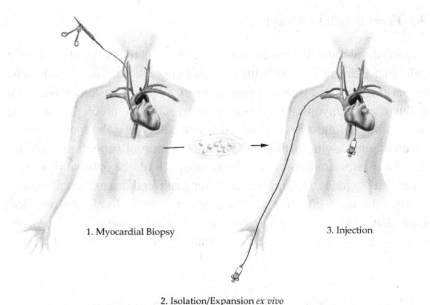

1. Myocardial Biopsy   3. Injection

2. Isolation/Expansion *ex vivo*

Figure 9.1. The highly probable process of cardiac stem/progenitor cell therapy in humans.

When sufficient number of cardiac progenitor cells in culture is reached, the patient can be offered the most appropriate route of cell delivery, depending on the underlying disease and patient anatomy. Cells may be injected intramuscularly with or without concomitant surgical coronary revascularization. Modern surgical techniques can be applied, such as minimally invasive direct revascularization or robotic surgery. If surgery is not feasible or required, cells may be injected directly into the coronary arteries during coronary catheterization.

The notion that the heart possesses the ability to regenerate itself is one of the most important discoveries of the last decade. Once viewed as a fully differentiated organ, the heart is now perceived as an ever changing complex, where myocytes are in a slow but constant cycle of life and death (Urbanek et al., 2005). CSC carry the potential for the future regenerative therapy of the heart. When properly extracted by surgeon or cardiologist via a surgical or percutaneous biopsy, and expanded *in vitro*, CSC become a powerful, and non-immunogenic solution for the infarcted or failing myocardium.

9.3 From Bench to Bedside

Experimental studies have demonstrated the functional benefits of stem cell transplantation. The ultimate challenge – to successfully and everlastingly cure a diseased human heart, is yet to be undertaken. For cellular cardiomyoplasty to occur, many clinical problems must be solved. First, it must be determined which cell type is the most effective given the underlying pathology. Second, a group of patients suitable for cellular transplantation needs to be defined. Third, the optimal timing, or so called "window of opportunity" for each cell/disease combination. Fourth, the most effective and safe delivery method must be resolved. Last, but not least, the question of long-term side-effects must be addressed, as none of the experimental studies have provided a clear answer.

9.3.1 *Cell type – where multitude brings confusion*

As of first quarter of 2007, bone-marrow derived cells together with skeletal myoblasts dominate the clinical arena of stem cell transplantation (Fig. 9.2). The evidence supporting their role in myocardial regeneration is encouraging. Importantly, both cell types can be obtained in sufficient quantities from every patient scheduled to undergo a cellular transplantation as the harvesting process requires only local anesthesia and is nearly risk-free. Harvested cells can be effortlessly processed *ex vivo*, where further isolation and expansion of specific cell lineages may take place. However, in a vast majority of clinical studies bone marrow mononuclear cells (BMMNC) have been utilized. This unfractioned pool of bone marrow cells contains hematopoietic (HSC), mesenchymal (MSC), as well as endothelial progenitor cells (EPC). Although controversies surrounding HSC plasticity are still to be resolved, MSC are known to transdifferentiate into cardiomyocytes *in vivo* and *ex vivo*. Unfortunately they represent only 1% of entire BMMNC population. Moreover, keep in mind that their potential is limited, and only 40% of MSC are capable of successful transdifferentiation into cardiac muscle cells.

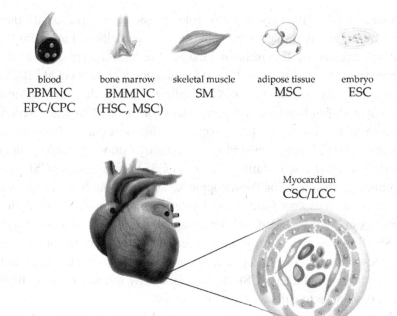

blood   bone marrow   skeletal muscle   adipose tissue   embryo
PBMNC   **BMMNC**   **SM**   **MSC**   **ESC**
EPC/CPC   **(HSC, MSC)**

Myocardium
CSC/LCC

Figure 9.2. All currently known sources of undifferentiated cells used in myocardial regeneration. Black dots on the heart point locations dense in cardiac stem/progenitor cells. A niche is visible in the magnification.

Although the majority of MSC studies currently performed focus on non-cardiac related disorders, such as Crohn's disease and osteogenesis imperfecta, the potential for a significant breakthrough in the field of myocardial regeneration remains. As described earlier in this chapter, MSC lack major histocompatibility complex (MHC-II) molecules and thus are not recognized by the hosts' immune system. Therefore it is feasible to use MSC as "universal" cells in cellular transplantation without the need for immunosupression. Vast availability and entrusted culture methodology, supported by very promising experimental data, suggest that MSC will play an important role in myocardial regeneration within next few years.

The third major subpopulation of mononuclear cells is endothelial progenitors (EPC/CPC). These circulating peripheral blood multipotent cells are partially committed to the endothelial lineage. EPC, as discussed previously, play the key role in neovascularization as they transdifferentiate into mature vascular endothelial cells and augment the capillary density of the ischemic tissue. Successful engraftment and regenerative potential has also been documented (Murasawa et al., 2005). A recent discovery of the EPC's ability to transdifferentiate into cardiomyocytes unfolds a novel perspective for myocardial regeneration. The ease of harvesting is what makes EPC the most patient-friendly, as cells are isolated from peripheral blood, although prior administration of granulocyte colony stimulating factor (G-CSF) is desired. G-CSF is a glycoprotein that acts on hematopoietic cells by binding to specific cell surface receptors and stimulating proliferation, differentiation commitment, and some end-cell functional activation. Pre-treatment with G-CSF allows for a greater number of EPC/CPC cells to be collected as the bone-marrow resident progenitors are recruited into the blood stream. Commercially available G-CSF is subcutaneously injected on daily basis for 3-5 days prior to cell harvesting procedure.

Driven by the promising results achieved in animal models of heart failure, human autologous skeletal myoblast transplantation has been undertaken in both Europe and the United States. SM can be easily and safely obtained from small amounts of the patient's own skeletal muscle and expanded readily in culture, overcoming the shortages of donor tissue. Therefore the use of autologous cells avoids the ethical issues currently constraining stem cell research, and obviates the need for immunosupression. A number of Phase I clinical trials assessing the safety and feasibility of SM transplantation have been completed in the US and Europe.

9.3.2 *Cell delivery – shipping matters*

Cells can be delivered to the myocardium in 2 distinct ways, by intravascular or by intramuscular injection (Fig. 9.3). Although a relatively safe and straightforward procedure, intracoronary, catheter-based delivery (PCI) has some important drawbacks – cells are subject to a "washout" effect that ruthlessly limits engraftment efficiency. Moreover, cells may be unable to reach the microcirculation when a no-reflow phenomenon occurs in the freshly reperfused vessel. Furthermore,

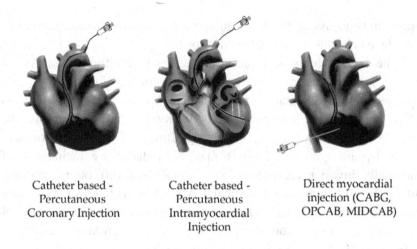

Catheter based -   Catheter based -   Direct myocardial
Percutaneous   Percutaneous   injection (CABG,
Coronary Injection   Intramyocardial   OPCAB, MIDCAB)
Injection

Figure 9.3. The most commonly used delivery routes.

compromised flow and fragility of unstable atherosclerotic plaques may represent a formidable risk of rupture and platelet aggregation when suspended cells are injected into a severely diseased artery. Despite these limitations, two mainstream approaches involving intracoronary delivery prevail, one aiming at the early repair of ischemic myocardium and the second as an alternative in severely diseased patients with no options for conventional treatment. In the former, with PCI as a treatment of choice, cellular material can be rapidly, safely and effectively introduced to the infarct-related artery within the first hour after the onset of chest pain. In the latter, percutaneously performed intracoronary injection represents the least invasive option with great potential for success. Moreover it avoids the focal accumulation of cells associated with a direct injection strategy.

On the other hand, the surgical approach offers the most precise method of cell delivery via direct intramuscular injection. Intramuscular injection is also feasible with a catheter-based needle. Inserted percutaneously via the femoral artery, the catheter-based needle enters the left ventricle and punches the myocardium from the inside. However, such an approach is severely limited by the lack of direct visualization of the fibrous scar and its complexity. The surgeon has the unrivaled opportunity to assess the heart anatomy and repeatedly and accurately introduce cells into the infarct border zone.

The surgical route is preferred in patients with diffused, multivessel coronary artery disease and poor left ventricular function. In such settings cell transplantation is augmented by coronary artery bypass grafts that restore previously limited blood supply, increasing the chances of the cells' survival and engraftment. The risk of coronary artery bypass grafting (CABG) may be reduced by facilitation of minimally invasive techniques such as OPCAB (off pump coronary artery bypass grafting) and MIDCAB (minimally invasive direct coronary artery bypass). While both techniques alleviate the use of extracorporeal circulation, thus reducing risk of neurological and renal complications, MIDCAB is, in addition, performed via a small thoracic incision. Robotic surgery, also known as TECAB (Totally Endoscopic Coronary Artery Bypass), is currently being explored as another option in various areas of cardiothoracic surgery such as coronary artery revascularization and mitral valve repair. This highly sophisticated approach may also be used to deliver stem cells to a specific area of the myocardium with concurrent coronary revascularization or valve repair in the near future.

Technical issues are secondary to cell properties, as the unique cell properties dictate the delivery route. For intracoronary injection, the cells must have the ability to migrate through the vessel wall into the interstitium within a very limited time. Furthermore, the cell's diameter is important, as large cells may clot and embolize distal capillaries. BMMNC, including MSC and EPC, have been successfully injected into the coronary vasculature in both experimental and clinical settings. However, initial studies on MSC by Richard Vulliet and colleagues (Vulliet et al., 2004) cast a shadow on the safety of intracoronary MSC injection, when cells were found to cause myocardial ischemia in all of the treated canine hearts. Vulliet's findings have not been confirmed in human studies, as intracoronary MSC injection is now considered to be feasible and safe.

On the other hand, skeletal myoblasts may only be transplanted using direct myocardial injections, as their ability to cross the vascular wall is limited. This shortcoming has been overcome by a transvenous coronary sinus approach. With a specially designed catheter introduced percutaneously, the coronary sinus and great cardiac veins are accessed. The catheter is equipped with an endovascular ultrasound transducer, which provides unparalleled identification of the target area. Its' tip acts as a pierce that tunnels through the vessel wall into the myocardial tissue. Cellular material is then injected directly into the myocardium.

9.3.3 *Patient selection – Is it the only option for "no-option"?*

Which patient population will benefit most from cellular transplantation? The previously accepted concept of delivering angiogenic growth factors and cells into a severely diseased, failing heart with little or no alternative in conventional treatment (so called "no-option" patients) is now challenged by a novel approach where myocardial restoration begins at the time of injury. Acute myocardial infarction (AMI), and congestive heart failure (CHF) as its unavoidable consequence, remains an utmost priority as they account for a steadily increasing mortality and morbidity. The goals of cellular therapy shortly after the onset of an acute myocardial infarction are to replace deceased cardiomyocytes with viable, contractile and synchronized tissue, able to preserve left ventricular function and prevent chamber dilatation and remodeling. Animal and human studies have demonstrated that an ischemic insult of the myocardium results in bone marrow stem cells homing to the site of injury. This "self-defense" mechanism seems inadequate, as it does not prevent functional and geometrical deterioration. Therefore the idea of supplying myocardium with a large number of allogenic, multipotent cells directly into coronary vasculature at the time of or shortly after primary coronary intervention gains strong attention. In 2002, Bodo Strauer (Strauer et al., 2002) successfully conducted the first clinical study using bone-marrow derived stem cells to repair myocardium shortly after an ischemic insult. In 10 patients with an acute coronary syndrome, bone marrow biopsy was performed 7 days after percutaneous coronary intervention. Mononuclear cells (BMMNC) were isolated and expanded *ex vivo*, and injected into the infarct related artery three days later. After 3 months of observation, patients treated with BMMNC demonstrated significant improvements in left ventricular dynamics and geometry. It is worth mentioning that no adverse events related to bone marrow aspiration and transplantation were noted.

At the same time, Assmus and collaborators (Assmus et al., 2002) carried out a randomized, open-label clinical trial assessing the safety, feasibility and efficacy of bone marrow-derived stem cells and circulating blood-derived progenitor cells transplantation in acute myocardial infarction (TOPCARE-AMI). A total of 20 patients were enrolled in the study, and randomly assigned to receive either BMMNC or CPC. Within a mean time of 4.3 days after AMI, cells were successfully injected into the previously stented, infarct related artery. After 4 months of observation left ventricular ejection fraction had increased by 14% (from 51.6 to 60%) in patients in whom cellular transplantation was carried out, while such augmentation in the control group was not noted. Furthermore, profound improvement in wall motion abnormalities in the infarct area and a significant reduction in end-systolic left ventricular volume was seen, indicating a valuable impact on postinfarction remodeling. Surprisingly, there was no difference in LV function between the two groups receiving BMMNC or CPC. Again, a pure progenitor cell population was not used in the study, with less than 3% of CD34(+) cells detected in the infused BMMNC. The population of blood-derived progenitors was more homogenous, with the majority of cells being endothelial progenitor cells. A subgroup of patients enrolled to TOPCARE-AMI trial, was evaluated by contrast-enhanced MRI (Britten et al., 2003), which also revealed an increased LVEF and reduced infarct size. Moreover, increased coronary flow reserve in patients receiving progenitor cells was noted, strongly supporting their role in neovascularization. Furthermore, the migratory capacity of the infused cells was found to be the most important predictor of infarct remodeling.

Results of the TOPCARE-AMI trial were reconfirmed by Wollert and collaborators (Wollert et al., 2004), who directed a Phase II randomized, controlled clinical trial on a larger population of patients. BOne marrOw transfer to enhance ST-elevation infarct regeneration (or BOOST Trial) enlisted 60 patients, randomly assigned to receive either BMMNC or standard therapy. Interestingly, BMMNC were injected into the infarct related artery only 6 to 8 hours after being harvested from the ilia. This "fast track" approach did not allow for cell culture and *ex vivo* expansion, therefore a significant volume of bone marrow was necessary (an average of 128ml per patient) in order to obtain the desired number of progenitor cells. Compared with the control group, patients receiving BMMNC had augmented regional and global LVEF and systolic wall motion in the infarct border zone at 6 months. Again, careful safety evaluation of BMMNC administration was undertaken, and revealed no adverse events throughout duration of the study.

Everyone does not share this optimism. In a recently released publication in the New England Journal of Medicine, Ketil Lunde and coworkers (Lunde et al., 2006) noted no improvement in left ventricular function six months after intracoronary injection of BMMNC into infarcted myocardium. Similar to previously mentioned studies, cells were injected into the infarct related artery 6 days after the onset of ischemia. One hundred patients were enrolled into this meticulously designed study, and randomly selected to receive either BMMNC or standard medical therapy. Despite similar methods used to assess myocardial geometry and performance, Lunde was unable to show statistically significant differences between the two groups of patients.

The question arises why he was unable to confirm previous findings, despite a similar protocol, group of patients, pathology and most of all, the same type of cells. Is cell number important? Or is it a matter of study duration? The number of injected BMMNC varies among studies. The range extends from 1.5×10^6 cells/ml through 7.35×10^6 (TOPCARE-AMI) up to 24×10^8 (BOOST) and the total number of injected CD34+ cells has not been found to correlate with treatment efficacy. Surprisingly, an effect on myocardial function has been confirmed in studies using similar to Lunde's number of CD34+ cells. At the same time, investigators of the BOOST Trial announced completion of the 18 month follow up of their trial (Meyer et al., 2006). To general disbelief, they concluded that a single dose of intracoronary BMMNC did not provide long-term benefit on LV systolic function after myocardial infarction compared with a randomized control group.

Investigators noticed however, that BMMNC therapy accelerated LV ejection fraction recovery shortly after AMI.

Meanwhile Chen (Chen et al., 2004) and collaborators published the first clinical trial to utilize a more defined group of multipotent cells. Mesenchymal stem cells (MSC) were tested to restore left ventricular function shortly after myocardial infarction. A large (n=69) cohort of patients was enrolled in the study, and randomized to receive either intracoronary injection of MSC or placebo (saline). A total of 60 ml of bone marrow was aspirated from the ilia. MSC were isolated by density gradient centrifugation and cultured for 10 days. A mean of $8-10 \times 10^9$ cells/ml were injected into the lumen of infarct related artery, 18 days after onset of myocardial infarction. After 6 months of follow-up, left ventricular geometry, dynamics and perfusion were assessed using echocardiography, positron emission tomography and electromechanical mapping, respectively. Left ventricular ejection fraction and wall movement velocity in patients randomized to the cell therapy group significantly improved. Moreover, patients treated with MSC had fewer hypokinetic, akinetic and dyskinetic segments of the left ventricle than matched controls. Interestingly, improvements in LV function were noted as early as 3 months after MSC injection, and remained constant for the next 3 months. Late results will reveal whether MSC induced myocardial regeneration is a long-lasting effect or transient but desirable acceleration of recovery.

Cellular transplantation still represents an important opportunity for patients with angiographically proven coronary artery disease but without viable percutaneous or surgical treatment options. These include subjects with diffuse small-vessel disease, in-stent restenosis (ISR), chronic total occlusions, and degenerated vein grafts. There is also an increasing number of patients with a severely damaged heart and advanced atherosclerosis following AMI. For this group of patients, with severely dilated left ventricles and impaired ejection fractions of lower than 30%, cardiac transplantation and/or mechanical support remains the main therapeutic choices limited by availability and efficiency. Although novel approaches are explored (surgical ventricular remodeling (SVR)) this group of "no-option" patients is in urgent need for an effective and long lasting cure.

In 2004 Mustafa Ozbaran and collaborators (Ozbaran et al., 2004) undertook a clinical study aimed at cellular regeneration of the failing heart. Six patients were included in the study, all with ejection fractions lower than 25%, and poor distal coronary beds not suitable for coronary revascularization. Bone marrow derived mononuclear cells were mobilized with G-CSF and collected by apheresis from the peripheral circulation. Twenty-four hours later, cells were injected directly into the myocardium, with subsequent coronary artery by-pass grafting. Six months after cellular transplantation five patients showed clinical improvement, but only in three was an increased ejection fraction noted. Out of these three, two had significantly improved myocardial viability on perfusion scintigraphy and PET when compared to preoperative values. Interestingly, the patients who benefited most were the ones with recent myocardial infarctions. The concomitant surgical revascularization raised concerns whether improvement was due to cellular regeneration or restored blood supply to the myocardium. Just recently, Losordo et al. (Losordo et al., 2007) reported results of a prospective, randomized, double-blind, placebo controlled, dose-escalating clinical trial of intramyocardial injection of autologous CD34+ cells in patients with intractable angina. Cells were mobilized from peripheral blood after 5 days of growth inducement with G-CSF, and injected into ischemic, but viable myocardium. Efficacy parameters including chest pain frequency, nitroglycerine usage, exercise time etc. showed trends that favored CD34+ cell treated patients. Larger and longer observational studies are currently under way to further evaluate this therapy.

Skeletal muscle transplantation plays an important role in attempts to recover once lost myocardial contractility. As part of the first Phase one trial in Europe, Menasché and collaborators (Menasche et al., 2003) reported on 10 patients who underwent cell grafting at the time of surgical coronary revascularization. Inclusion criteria included ejection fractions lower than 35%, non-viable scar, and an indication for coronary artery bypass surgery. After an average follow-op of 10.9 months, the mean New York Heart Association (NYHA) functional class improved from 2.7 ± 0.2 to 1.6 ± 0.1. Objectively the group's average left ventricular ejection fraction improved from 24 ± 1% to 32 ± 1% and blinded echocardiographic assessment of regional wall function demonstrated improvement in 63% of implanted scars. These encouraging results, however, were tempered by a disturbing number of ventricular arrhythmias necessitating the implantation of automatic cardioverter-defibrillator (ICD) in four patients. Again, the improvements in post-operative wall motion attributable to the grafted cells were difficult to interpret in the setting of concomitant CABG. Despite these limitations, the investigators demonstrated the feasibility and relative safety of this technique, justifying further investigation.

Herreros and colleagues (Herreros et al., 2003). using a similar study design reported comparable findings. This European Phase I study enrolled 12 patients with a mean follow-up of 6.5 months. Inclusion criteria were remote history (greater than 4 weeks) of myocardial infarction (MI), presence of akinetic or dyskinetic non-viable scar, indication for surgical revascularization, and left ventricular ejection fraction greater than 25%. A total of 11 patients were treated with a mean of 211 ± 10^7 x 10^6 skeletal myoblasts. Left ventricular ejection fraction improved from 35.5 ± 2.3% to 53.5 ± 4.98% at 3 months. Furthermore, in the 7 patients in whom ^{18}F-FDG PET imaging was performed both pre- and postoperatively, glucose uptake was significantly increased in both the whole myocardium and the infarct areas. Importantly, only one of the treated patients experienced ventricular arrhythmias during the follow-up period and this patient underwent a concomitant anuerysmectomy at the time of surgery. The authors speculate that a major complication is altered immunogenecity on the implanted cells by prolonged *ex vivo* culture conditions and the use of autologous serum in the cellular preparation prevents the immunologic inflammatory reaction that triggers arrhythmias.

The findings of a third clinical trial were reported by Siminiak (Siminiak et al., 2004). Inclusion criteria for this study were prior history of MI (minimum of 3 months before surgery), suitable anatomy for bypass surgery, and impaired ejection fraction between 25% and 40% with one or more dyskinetic segments on echocardiography and lack of myocardial viability on dobutamine echocardiography. The investigators documented improved ejection fraction in all 9 patients. While the first two treated patients did suffer ventricular arrhythmias, the addition of amiodarone prevented further episodes in these and subsequent patients.

In all the aforementioned clinical trials myoblast transplantation was performed in conjunction with surgical revascularization. The benefit attributable to the transplanted cells is thus disputable.

Smits and colleagues (Smits et al., 2003) designed and reported on the first study to evaluate safety and feasibility of autologous myoblast transplantation as stand-alone therapy. Five patients were enrolled to the study, based on similar inclusion criteria to used in abovementioned studies. However surgical revascularization was not attempted due to bad peripheral vasculature. The authors demonstrated a change in left ventricular ejection fraction from 36 ± 11% to 45 ± 8% by 6 months. Ventricular arrhythmias were only problematic in one patient in their series in whom a prophylactic ICD was eventually implanted.

Recently Siminiak and others (Siminiak et al., 2005) reported their initial findings in a Phase I clinical trial in which myoblasts were administered as sole therapy in post MI patients using a percutaneous delivery system. Designed to evaluate feasibility and safety, investigators enrolled 10 patients and reported on 6-month follow-up. Inclusion criteria were preserved from Siminiak's first study (Siminiak et al., 2004). While only modest improvements in left ventricular ejection fraction was found (3-8% improvement in 6 of 9 patients treated), there was symptomatic improvement in all 9 patients treated with skeletal myoblasts, with all nine improving to NYHA class I by 6 months. In contrast, the one patient who was not successfully grafted showed no change in either his ejection fraction or NYHA class.

While far from conclusive, these reports suggest that skeletal myoblast transplantation may be beneficial in the absence of surgical revascularization. They further validate minimally invasive techniques that could significantly broaden the applicability of this burgeoning technology. Histopathological analysis of transplanted cells in humans is limited to date. Menasché and colleagues (Menasche et al., 2003) reported on one patient who died of a stroke 17.5 months after skeletal myoblast transplantation. On post-mortem examination myotubes were found embedded in the scar tissue. No gap junctions or other evidence of cardiomyogenic differentiation was appreciated. The percentages of cells staining positive for slow myosin heavy chain isoforms was evaluated, demonstrating over half of the surviving cells staining positive with 33% of cells coexpressing fast and slow isoforms. This is in contrast to native skeletal muscle populations in which only 0.6% expresses both isoforms.

Pagani and collaborators (Pagani et al., 2003) reported on the outcomes in four patients who received cellular grafts at the time of LVAD implantation. In three patients in whom a dose of 300×10^6 cells were transplanted, surviving autologous skeletal muscle cells were identified by trichrome staining. The majority of skeletal myofibers were aligned in parallel with the resident myocardial fibers. Additionally, investigators noted expression of slow-twitch myosin isoforms - the evidence of myoblast differentiation. This study did not investigate the presence of gap junctions in the grafted cells. Authors estimate that the survival of transplanted myoblasts was less than 1% of the total cells grafted based on their histological analysis. Furthermore, they noted surviving cells in the epicardial fat presumably resulting from post-injection leakage of transplanted cells. A similar study was undertaken by Dib and collaborators (Dib et al., 2005), where 6 patients were treated with LVAD as a bridge to transplantation, with concurrent autologous skeletal myoblasts transplantation. Native hearts were excised at the time of transplantation and subject to careful histological evaluation. In 4 of 6 patients evident signs of cells' engraftment were documented, demonstrating survival, feasibility and safety of SM transplantation.

These findings further support the viability and possible functionality of these transplanted myoblasts but also suggest limitations to their ultimate ability to differentiate into functional cardiomyocytes. Such imperfection often results in impaired electrical coupling of engrafted cells, and contributes to ventricular arrhythmias (VT). Based on results of abovementioned Phase I clinical studies, incidence of VT after SM transplantation is estimated to be as high as 45% (Menasche et al., 2003; Siminiak et al., 2005). Therefore most of the treated patients undergo simultaneous implantation of cardiac defibrillators.

9.4 Future Possibilities

Cell transplantation for the treatment of heart disease is a promising field but many questions remain. The idea of supplying damaged myocardium with a cocktail of stem/progenitor cells able to transdifferentiate into cardiac muscle and vascular cells is safe and feasible, but its' effectiveness requires further investigation. Multipotent cells injected shortly after onset of myocardial ischemia seem to have better chance to survive, differentiate and maturate, as they are exposed to elevated concentrations of hypoxia-inducible growth factors released by cells undergoing apoptosis/necrosis. Such stimulation is feasible with exogenously introduced growth factors at the time of stem cell injection. However, our knowledge on complexity of homing/activating factors affecting these multipotent cells is far from being complete.

The aggregate findings of multiple studies suggest a modest beneficial effect from the autologous transplantation of skeletal myoblasts in patients who suffer from heart failure. The mechanisms through which these cells exert their effect remain, once again, elusive. The notion that these cells provide a significant contractile force in the absence of gap junctions seems simplistic. Alternative explanations include a potential role in limiting post-infarction remodeling to possible paracrine effects on host tissue (Menasche, 2005).

Future studies will need to better evaluate the safety and efficacy of a wider range of cell numbers and delivery techniques. Furthermore, issues about the optimal timing of delivery will need to be addressed. We might expect that through continuing collaborative efforts combining insights derived form animal studies and well-designed clinical trials, multipotent cells will be a useful and effective part of a clinical armamentarium to treat heart disease.

9.5 References

Alvarez-Dolado, M., Pardal, R., Garcia-Verdugo, J. M., Fike, J. R., Lee, H. O., Pfeffer, K., Lois, C., Morrison, S. J., and Alvarez-Buylla, A. (2003). Fusion of bone-marrow-derived cells with Purkinje neurons, cardiomyocytes and hepatocytes. *Nature*, 425(6961), pp. 968-973.

Antman, E. M. (2004). Coronary Care Medicine: It's Not Your Father's CCU Anymore. *Trans Am Clin Climatol Assoc,* 115. pp. 123-135.

Anversa, P., Kajstura, J., Leri, A., and Bolli, R. (2006). Life and death of cardiac stem cells: a paradigm shift in cardiac biology. *Circulation,* 113(11), pp. 1451-1463.

Asahara, T., Bauters, C., Zheng, L. P., Takeshita, S., Bunting, S., Ferrara, N., Symes, J. F., and Isner, J. M. (1995). Synergistic effect of vascular endothelial growth factor and basic fibroblast growth factor on angiogenesis in vivo. *Circulation*, 92(9 Suppl), pp. II365-371.

Asahara, T., Murohara, T., Sullivan, A., Silver, M., van der Zee, R., Li, T., Witzenbichler, B., Schatteman, G., and Isner, J. M. (1997). Isolation of putative progenitor endothelial cells for angiogenesis. *Science,* 275(5302), pp. 964-967.

Assmus, B., Schachinger, V., Teupe, C., Britten, M., Lehmann, R., Dobert, N., Grunwald, F., Aicher, A., Urbich, C., Martin, H., Hoelzer, D., Dimmeler, S., and Zeiher, A. M. (2002). Transplantation of Progenitor Cells and Regeneration Enhancement in Acute Myocardial Infarction (TOPCARE-AMI). *Circulation,* 106(24), pp. 3009-3017.

Balsam, L. B., Wagers, A. J., Christensen, J. L., Kofidis, T., Weissman, I. L., and Robbins, R. C. (2004). Haematopoietic stem cells adopt mature haematopoietic fates in ischaemic myocardium. *Nature,* 428(6983), pp. 668-673.

Beltrami, A. P., Barlucchi, L., Torella, D., Baker, M., Limana, F., Chimenti, S., Kasahara, H., Rota, M., Musso, E., Urbanek, K., Leri, A., Kajstura, J., Nadal-Ginard, B., and Anversa, P. (2003). Adult cardiac stem cells are multipotent and support myocardial regeneration. *Cell,* 114(6), pp. 763-776.

Boheler, K. R., Czyz, J., Tweedie, D., Yang, H. T., Anisimov, S. V., and Wobus, A. M. (2002). Differentiation of pluripotent embryonic stem cells into cardiomyocytes. *Circ Res,* 91(3), pp. 189-201.

Britten, M. B., Abolmaali, N. D., Assmus, B., Lehmann, R., Honold, J., Schmitt, J., Vogl, T. J., Martin, H., Schachinger, V., Dimmeler, S., and Zeiher, A. M. (2003). Infarct remodeling after intracoronary progenitor cell treatment in patients with acute myocardial infarction (TOPCARE-AMI): mechanistic insights from serial contrast-enhanced magnetic resonance imaging. *Circulation,* 108(18), pp. 2212-2218.

Buhring, H. J., Seiffert, M., Bock, T. A., Scheding, S., Thiel, A., Scheffold, A., Kanz, L., and Brugger, W. (1999). Expression of novel surface antigens on early hematopoietic cells. *Annals of the New York Academy of Sciences,* 872, pp. 25-38; Discussion, pp. 38-39.

Castro-Malaspina, H,. Gay, R. E., Resnick, G., Kapoor, N., Meyers, P., Chiarieri, D., McKenzie, S., Broxmeyer, H. E., and Moore, M. A. (1980). Characterization of human bone marrow fibroblast colony-forming cells (CFU-F) and their progeny. *Blood,* 56(2), pp. 289-301.

Chen, S. L., Fang, W. W., Ye, F., Liu, Y. H., Qian, J., Shan, S. J., Zhang, J. J., Chunhua, R. Z., Liao, L. M., Lin, S., and Sun, J. P. (2004). Effect on left ventricular function of intracoronary transplantation of autologous bone marrow mesenchymal stem cell in patients with acute myocardial infarction. *Am J Cardiol,* 94(1), pp. 92-95.

Dawn, B., Stein, A. B., Urbanek, K., Rota, M., Whang, B., Rastaldo, R., Torella, D., Tang, X. L., Rezazadeh, A., Kajstura, J., Leri, A., Hunt, G., Varma, J., Prabhu, S. D., Anversa, P., Bolli, R. (2005). Cardiac stem cells delivered intravascularly traverse the vessel barrier, regenerate infarcted myocardium, and improve cardiac function. *Proc Natl Acad Sci USA,* 102(10), pp. 3766-3771.

Di Donato, M., Toso, A., Dor, V., Sabatier, M., Barletta, G., Menicanti, L., and Fantini, F.. (2004). Surgical ventricular restoration improves mechanical intraventricular dyssynchrony in ischemic cardiomyopathy. *Circulation,* 109(21), pp. 2536-2543.

Dib, N., Michler, R. E., Pagani, F. D., Wright, S., Kereiakes, D. J., Lengerich, R., Binkley, P., Buchele, D., Anand, I., Swingen, C., Di Carli, M. F., Thomas, J. D., Jaber WA, Opie SR, Campbell A, McCarthy P, Yeager M, Dilsizian V, Griffith BP, Korn, R., Kreuger, S. K., Ghazoul, M., MacLellan, W. R., Fonarow, G., Eisen, H. J., Dinsmore, J., and Diethrich, E. (2005). Safety and feasibility of autologous myoblast transplantation in patients with ischemic cardiomyopathy: four-year follow-up. *Circulation,* 112(12), pp. 1748-1755.

Ferrari, G., Cusella-De Angelis, G., Coletta, M., Paolucci, E., Stornaiuolo, A., Cossu, G., and Mavilio, F. (1998). Muscle regeneration by bone marrow-derived myogenic progenitors. *Science,* 279(5356), pp. 1528-1530.

Formigli, L., Francini, F., Tani, A., Squecco, R., Nosi, D., Polidori, L., Nistri, S., Chiappini, L., Cesati, V., Pacini, A., Perna, A. M., Orlandini, G. E., Zecchi, P., Orlandini, S., and Bani, D. (2005). Morphofunctional integration between skeletal myoblasts and adult cardiomyocytes in coculture is favored by direct cell-cell contacts and relaxin treatment. *Am J Physiol Cell Physiol,* 288(4), pp. C795-804.

Fukuhara, S., Tomita, S., Yamashiro, S., Morisaki, T., Yutani, C., Kitamura, S., and Nakatani, T. (2003). Direct cell-cell interaction of cardiomyocytes is key for bone marrow stromal cells to go into cardiac lineage in vitro. *J Thorac Cardiovasc Surg,* 125(6), pp. 1470-1480.

Furness, S. G., and McNagny, K. (2006). Beyond mere markers: functions for CD34 family of sialomucins in hematopoiesis. *Immunol Res.,* 34(1), pp. 13-32.

Gao, S. Z., Chaparro, S. V., Perlroth, M., Montoya, J. G., Miller, J. L., DiMiceli, S., Hastie, T., Oyer, P. E., and Schroeder, J. (2003). Post-transplantation lymphoproliferative disease in heart and heart-lung transplant recipients: 30-year experience at Stanford University. *J Heart Lung Transplant,* 22(5), pp. 505-514.

Garcia, J., Tanabe, T., and Beam, K. G. (1994). Relationship of calcium transients to calcium currents and charge movements in myotubes expressing skeletal and cardiac dihydropyridine receptors. *J Gen Physiol,* 103(1), pp. 125-147.

Ghostine, S., Carrion, C., Souza, L. C., Richard, P., Bruneval, P., Vilquin, J. T., Pouzet, B., Schwartz, K., Menasche, P., and Hagege, A. A. (2002). Long-term efficacy of myoblast transplantation on regional structure and function after myocardial infarction. *Circulation,* 106(12 Suppl 1), pp. I131-136.

Goldstein, D. J., and Beauford, R. B. (2003). Left ventricular assist devices and bleeding: adding insult to injury. *Ann Thorac Surg,* 75(6 Suppl), pp. S42-47.

Goldstein, D. J., Smego, D., and Michler, R. E. (2006). Surgical aspects of congestive heart failure. *Heart Fail Rev,* 11(2), pp. 171-192.

Goldstein, D. J., Oz, M. C., and Rose, E. A. (1998). Implantable left ventricular assist devices. *N Engl J Med.*, 339(21), pp. 1522-1533.

Hakuno, D., Fukuda, K., Makino, S., Konishi, F., Tomita, Y., Manabe, T., Suzuki, Y., Umezawa, A., and Ogawa, S. (2002). Bone marrow-derived regenerated cardiomyocytes (CMG Cells) express functional adrenergic and muscarinic receptors. *Circulation,* 105(3), pp. 380-386.

Herreros, J., Prosper, F., Perez, A., Gavira, J. J., Garcia-Velloso, M. J., Barba, J., Sanchez, P. L., Canizo, C., Rabago, G., Marti-Climent, J. M., Hernandez, M., Lopez-Holgado, N., Gonzalez-Santos, J. M., Martin-Luengo, C., and Alegria, E. (2003). Autologous intramyocardial injection of cultured skeletal muscle-derived stem cells in patients with non-acute myocardial infarction. *Eur Heart J,* 24(22), pp. 2012-2020.

Hur, J., Yoon, C. H., Kim, H. S., Choi, J. H., Kang, H. J., Hwang, K. K., Oh, B. H., Lee, M. M., and Park, Y. B. (2004). Characterization of two types of endothelial progenitor cells and their different contributions to neovasculogenesis. *Arterioscler Thromb Vasc Bio,* 24(2), pp. 288-293.

Jackson, K. A., Majka, S. M., Wang, H., Pocius, J., Hartley, C. J., Majesky, M. W., Entman, M. L., Michael, L. H., Hirschi, K. K., and Goodell, M. A. (2001). Regeneration of ischemic cardiac muscle and vascular endothelium by adult stem cells. *J Clin Invest,* 107(11), pp. 1395-1402.

Kawashima, I., Zanjani, E. D., Almaida-Porada, G., Flake, A. W., Zeng, H., and Ogawa, M. (1996). CD34+ human marrow cells that express low levels of Kit protein are enriched for long-term marrow-engrafting cells. *Blood,* 87(10), pp. 4136-4142.

Kocher, A. A., Schuster, M. D., Szabolcs, M. J., Takuma, S., Burkhoff, D., Wang, J., Homma, S., Edwards, N. M., and Itescu, S. (2001). Neovascularization of ischemic myocardium by human bone-marrow-derived angioblasts prevents cardiomyocyte apoptosis, reduces remodeling and improves cardiac function. *Nat Med,* 7(4), pp. 430-436.

Kraitchman, D. L., Tatsumi, M., Gilson, W.D., Ishimori, T., Kedziorek, D., Walczak, P., Segars, W. P., Chen, H. H., Fritzges, D., Izbudak, I., Young, R. G., Marcelino, M., Pittenger, M. F., Solaiyappan, M., Boston, R. C., Tsui, B. M., Wahl, R. L., and Bulte, J. W. (2005). Dynamic imaging of allogeneic mesenchymal stem cells trafficking to myocardial infarction. *Circulation,* 112(10), pp. 1451-1461.

Lagasse, E., Connors, H., Al-Dhalimy, M., Reitsma, M., Dohse, M., Osborne, L., Wang, X., Finegold, M., Weissman, I. L., and Grompe, M. (2000). Purified hematopoietic stem cells can differentiate into hepatocytes in vivo. *Nat Med,* 6(11), pp. 1229-1234.

Lenzen, M. J., Boersma, E., Bertrand, M. E., Maier, W., Moris, C., Piscione, F., Sechtem, U., Stahle, E., Widimsky, P., de Jaegere, P., Scholte op Reimer, W. J. M., Mercado, N., and Wijns, W. (2005). Management and outcome of patients with established coronary artery disease: the Euro Heart Survey on coronary revascularization. *Euro Heart J,* 26(12), pp. 1169-1179.

Leobon, B., Garcin, I., Menasche, P., Vilquin, J. T., Audinat, E., and Charpak, S. (2003). Myoblasts transplanted into rat infarcted myocardium are functionally isolated from their host. *Proc Natl Acad Sci USA,* 100(13), pp. 7808-7811.

Linke, A., Muller, P., Nurzynska, D., Casarsa, C., Torella, D., Nascimbene, A., Castaldo, C., Cascapera, S., Bohm, M., Quaini, F., Urbanek, K., Leri, A., Hintze, T. H., Kajstura, J., and Anversa, P. (2005). Stem cells in the dog heart are self-renewing, clonogenic, and multipotent and regenerate infarcted myocardium, improving cardiac function. *Proc Natl Acad Sci USA,* 102(25), pp. 8966-8971.

Losordo, D. W., Schatz, R. A., White, C. J., Udelson J. E., Veereshwarayya, V., Durgin, M., Poh, K. K., Weinstein, R., Kearney, M., Chaudhry, M., Burg, A., Eaton, L., Heyd, L., Thorne, T., Shturman, L., Hoffmeister, P., Story, K., Zak, V., Dowling, D., Traverse, J. H., Olson, R. E., Flanagan, J., Sodano, D., Murayama, T., Kawamoto, A., Kusano, K. F., Wollins, J., Welt, F., Shah, P., Soukas, P., Asahara, T., and Henry. T. D. (2007). Intramyocardial transplantation of autologous CD34+ stem cells for intractable angina: a phase I/IIa double-blind, randomized controlled trial. *Circulation,* 115(25), pp. 3165-3172.

Lunde, K., Solheim, S., Aakhus, S., Arnesen, H., Abdelnoor, M., Egeland, T., Endresen, K., Ilebekk, A., Mangschau, A., Fjeld, J. G., Smith, H. J., Taraldsrud, E., Grogaard, H. K., Bjornerheim, R., Brekke, M., Muller, C., Hopp, E., Ragnarsson, A., Brinchmann, J. E., and Forfang, K. (2006). Intracoronary injection of mononuclear bone marrow cells in acute myocardial infarction. *N Engl J Med,* 355(12), pp. 1199-1209.

MacLellan, W. R., and Schneider, M. D. (2000). Genetic dissection of cardiac growth control pathways. *Annu Rev Physiol.,* 62, pp. 289-319.

Makino, S., Fukuda, K., Miyoshi, S., Konishi, F., Kodama, H., Pan, J., Sano, M., Takahashi, T., Hori, S., Abe, H., Hata, J., Umezawa, A., and Ogawa, S. (1999). Cardiomyocytes can be generated from marrow stromal cells in vitro. *J Clin Invest,* 103(5), pp. 697-705.

Mangi, A. A., Noiseux, N., Kong, D., He, H., Rezvani, M., Ingwall, J. S., and Dzau, V. J. (2003). Mesenchymal stem cells modified with Akt prevent remodeling and restore performance of infarcted hearts. *Nat Med,* 9(9), pp. 1195-1201.

Mauro, A. (1961). Satellite cell of skeletal muscle fibers. *J Biophys Biochem Cytol,* 9, pp. 493-495.

McConnell, P. I., del Rio, C. L., Jacoby, D. B., Pavlicova, M., Kwiatkowski, P., Zawadzka, A., Dinsmore, J. H., Astra, L., Wisel, S., and Michler, R. E. (2005). Correlation of autologous skeletal myoblast survival with changes in left ventricular remodeling in dilated ischemic heart failure. *J Thorac Cardiovasc Surg,* 130(4), pp. 1001.

Menasche, P., Hagege, A. A., Vilquin, J. T., Desnos, M., Abergel, E., Pouzet, B., Bel, A., Sarateanu, S., Scorsin, M., Schwartz, K., Bruneval, P., Benbunan, M., Marolleau, J. P., and Duboc, D. (2003). Autologous skeletal myoblast transplantation for severe postinfarction left ventricular dysfunction. *J Am Coll Cardiol,* 41(7), pp. 1078-1083.

Menasche, P. (2005). Skeletal myoblast for cell therapy. *Coron Artery Dis,* 16(2), pp. 105-110.

Menicanti, L., and Di Donato, M. (2004). Surgical left ventricle reconstruction, pathophysiologic insights, results and expectation from the STICH trial. *Eur J Cardiothorac Surg,* 26 Suppl 1, pp. S42-46; Discussion, pp. S46-47.

Meyer, G. P., Wollert, K. C., Lotz, J., Steffens, J., Lippolt, P., Fichtner, S., Hecker, H., Schaefer, A., Arseniev, L., Hertenstein, B., Ganser, A., and Drexler, H. (2006). Intracoronary bone marrow cell transfer after myocardial infarction: eighteen months' follow-up data from the randomized, controlled BOOST (BOne marrOw transfer to enhance ST-elevation infarct regeneration) trial. *Circulation,* 113(10), pp. 1287-1294.

Mezey, E., Chandross, K. J., Harta, G., Maki, R. A., and McKercher, S. R. (2000). Turning blood into brain: cells bearing neuronal antigens generated in vivo from bone marrow. *Science,* 290(5497), pp. 1779-1782.

Min, J. Y., Yang, Y., Converso, K. L., Liu, L., Huang, Q., Morgan, J. P., and Xiao, Y. F. (2002). Transplantation of embryonic stem cells improves cardiac function in postinfarcted rats. *J Appl Physio,* 92(1), pp. 288-296.

Mocini, D., Colivicchi, F., and Santini, M.. (2005). Stem cell therapy for cardiac arrhythmias. *Ital Heart J,* 6(3), pp. 267-271.

Morishita, R., Aoki, M., Hashiya, N., Makino, H., Yamasaki, K., Azuma, J., Sawa, Y., Matsuda, H., Kaneda, Y., and Ogihara, T. (2004). Safety evaluation of clinical gene therapy using hepatocyte growth factor to treat peripheral arterial disease. *Hypertension,* 44(2), pp. 203-209.

Murasawa, S., Kawamoto, A., Horii, M., Nakamori, S., and Asahara, T. (2005). Niche-dependent translineage commitment of endothelial progenitor cells, not cell fusion in general, into myocardial lineage cells. *Arterioscler Thromb Vasc Biol.,* 25(7), pp. 1388-1394.

Murdoch, D. R., Love, M. P., Robb, S. D., McDonagh, T. A., Davie, A. P., Ford, I., Capewell, S., Morrison, C. E., and McMurray, J. J. (1998). Importance of heart failure as a cause of death. Changing contribution to overall mortality and coronary heart disease mortality in Scotland 1979-1992. *Eur Heart J,* 19(12), pp. 1829-1835.

Nelson, T. J, Ge, Z. D., Van Orman, J., Barron, M., Rudy-Reil, D., Hacker, T. A., Misra, R., Duncan, S. A., Auchampach, J. A., and Lough, J. W. (2006). Improved cardiac function in infarcted mice after treatment with pluripotent embryonic stem cells. *Anat Rec A Discov Mol Cell Evol Biol,* 288(11), pp. 1216-1224.

Ochiai, Y., McCarthy, P. M., Smedira, N. G., Banbury, M. K., Navia, J. L., Feng, J., Hsu, A. P., Yeager, M. L., Buda, T., Hoercher, K. J., Howard, M. W., Takagaki, M., Doi, K., and Fukamachi, K. (2002). Predictors of severe right ventricular failure after implantable left ventricular assist device insertion: analysis of 245 patients. *Circulation,* 106(12 Suppl 1), pp. I198-202.

O'Connell, J. B., and Bristow, M. R. (1994). Economic impact of heart failure in the United States: time for a different approach. *J Heart Lung Transplant,* 13(4), pp. S107-112.

Ohno, N., Fedak, P. W., Weisel, R. D., Mickle, D. A., Fujii, T., and Li, R.K. (2003). Transplantation of cryopreserved muscle cells in dilated cardiomyopathy: effects on left ventricular geometry and function. *J Thorac Cardiovasc Surg,* 126(5), pp. 1537-1548.

Orlic, D., Kajstura, J., Chimenti, S., Jakoniuk, I., Anderson, S. M., Li, B., Pickel, J., McKay, R., Nadal-Ginard, B., Bodine, D. M., Leri, A., and Anversa, P. (2001). Bone marrow cells regenerate infarcted myocardium. *Nature,* 410(6829), pp. 701-705.

Ozbaran, M., Omay, S. B., Nalbantgil, S., Kultursay, H., Kumanlioglu, K., Nart, D., and Pektok, E. (2004). Autologous peripheral stem cell transplantation in patients with congestive heart failure due to ischemic heart disease. *Eur J Cardiothorac Surg,* 25(3), pp. 342-350; Discussion, pp. 350-351.

Pagani, F. D., DerSimonian, H., Zawadzka, A., Wetzel, K., Edge, A. S., Jacoby, D. B., Dinsmore, J. H., Wright, S., Aretz, T. H., Eisen, H. J., and Aaronson, K. D. (2003). Autologous skeletal myoblasts transplanted to ischemia-damaged myocardium in humans. Histological analysis of cell survival and differentiation. *J Am Coll Cardiol,* 41(5), pp. 879-888.

Perriard, J. C., Hirschy, A., and Ehler, E. (2003). Dilated cardiomyopathy: a disease of the intercalated disc? *Trends Cardiovasc Med,* 13(1), pp. 30-38.

Pittenger, M. F., Mackay, A. M., Beck, S. C., Jaiswal, R. K., Douglas, R., Mosca, J. D., Moorman, M. A., Simonetti, D. W., Craig, S., and Marshak, D. R. (1999). Multilineage potential of adult human mesenchymal stem cells. *Science,* 284(5411), pp. 143-147.

Reinecke, H., MacDonald, G. H., Hauschka, S. D., and Murry, C. E. (2000). Electromechanical coupling between skeletal and cardiac muscle. Implications for infarct repair. *J Cell Biol,* 149(3), pp. 731-740.

Rolletschek, A., Blyszczuk, P., and Wobus, A. M. (2004). Embryonic stem cell-derived cardiac, neuronal and pancreatic cells as model systems to study toxicological effects. *Toxicol Lett,* 149(1-3), pp. 361-369.

Siminiak, T., Kalawski, R., Fiszer, D., Jerzykowska, O., Rzezniczak, J., Rozwadowska, N., and Kurpisz, M. (2004). Autologous skeletal myoblast transplantation for the treatment of postinfarction myocardial injury: phase I clinical study with 12 months of follow-up. *Am Heart J,* 148(3), pp. 531-537.

Siminiak, T., Fiszer, D., Jerzykowska, O., Grygielska, B., Rozwadowska, N., Kalmucki, P., and Kurpisz, M. (2005). Percutaneous trans-coronary-venous transplantation of autologous skeletal myoblasts in the treatment of post-infarction myocardial contractility impairment: the POZNAN trial. *Eur Heart J,* 26(12), pp. 1188-1195.

Smith, R. R., Barile, L., Cho, H. C., Leppo, M. K., Hare, J. M., Messina, E., Giacomello, A., Abraham, M. R., and Marban, E. (2007). Regenerative potential of cardiosphere-derived cells expanded from percutaneous endomyocardial biopsy specimens. *Circulation,* 115(7), pp. 896-908.

Smits, P. C., van Geuns, R. J., Poldermans, D., Bountioukos, M., Onderwater, E. E., Lee, C. H., Maat, A. P., and Serruys, P. W. (2003). Catheter-based intramyocardial injection of autologous skeletal myoblasts as a primary treatment of ischemic heart failure: clinical experience with six-month follow-up. *J Am Coll Cardiol,* 42(12), pp. 2063-2069.

Strauer, B. E., Brehm, M., Zeus, T., Kostering, M., Hernandez, A., Sorg, R. V., Kogler, G., and Wernet, P. (2002). Repair of infarcted myocardium by autologous intracoronary mononuclear bone marrow cell transplantation in humans. *Circulation,* 106(15), pp. 1913-1918.

Tang, J., Xie, Q., Pan, G., Wang, J., and Wang, M. (2006). Mesenchymal stem cells participate in angiogenesis and improve heart function in rat model of myocardial ischemia with reperfusion. *Eur J Cardiothorac Surg,* 30(2), pp. 353-361.

Terrovitis, J. V., Bulte, J. W., Sarvananthan, S., Crowe, L. A., Sarathchandra, P., Batten, P., Sachlos, E., Chester, A. H., Czernuszka, J. T., Firmin, D. N., Taylor, P. M., and Yacoub, M. H. (2006). Magnetic Resonance Imaging of Ferumoxide-Labeled Mesenchymal Stem Cells Seeded on Collagen Scaffolds-Relevance to Tissue Engineering. *Tissue Eng.*

Thom, T., Haase, N., Rosamond, W., Howard, V. J., Rumsfeld, J., Manolio, T., Zheng, Z. J., Flegal, K., O'Donnell, C., Kittner, S., Lloyd-Jones, D., Goff, D. C., Jr., Hong, Y., Adams, R., Friday, G., Furie, K., Gorelick, P., Kissela, B., Marler, J., Meigs, J., Roger, V., Sidney, S., Sorlie, P., Steinberger, J., Wasserthiel-Smoller, S., Wilson,

M., and Wolf, P. (2006). Heart disease and stroke statistics--2006 update: a report from the American Heart Association Statistics Committee and Stroke Statistics Subcommittee. *Circulation,* 113(6), pp. e85-151.

Toma, C., Pittenger, M. F., Cahill, K. S., Byrne, B. J., and Kessler, P. D. (2002). Human mesenchymal stem cells differentiate to a cardiomyocyte phenotype in the adult murine heart. *Circulation,* 105(1), pp. 93-98.

Urbanek, K., Quaini, F., Tasca, G., Torella, D., Castaldo, C., Nadal-Ginard, B., Leri, A., Kajstura, J., Quaini, E., and Anversa, P. (2003). Intense myocyte formation from cardiac stem cells in human cardiac hypertrophy. *Proc Natl Acad Sci USA,* 100(18), pp. 10440-10445.

Urbanek, K., Torella, D., Sheikh, F., De Angelis, A., Nurzynska, D., Silvestri, F., Beltrami, C. A., Bussani, R., Beltrami, A. P., Quaini, F., Bolli, R., Leri, A., Kajstura, J., and Anversa, P. (2005). Myocardial regeneration by activation of multipotent cardiac stem cells in ischemic heart failure. *Proc Natl Acad Sci USA,* 102(24), pp. 8692-8697.

Urbanek, K., Rota, M., Cascapera, S., Bearzi, C., Nascimbene, A., De Angelis, A., Hosoda, T., Chimenti, S., Baker, M., Limana, F., Nurzynska, D., Torella, D., Rotatori, F., Rastaldo, R., Musso, E., Quaini, F., Leri, A., Kajstura, J., and Anversa, P. (2005).Cardiac stem cells possess growth factor-receptor systems that after activation regenerate the infarcted myocardium, improving ventricular function and long-term survival. *Circ Res,* 97(7), pp. 663-673.

Vulliet, P. R., Greeley, M., Halloran, S. M., MacDonald, K. A., and Kittleson, M. D. (2004). Intra-coronary arterial injection of mesenchymal stromal cells and microinfarction in dogs. *Lancet,* 363(9411), pp. 783-784.

Wollert, K. C., Meyer, G. P., Lotz, J., Ringes-Lichtenberg, S., Lippolt, P., Breidenbach, C., Fichtner, S., Korte, T., Hornig, B., Messinger, D., Arseniev, L., Hertenstein, B., Ganser, A., and Drexler, H. (2004). Intracoronary autologous bone-marrow cell transfer after myocardial infarction: the BOOST randomised controlled clinical trial. *Lancet,* 364(9429), pp. 141-148.

9.6 Review Questions

Q9.1   What is congestive heart failure?

Q9.2   Why is research into the regeneration of damaged myocardium important?

Q9.3   True or False: The heart is a terminally differentiated organ.

Q9.4   The heart likely replaces its entire cell population every:
A. month
B. year
C. 4-5 years
D. 20-25 years
E. never

Q9.5   Possible sources of stem cells include:
A. embryonic cells
B. skeletal myoblasts
C. bone morrow cells
D. endothelial cells
E. cardiac cells
F. all of the above

Q9.6   What are cardiac stem cells?

Q9.7   What is a major obstacle to the use of cardiac stem cells for theraputic purposes and how can it be overcome?

Q9.8   How can stem cells be delivered to the heart for theraputic purposes?

Q9.9   Which of the following issues must be resolved prior to widespread clinical applications of cell based therapy for cardiovascular disease?
A. Which cell type is most effective?
B. Who are appropriate patients?
C. When is the optimal timing for therapy?
D. What is the best delivery method?
E. What are the side effects?
F. All of the above

Chapter 10

Gene Therapy for the Heart

Christian Spies, M.D.[1] and Gary L. Schaer, M.D.[2]

[1] The Queen's Medical Center, Queen's Heart
550 S. Beretania St., Suite 300, Honolulu, HI 96813
PH: 808-545-8900; FX: 808-545-8919; EM: cspies@queens.org

[2] Rush University Medical Center, Section of Cardiology
1653 W. Congress Parkway, Jelke 1035, Chicago, IL 60612
PH: 312-942-4655; FX: 312-563-3213; EM: gary.schaer@sbcglobal.net

10.1 Introduction - Rationale for Gene Therapy for Heart Disease, a Clinician's Perspective

A gene is the fundamental physical and functional unit of heredity. The complete set of genes of an organism is called the genome. Genes consist of deoxyribonucleic acid (DNA) organized into 23 pairs of chromosomes in humans. DNA is composed of two long strands of millions of nucleotides. Each gene is composed of an individual sequence of nucleotides that contains information needed to encode one of the 24,000 human proteins (Pennisi, 2003; Ginsburg et al., 2005). The central dogma of molecular biology states that one gene contained in the DNA is transcribed to ribonucleic acid (RNA), which then is translated to a protein (Fig 10.1). Since the genome is located in the nucleus of the cell, transcription takes place inside the nucleus. Following transfer of the RNA into the cytoplasm of the cell, the RNA is translated into a protein. Proteins are key players within the cell. Their duties include functioning as structural elements, serving as enzymes, participate in the communication and development of a cell as either a cell surface receptor or as a secretory signal, such as hormones, cytokines or growth factors. The latter has been mainly used in gene therapy attempts in the past.

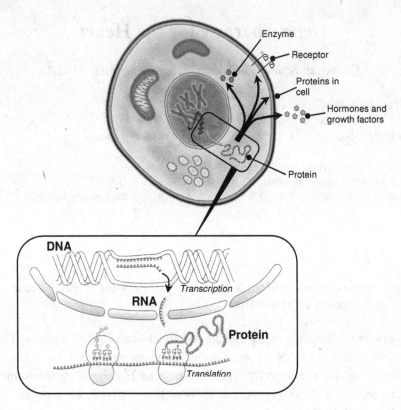

Figure 10.1. Protein biosynthesis (see text).

The transcription process of the DNA of course needs to be regulated, since not all genes or proteins are required at all times in all cells. Although regulation of gene expression can occur on several levels during the process of transcription and translation, certain regulatory DNA sequences play a major role in this context. Rather than get transcribed, these control sequences function to control the expression pattern of an individual gene depending on the cell type in response to different extra cellular signals such as growth factors or hormones. This regulatory DNA, called promoter, enhancer or silencer, according to their primary function, is recognized and bound by specialized nuclear proteins named transcription factors (Novina and Roy, 1996; Kadonaga, 1998). Binding of a transcription factor leads to either promotion or inhibition of gene transcription. Transcription factors have also been targets of gene therapy attempts in the past. The fact that all of the 200 different cell types in the human body originate from a single pluripotent stem cell underlines the complicated task of gene expression. All cells are programmed by their genes to become what they are and to perform with highly specialized functions.

Generally one can categorize genes according to their expression behavior and gene product function. First, genes which are largely concerned with maintenance of cell integrity are expressed in almost all cells are called housekeeping genes. Second, a subset of genes is expressed only in differentiated cells, called lineage-specific genes, which ultimately gives the cell its unique identity and function as a particular cell type. An example for lineage-specific genes are genes encoding for cardiac troponins which are only required in the cardiomyocyte. Third, certain genes are expressed only in response to specific stimuli, what results in a temporal pattern of gene expression tailored to the individual needs of the cell. One example of such a gene, pertinent to potential strategies of gene therapy for the heart, are growth factors such as vascular endothelial growth factor (VEGF) or fibroblast growth factor (FGF). These substances are released as a response to profound ischemia enabling development of new vasculature to overcome ischemia and imminent cell death (Folkman, 1995).

Gene therapy can be defined as the ability to introduce genetic material into cells to produce a therapeutic effect. It can be separated into somatic and germline gene therapy. Gene therapy attempts in humans have been directed at somatic cells, as germline gene therapy remains highly controversial. Somatic gene therapy can be divided into two categories based on the location of cell transduction. During the ex vivo approach cells are transduced with the therapeutic gene outside the body and then re-transplanted into the recipient host. In contrast, in vivo gene therapy involves the transduction of the target cell type in vivo without any cell isolation process or transplantation. This method represents the dominant technique for gene therapy used these days.

Cardiovascular disease is the leading cause of death in the western world (Thom et al., 2006). Despite improved prevention strategies, better medical and surgical therapies, morbidity and mortality of cardiovascular disease remains high. Gene therapy might offer new treatment strategies, specifically for patients not adequately treated with current standard therapy. Potential areas within the spectrum of heart disease are gene therapy for myocardial ischemia, involving therapeutic angiogenesis, the formation of new blood vessels (Isner, 2002). Gene therapy for rescue of contractile function in patients with heart failure is another potential application for this new technology (Nayak and Rosengart, 2005). Inherited genetic disorders leading to premature coronary artery disease (CAD) or congenital heart diseases, such as certain forms of inherited cardiomyopathy or long-QT syndromes are additional possible targets for gene therapy (Baartscheer, 2001; Ikeda et al., 2002). Finally, gene therapy can be used for prevention of intimal hyperplasia following percutaneous intervention (angioplasty procedure) or to prevent vein graft disease following coronary artery bypass surgery (Simons et al., 1992; Mann, 2000). The largest body of evidence of gene therapy for the heart to date has focused on the treatment of chronic myocardial ischemia, which this chapter will focus on.

10.2 The "Limited Option" Patient with Severe Angina

Angina pectoris is caused by a mismatch between supply and demand of oxygen to the heart muscle. It may manifest as pain or discomfort, heaviness, tightness or pressure sensation in the chest, back, neck, throat, jaw or arms. Most commonly, angina is caused by one or more severely blocked coronary arteries due to CAD. Depending on the presentation angina can be separated into unstable or stable angina. Unstable angina is being treated like an acute heart attack, while stable angina is a chronic disease, which is treated more conservatively. Chronic stable angina is more prevalent than the acute coronary syndromes (unstable angina and myocardial infarction). It is estimated, that at least 16 Million Americans suffer from chronic angina (Gibbons et al., 2003). Stable angina can be categorized according to level of physical activity leading to angina pectoris symptoms. The Canadian Cardiovascular Society Functional Classification of stable angina differentiates four classes, of which class 3 and 4 are defined by marked limitation of ordinary physical activity due to angina or even anginal symptoms occurring at rest (Goldmano et al., 1981).

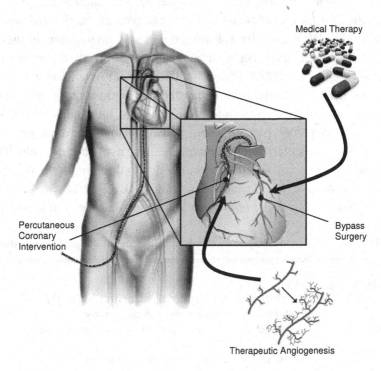

Figure 10.2. Therapeutic options for patients with chronic stable angina.

Stable angina can be treated medically with medications that either improve the oxygen supply or reduce the oxygen demand of the myocardium. The mainstay of medical therapy includes nitrates, beta blockers, calcium channel blockers and more recently ranolazine (Goldman et al., 1981; Chaitman et al., 2004). Revascularization completes the armamentarium available to the treating physician.

Coronary artery bypass surgery and percutaneous coronary intervention are the two revascularization strategies utilized (Fig 10.2).

However, a significant portion of patients may not be candidates for either of these strategies. Common reasons for the inability to perform bypass surgery or percutaneous interventions are largely technical due to unfavorable lesion characteristics or poor, meaning small and calcified, targets for bypass grafts. It is estimated that approximately 5 percent of patients undergoing coronary angiography for angina may not be candidates for those traditional methods of revascularization (Mukherjee et al., 1999). With annually 1.4 million coronary angiograms in the US, around 70,000 patients per year may have significant unmet medical needs (Thom et al., 2006). Patients suffering from severe angina despite maximal medical therapy with exhausted conventional revascularization strategies are referred to as "no-option" patients, although we prefer the term "limited-option" patient. These patients actually have an option of alternative revascularization strategies such as gene or cell based therapies. Besides considering morbidity due to disabling ischemia, these patients also have a high annual mortality of 17 percent (Mukherjee et al., 2001). Table 10.1 summarizes key features of the "limited-option"

Table 10.1. Inclusion and exclusion criteria for candidacy in prior gene therapy trials.

Inclusion Criteria
  o   Stable Canadian Cardiovascular Class 3-4 angina
  o   Refractory to maximum medical therapy
  o   Area of ischemic myocardium on an imaging stress study
  o   Severe coronary artery disease not amenable to traditional revascularization

Exclusion Criteria
  o   Fundoscopic signs of diabetic retinopathy
  o   Severe left ventricular systolic dysfunction
  o   Unstable angina
  o   Concurrent illness with markedly reduced life-expectancy

patient, commonly used as inclusion criteria for gene therapy trials for ischemic heart disease. Maximal medical therapy includes anti-platelet therapy, aggressive lipid lowering strategies, control of hyperglycemia, and of course at all three anti-anginal medications (nitrates, beta blockers and calcium channel blockers), unless contraindicated.

10.3 Therapeutic Angiogenesis – Is this Feasible?

Three different processes result in the growth of new blood vessels: angiogenesis, arteriogeneis and vasculogenesis (Risau, 1997; Simons et al., 2000). The term angiogenesis is used liberally in the cardiovascular community, commonly lumping every form of new vessel growth together. However, one needs to distinguish among those three different aspects of neovascularization. Angiogenesis in its strictest definition describes capillary growth from post-capillary venules, and is mainly stimulated by tissue hypoxia or ischemia involving several mediators, including the transcription factor hypoxia-inducible factor (HIF)-1 (Carmeliet, 2000; Wang et al., 1995). Arteriogensis is a process that produces fully developed arteries, in contrast to angiogenesis, usually sufficiently large to be visualized with angiography (Helisch and Schaper, 2003; de Muinck and Simons, 2004). This process occurs mainly by maturation of preexisting arteriolar collateral connections by remodeling or, perhaps, via de novo growth of collateral conduits (Arras et al., 1998). Among the factors involved in this process are VEGF, FGF and platelet-derived growth factor (PDGF) (Helisch and Schaper, 2003; Carmeliet, 2000). Finally, vasculogenesis is the formation of new vessels in situ directly from endothelial progenitor cells and angioblasts (Flamme and Risau, 1992; Risau and Flamme, 1995). Until recently, vasculogenesis was thought to be restricted to embryonic development. However, recent data suggests that postnatal vasculogenesis occurs (Asahara et al., 1997; Asahara et al., 1999; Takahashi et al., 1999; Kalka et al., 2000). It is now believed that angiogenesis together with vasculogensis contributes to neovascularization in adult cardiac tissues (Luttun and Carmeliet, 2003). A well known fact is that the native biologic response to vascular occlusion is development of collaterals and up-regulation of naturally occurring angiogens. Therapeutic angiogenesis is defined very broadly as a therapeutic intervention which seeks to induce growth of new vessels in tissues compromised by arterial occlusions in order to improve blood supply and relieve ischemia. These interventions may include: (A) delivery of angiogenic factors as a protein or gene to the ischemic area; (B) supply of endothelial progenitor cells; or (C) mobilization of endogenous progenitor cells (Tirziu and Simons, 2005).

With current technology, gene therapy-derived blood vessels are usually about 100 micrometers in diameter. The larger through gene therapy generated vessels are visible on conventional angiography. However, the majority of smaller gene therapy-derived blood vessels are likely to be missed on angiograms. Further, whether these artificially grown arteries have the same features of regular arteries in terms of endothelial function, compliance and resistance is unclear.

Besides the prior elucidated potential benefits of therapeutic angiogenesis for the treatment of ischemic heart disease, potential risks of the use of angiogens needs to be considered as well. Much concern was expressed initially because of the possible detrimental pro-angiogenic effect on atherosclerosis and malignancies. Pathologic angiogenesis plays a critical role in the development and progression of these diseases (Folkman, 1971; Barger et al., 1984). Further, supra-physiologic doses of VEGF were found to cause angiomas in rodents. Neither of these concerns was found to occur in humans, albeit patients with a history of cancer or active malignancy were excluded from trials (van der, Murohara et al., 1997; Lee et al., 2000) (Tab. 10.1). Another field of possible "off-target" angiogenesis is the development of proliferative retinopathy by angiogenic growth factors (Aiello et al., 1994). Clinical studies to date have not supported that exacerbation of proliferative retinopathy is a potential side effect of therapeutic angiogenesis in humans.

10.4 Which Gene Product to Choose?

Different classes of gene products are involved in the physiologic process of angiogenesis, which are potential candidates for gene therapy. These include growth factors, transcription factors, certain chemokines and extracellular matrix proteins. The group best studied to date is the growth factors. Among those, VEGF and FGF are the best characterized angiogens. The VEGF family comprises 5 closely related genes: VEGF-A to –D, and placenta-derived growth factor (PDGF) (Yancopoulos et al., 2000; Ferrara et al., 2003). VEGF-A has several isoforms that differ by their amino acid length, of which VEGF-A121 and VEGF-A165 are most widely studied in clinical trials. Since VEGF-A and VEGF-B preferentially bind to the VEGF receptors 1 and 2, expressed on endothelial cells and hematopoetic stem cells, their potential for clinical relevant therapeutic angiogenesis was judged to be highest. Contrarily, VEGF-C and –D binds mainly to the receptor types 2 and 3, contributing to lymphangiogenesis. Placenta growth factor (PIGF) was also found to be a potent activator of VEGF receptor 1 and an amplifier of the VEGF receptor 2 signaling cascade, for which reason PIGF can also be considered an attractive target for gene therapy (Park et al., 1994; Walsh and Grant, 1997).

Of the 23 different FGF family members, FGF-1, FGF-2, and FGF-4 are highly angiogenic and thus have been the focus of attention in recent clinical trials of therapeutic angiogenesis (Horowitz et al., 2002; Friesel and Maciag, 1995). FGF receptors are found on endothelial cells, smooth muscle cells and myoblasts. Their activation leads to proliferation of the respective cell type (Presta et al., 2005). Physiologically, FGF likely acts synergistically with VEGF in the process of arteriogenesis. Other angiogens include hepatocyte growth factor, which exhibits its angiogenic activity via induction of VEGF (Hayashi et al., 1999; Mukherjee, 2004). Angiopoetin-1, as well as neurotrophin nerve growth factor, erythropoietin, and insulin-like growth factor are further potential candidates for therapeutic angiogenesis (Fig 10.3) (Shyu et al., 1998).

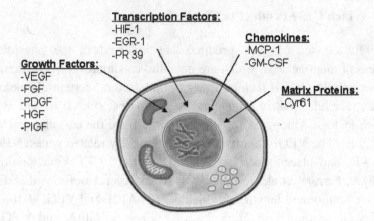

Figure 10.3. Potential candidate genes for therapeutic angiogenesis. For explanation of abbreviations see text.

A second class of candidate genes represents chemokines, such as monocyte chemoattractant protein-1 and granulocyte-macrophage colony stimulating factors, both acting on monocytic cells involved in angiogenesis (Ito et al., 1997; Schaper and Scholz, 2003). Finally, transcription factors like HIF-1 or early growth response protein (EGR-1) can upregulate the expression of angiogens (Fahmy et al., 2003). HIF-1 activates the transcription of several genes involved in the angiogenesis and arteriogenesis including VGEF, thus it is another promising target for gene therapy (Guillemin and Krasnow, 1997). PR39, which increases HIF-1 or extracellular matrix proteins, such as Cyr61 may also be useful targets for human gene therapy given their possible involvement in the complex mechanism of neovascularization (Schaper and Scholz, 2003; Li et al., 2000; Babic et al., 1998).

When considering therapeutic angiogenesis approaches, one needs to consider the vehicles used for delivery of the DNA. Four vector systems can be differentiated: (1) "naked" plasmid DNA, (2) replication defective adenoviruses, (3) replication defective adeno-associated viruses (AAV) and (4) retro- or lentiviruses. Each vector system has its advantages and disadvantages. Naked DNA vectors require direct intramuscular injection, because degradation by circulating nucleases prohibits its systemic or intravascular administration (Wolff et al., 1992; Tsurumi et al., 1996). Simplicity of their production and their inability to produce off-target transduction following their intramyocardial delivery are advantages. However, the very poor transduction efficacy of cardiomyocytes on the other hand is a major disadvantage of this vehicle (Lin et al., 1990; Kitsis et al., 1991). Adenoviral vectors are double-stranded DNA viruses. They can be readily produced as replication deficient mutants for gene transfer applications (Kozarsky and Wilson, 1993). Their advantages include very high transfection efficiency, although more complicated than naked DNA, a relatively simple production of large amounts of virus and the ability to deliver adenoviruses via the vascular system (intravenous or intracoronary). However, neutralizing antibodies are common in humans and may elicit an inflammatory response compromising gene incorporation and expression (Gilgenkrantz et al., 1995). Adeno-associated viruses are single-stranded DNA viruses that are by its nature nonpathogenic to humans (Rabinowitz and Samulski, 1998). Unlike adenoviruses, AAV vectors do not cause significant inflammatory or immune responses. Transfection rates appear comparable to adenoviruses. The major limitation of AAVs is the difficulty to produce large amounts of vectors and the relative small size of foreign gene product the virus can accommodate (Lynch et al., 1997). Retroviruses and lentiviruses are RNA viruses that actually integrate their reverse transcribed DNA into the host genome, rather than keeping the transfected gene extrachromosomal as do the other vectors. Generally this may lead to very long lasting expression, which simultaneously raises safety concerns related to its potential for overexpression (Simons et al., 2000). Further, since retroviruses require cell proliferation for efficient infection, their use in cardiovascular gene therapies will be very limited since cardiomyocytes are largely resting cells (Vile et al., 1996).

10.5 Modes of Gene Delivery

The therapeutic potency of therapeutic angiogenesis is largely affected by physical targeting, the specific delivery of the gene to the area of interest. When considering the mode of gene delivery one must consider not only the fact, that the gene needs to find its way into the cell, it also has to make it into the cell nucleus; a fact which can not be influenced by the general mode of delivery, rather than the vehicle used. Thus, identifying the right combination of gene vehicle and delivery method is crucial in order to enable optimal results. Until today, the right combination has not been found yet. Generally three routes of gene delivery are available: intravenous administration, intracoronary injection or intramuscular delivery (Fig 10.4).

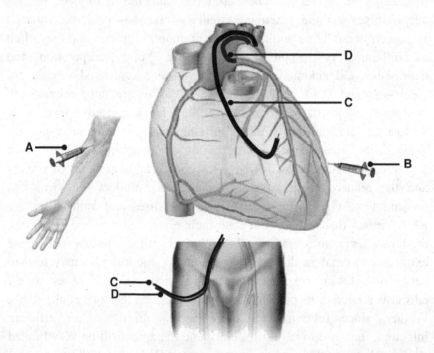

Figure 10.4. Modes of genes delivery. A: intravenous, B: direct intramyocardial, C: catheter delivered intramyocardial, D: intracoronary (intra-arterial).

It is true and intuitive to assume that systemic, intravenous application may result in the poorest delivery rate and outcome. Further, systemic exposure of viral vectors should be avoided in order to prevent transfection and potential harmful induction of angiogenesis in non-target tissue. More selective intra-coronary, transcatheter gene transfer has been safely performed in humans; although initial studies using this route of delivery administered the angiogenic protein rather than the gene (Grines et al., 2002; Simons et al., 2002; Henry et al., 2003).

Nevertheless, injection of gene vectors into the arterial circulation does not necessarily ensure transfection of the cardiomycocytes, which again mainly depends on the vehicle chosen. Whether intramycocardial injection of genes is advantageous to intra-coronary infusion needs to be determined. Although the vehicles do not have to overcome the endothelial barrier, the gene vectors are essentially sitting in the interstitium waiting to enter the surrounding myocytes. Several catheter systems have been developed for percutaneous delivery of the gene. These catheters have in common a deflectable tip to maneuver the catheter to the ischemic area of the myocardium. Once determined to be in the correct location, a needle can be extended out of the tip entering the cardiac muscle when the vector gets injected. Potential problems with these catheters include the risk for cardiac perforation, the production of local tissue damage when injecting into the myocardium and leak of vector into the systemic circulation.

To date, the optimal delivery mode remains unknown. Most investigators are committed to either the intracoronary infusion or intramyocardial injection; a head to head comparison of these methods has not been done. A modified approach of intramuscular gene delivery is injection of the vehicle under direct visualization as an adjunctive therapy at the time of coronary artery bypass surgery. This has already been done in human phase 1 trials (Schumacher et al., 1998; Laham et al., 1999). However, the patient collective for which this technology can be applied is clearly different then the limited option patient, given the fact that they are candidates for coronary artery bypass surgery. Another approach at the horizon is the injection of biodegradable microspheres coated with vectors of recombinant growth factors which can be targeted with ultrasonography techniques to the area of interest (Arras et al., 1998). These microspheres can be given intravenously and ultrasound waves, selectively applied to the heart region locally deliver the vector.

10.6 Results of Randomized Controlled Clinical Trials of Gene Therapy

Angiogenesis has been shown to work well in preclinical models. To date, several human phase 1 trials have also been reported. These studies are small, non-controlled and non-blinded, simply serving the purpose of proof-of-concept and establishing the safety profile of the study agent. In essence, all these trials revealed therapeutic angiogenesis to be safe, regardless of the vehicle or delivery route chosen (Hendel et al., 2000; Udelson et al., 2000; Unger et al., 2000; Vale et al., 2001; Losordo et al., 2002). Although these trials were not designed to evaluate efficacy of gene therapy in patients with heart disease, the data derived from these early trials showed promise that preclinical data will translate successfully into human experiments. The observed improvement in symptoms and myocardial function following gene therapy in patients with ischemic heart disease caused much excitement and let to the development of larger phase 2 trials. Although the field of therapeutic angiogenesis if a decade old only a handful of randomized controlled trials have been successfully completed to date. The first two such trials actually evaluated the effects of the protein-based gene products of VEGF in the Vascular endothelial growth factor in Ischemia for Vascular Angiogenesis "VIVA" trial and FGF in the FGF-2 Initiating Revascularization Support Trial "FIRST" (Henry et al., 2003; Simons et al., 2002). Both trials included limited option patients with chronic angina who received the angiogenic protein via intra-coronary infusion. Neither trial reached its primary endpoint, change in exercise tolerance, although the VIVA trial patients who received a higher protein dose had less angina.

Almost simultaneously, the first series using actual gene therapy for therapeutic angiogenesis in patients with chronic angina was published. The Angiogenic GENe Therapy "AGENT" 1 and 2 trials were small randomized, double-blind, placebo controlled trials of intra-coronary injection of adenoviruses encoding FGF-4 genes (Ad5FGF-4) (Grines et al., 2002; Grines et al., 2003). In AGENT 1, 79 limited option patients were treated with an escalating dose regimen. As with the protein based studies, a large placebo effect was noticed; nevertheless, the authors found in patients with poor exercise tolerance a statistically significant increase in exercise treadmill time in participants treated with the gene compared to those who received placebo. Following establishment of safety and possible efficacy of this methodology, the AGENT 2 trial was conducted. This more clinically oriented trial included 52 patients recruited from 13 U.S. centers. Inclusion criteria mandated nine percent of the left ventricle of patients with chronic stable angina to be ischemic, according to myocardial perfusion imaging studies. Patients underwent single dose intra-coronary administration of Ad5FGF-4. At eight weeks follow up, patients underwent repeat myocardial perfusion imaging. Although statistically non-significant, patients receiving the active treatment had a greater reduction in quantified ischemic burden compared to those who were treated with placebo (4.2% vs. 1.6% reduction in ischemic myocardium, p=0.14). Following exclusion of one outlier however, resulted in a significant difference (4.2% vs. 0.8% reduction, p<0.05). Somewhat unexpectedly, these encouraging results could not be transferred to the larger AGENT 3 trial. This 415 patients large trial has not been published yet. Preliminary results presented in 2005 revealed no difference in exercise treadmill time 12 weeks following therapy with Ad5FGF-4 or placebo. A pre-specified subgroup analysis, however, revealed that patients older than 55 years with more severe angina had a statistically significant greater increase in exercise treadmill time compared to those treated with placebo.

The first gene therapy trial completed to date evaluating the percutaneous intramyocardial delivery of a gene is the EUROINJECT-ONE trial (Kastrup et al., 2005; Gyongyosi et al., 2005). Eighty limited option patients with severe chronic stable angina underwent intramyocardial injection of a plasmid containing VEGF-A or placebo. Patients were required to have ischemia demonstrated with myocardial perfusion imaging, which was repeated 3 months following therapy. Despite a sophisticated mapping system to identify ischemic myocardium at the time of delivery, no difference in myocardial perfusion was found between the two study groups during follow up. However, as with prior trials certain aspects showed promising effects of gene therapy. In case of the EUROINJECT-ONE trial, there was an improvement in regional wall motion of the left ventricle seen in those patients treated with VEGF-A.

More recently, results of the NOGA Angiogenesis Revascularization Therapy "Northern" trial have been presented (Stewart and Kutryk, 2007). This was a multicenter, randomized, double blind, placebo controlled trial evaluating intramyocardial injections of VEGF165 in limited option patients with chronic angina. The injections were performed using a percutaneous catheter system which is able to detect areas of poor blood supply via electromechanical mapping (NOGA; Cordis, Warren, NJ). During 6 months follow up, there was no difference between the active treatment arm and placebo among the 120 patients in terms of myocardial perfusion, exercise tolerance or anginal symptom class; although all participants showed improvements compared to baseline. The improvement in myocardial perfusion in both placebo and treatment groups raises the question whether there is a pro-angiogenic therapeutic effect regardless of the substance injected, despite an apparent lack of efficacy of simple VEGF gene transfer.

The largest planned randomized controlled trial evaluating intramyocardial injection of VEGF in the U.S. to date has been the Genetic Angiogenic Stimlation Investigational Study "GENASIS". It was planned to enroll over 400 patients at approximately 20 sites. With inclusion criteria for patients similar to prior trials, participants underwent either percutaneous intramyocardial delivery of VEGF or placebo. After enrollment of 295 patients, the trial was stopped prematurely due to safety concerns related to the delivery catheter, since an unexpected high number of pericardial effusions following intramyocardial injections were seen. No results have not been published in manuscript format or presented at a scientific meeting yet. However, the study sponsor has issued a press release that the results from the GENASIS trial did not achieve a statistically significant difference from placebo in any active dose group for the primary efficacy endpoint. The primary efficacy endpoint in the GENASIS trial was an improvement of at least one minute in exercise tolerance time from baseline to three months. Again, the investigators found a pronounced placebo effect which was more significant and more sustained than anticipated in the initial design of the GENASIS trial.

10.7 Prior Shortcomings and Future Directions

The initial euphoria of therapeutic angiogenesis as a novel treatment option for patients with coronary artery disease triggered by the phase 1 trials partially subsided after publication of the negative phase 2 studies. This raises the question why the remarkably positive results from animal models as well as phase 1 trials did not translate into clinical practice. The first explanation for treatment failures relates to patient selection. Patients selected for trials of therapeutic angiogenesis tend to be older, often have previously undergone multiple revascularization attempts, usually have extensive disease and have exhausted standard therapeutic options. One can argue that these patients suffer from a failure of natural angiogenic responses, and thus represent the group least likely to respond to gene therapy. A possible mechanism is growth factor resistance from down-regulated receptors leading to a blunted or absent response to the administration of angiogenic factor. The choice of therapeutic agent and route of administration is another important aspect to consider in this context. Pharmacokinetics and pharmacodynamics of a variety of vectors and genes are largely unknown (Pislaru et al., 2002). Since several cofactors affect the optimal dose of the agents, such as the vehicle used, or the route of delivery chosen, identifying the optimal combination of agent, vehicle and route will take some time. Nevertheless, the excitement for therapeutic angiogenesis in patients with ischemic heart disease is ongoing. Obviously, trials with more participants and longer follow up times are needed. Eventually two general questions need to be answered which go beyond study design issues or the single evaluation of various potential candidate genes. First, to be effective in patients with CAD, should gene therapy induce angiogenesis or arteriogenesis? In other words, is the development of capillaries sufficient to improve blood flow and symptoms in patients with chronic angina, or are newly formed arterial conduits necessary to achieve this goal. Second, are we able to achieve clinical meaningful results in therapeutic angiogenesis with a single agent in general? Considering the complexity of physiologic angiogenesis, future research may need to focus on multiagent therapy to mimic the complex process of angiogenesis in humans.

10.8 References

Aiello, L. P., Avery, R. L., Arrigg, P. G., Keyt, B. A., Jampel, H. D., Shah, S. T., Pasquale, L. R., Thieme, H., Iwamoto, M. A., Park, J. E., . (1994). Vascular endothelial growth factor in ocular fluid of patients with diabetic retinopathy and other retinal disorders. N Engl J Med, 331, pp. 1480-7.

Arras, M., Ito, W. D., Scholz, D., Winkler, B., Schaper, J., Schaper, W. (1998). Monocyte activation in angiogenesis and collateral growth in the rabbit hindlimb. J Clin Invest, 101, pp. 40-50.

Arras, M., Mollnau, H., Strasser, R., Wenz, R., Ito, W. D., Schaper, J., Schaper, W. (1998). The delivery of angiogenic factors to the heart by microsphere therapy. Nat Biotechnol, 16, pp. 159-62.

Asahara, T., Murohara, T., Sullivan, A., Silver, M., van der, Z. R., Li, T., Witzenbichler, B., Schatteman, G., Isner, J. M. (1997). Isolation of putative progenitor endothelial cells for angiogenesis. Science, 275, pp. 964-7.

Asahara, T., Takahashi, T., Masuda, H., Kalka, C., Chen, D., Iwaguro, H., Inai, Y., Silver, M., Isner, J. M. (1999). VEGF contributes to postnatal neovascularization by mobilizing bone marrow-derived endothelial progenitor cells. EMBO J, 18, pp. 3964-72.

Baartscheer, A. (2001). Adenovirus gene transfer of SERCA in heart failure. A promising therapeutic approach ? Cardiovasc Res, 49, pp. 249-52.

Babic, A. M., Kireeva, M. L., Kolesnikova, T. V., Lau, L. F. (1998). CYR61, a product of a growth factor-inducible immediate early gene, promotes angiogenesis and tumor growth. Proc Natl Acad Sci USA, 95, pp. 6355-60.

Barger, A. C., Beeuwkes, R., III, Lainey, L. L., Silverman, K. J. (1984). Hypothesis: vasa vasorum and neovascularization of human coronary arteries. A possible role in the pathophysiology of atherosclerosis. N Engl J Med, 310, pp. 175-7.

Carmeliet, P. (2000). Mechanisms of angiogenesis and arteriogenesis. Nat Med, 6, pp. 389-95.

Chaitman, B. R., Pepine, C. J., Parker, J. O., Skopal, J., Chumakova, G., Kuch, J., Wang, W., Skettino, S. L., Wolff, A. A. (2004). Effects of ranolazine with atenolol, amlodipine, or diltiazem on exercise tolerance and angina frequency in patients with severe chronic angina: a randomized controlled trial. JAMA, 291, pp. 309-16.

de Muinck, E. D., Simons, M. (2004). Re-evaluating therapeutic neovascularization. J Mol Cell Cardiol, 36, pp. 25-32.

Fahmy, R. G., Dass, C. R., Sun, L. Q., Chesterman, C. N., Khachigian, L. M. (2003). Transcription factor Egr-1 supports FGF-dependent angiogenesis during neovascularization and tumor growth. Nat Med, 9, pp. 1026-32.

Ferrara, N., Gerber, H. P., LeCouter, J. (2003). The biology of VEGF and its receptors. Nat Med, 9, pp. 669-76.

Flamme, I., Risau, W. (1992). Induction of vasculogenesis and hematopoiesis in vitro. Development, 116, pp. 435-9.

Folkman, J. (1995). Angiogenesis in cancer, vascular, rheumatoid and other disease. Nat Med, 1, pp. 27-31.

Folkman, J. (1971). Tumor angiogenesis: therapeutic implications. N Engl J Med, 285, pp. 1182-6.

Friesel, R. E., Maciag, T. (1995). Molecular mechanisms of angiogenesis: fibroblast growth factor signal transduction. FASEB J, 9, pp. 919-25.

Gibbons, R. J., Abrams, J., Chatterjee, K., Daley, J., Deedwania, P. C., Douglas, J. S., Ferguson, T. B., Jr., Fihn, S. D., Fraker, T. D., Jr., Gardin, J. M., O'Rourke, R. A., Pasternak, R. C., Williams, S. V., Gibbons, R. J., Alpert, J. S., Antman, E. M., Hiratzka, L. F., Fuster, V., Faxon, D. P., Gregoratos, G., Jacobs, A. K., Smith, S. C., Jr. (2003). ACC/AHA 2002 guideline update for the management of patients with chronic stable angina--summary article: a report of the American College of Cardiology/American Heart Association Task Force on Practice Guidelines (Committee on the Management of Patients With Chronic Stable Angina). Circulation, 107, pp. 149-58.

Gilgenkrantz, H., Duboc, D., Juillard, V., Couton, D., Pavirani, A., Guillet, J. G., Briand, P., Kahn, A. (1995). Transient expression of genes transferred in vivo into heart using first-generation adenoviral vectors: role of the immune response. Hum Gene Ther, 6, pp. 1265-74.

Ginsburg, G. S., Donahue, M. P., Newby, L. K. (2005). Prospects for personalized cardiovascular medicine: the impact of genomics. J Am Coll Cardiol, 46, pp. 1615-27.

Goldman, L., Hashimoto, B., Cook, E. F., Loscalzo, A. (1981). Comparative reproducibility and validity of systems for assessing cardiovascular functional class: advantages of a new specific activity scale. Circulation, 64, pp. 1227-34.

Grines, C. L., Watkins, M. W., Helmer, G., Penny, W., Brinker, J., Marmur, J. D., West, A., Rade, J. J., Marrott, P., Hammond, H. K., Engler, R. L. (2002). Angiogenic Gene Therapy (AGENT) trial in patients with stable angina pectoris. Circulation, 105, pp. 1291-7.

Grines, C. L., Watkins, M. W., Mahmarian, J. J., Iskandrian, A. E., Rade, J. J., Marrott, P., Pratt, C., Kleiman, N. (2003). A randomized, double-blind, placebo-controlled trial of Ad5FGF-4 gene therapy and its effect on myocardial perfusion in patients with stable angina. J Am Coll Cardiol, 42, pp. 1339-47.

Guillemin, K., Krasnow, M. A. (1997). The hypoxic response: huffing and HIFing. Cell, 89, pp. 9-12.

Gyongyosi, M., Khorsand, A., Zamini, S., Sperker, W., Strehblow, C., Kastrup, J., Jorgensen, E., Hesse, B., Tagil, K., Botker, H. E., Ruzyllo, W., Teresinska, A., Dudek, D., Hubalewska, A., Ruck, A., Nielsen, S. S., Graf, S., Mundigler, G., Novak, J., Sochor, H., Maurer, G., Glogar, D., Sylven, C. (2005). NOGA-guided analysis of regional myocardial perfusion abnormalities treated with intramyocardial injections of plasmid encoding vascular endothelial growth factor A-165 in patients with chronic myocardial ischemia: subanalysis of the EUROINJECT-ONE multicenter double-blind randomized study. Circulation, 112, pp. I157-I165.

Hayashi, S., Morishita, R., Nakamura, S., Yamamoto, K., Moriguchi, A., Nagano, T., Taiji, M., Noguchi, H., Matsumoto, K., Nakamura, T., Higaki, J., Ogihara, T. (1999). Potential role of hepatocyte growth factor, a novel angiogenic growth factor, in peripheral arterial disease: downregulation of HGF in response to hypoxia in vascular cells. Circulation, 100, pp. II301-II308.

Helisch, A., Schaper, W. (2003). Arteriogenesis: the development and growth of collateral arteries. Microcirculation, 10, pp. 83-97.

Hendel, R. C., Henry, T. D., Rocha-Singh, K., Isner, J. M., Kereiakes, D. J., Giordano, F. J., Simons, M., Bonow, R. O. (2000). Effect of intracoronary recombinant human vascular endothelial growth factor on myocardial perfusion: evidence for a dose-dependent effect. Circulation, 101, pp. 118-21.

Henry, T. D., Annex, B. H., McKendall, G. R., Azrin, M. A., Lopez, J. J., Giordano, F. J., Shah, P. K., Willerson, J. T., Benza, R. L., Berman, D. S., Gibson, C. M., Bajamonde, A., Rundle, A. C., Fine, J., McCluskey, E. R. (2003). The VIVA trial: Vascular endothelial growth factor in Ischemia for Vascular Angiogenesis. Circulation, 107, pp. 1359-65.

Horowitz, A., Tkachenko, E., Simons, M. (2002). Fibroblast growth factor-specific modulation of cellular response by syndecan-4. J Cell Biol, 157, pp. 715-25.

Ikeda, Y., Gu, Y., Iwanaga, Y., Hoshijima, M., Oh, S. S., Giordano, F. J., Chen, J., Nigro, V., Peterson, K. L., Chien, K. R., Ross, J., Jr. (2002). Restoration of deficient membrane proteins in the cardiomyopathic hamster by in vivo cardiac gene transfer. Circulation, 105, pp. 502-8.

Isner, J. M. (2002). Myocardial gene therapy. Nature, 415, pp. 234-9.

Ito, W. D., Arras, M., Winkler, B., Scholz, D., Schaper, J., Schaper, W. (1997). Monocyte chemotactic protein-1 increases collateral and peripheral conductance after femoral artery occlusion. Circ Res, 80, pp. 829-37.

Kadonaga, J. T. (1998). Eukaryotic transcription: an interlaced network of transcription factors and chromatin-modifying machines. Cell, 92, pp. 307-13.

Kalka, C., Masuda, H., Takahashi, T., Kalka-Moll, W. M., Silver, M., Kearney, M., Li, T., Isner, J. M., Asahara, T. (2000). Transplantation of ex vivo expanded endothelial progenitor cells for therapeutic neovascularization. Proc Natl Acad Sci USA, 97, pp. 3422-7.

Kastrup, J., Jorgensen, E., Ruck, A., Tagil, K., Glogar, D., Ruzyllo, W., Botker, H. E., Dudek, D., Drvota, V., Hesse, B., Thuesen, L., Blomberg, P., Gyongyosi, M., Sylven, C. (2005). Direct intramyocardial plasmid vascular endothelial growth factor-A165 gene therapy in patients with stable severe angina pectoris A randomized double-blind placebo-controlled study: the Euroinject One trial. J Am Coll Cardiol, 45, pp. 982-8.

Kitsis, R. N., Buttrick, P. M., McNally, E. M., Kaplan, M. L., Leinwand, L. A. (1991). Hormonal modulation of a gene injected into rat heart in vivo. Proc Natl Acad Sci USA, 88, pp. 4138-42.

Kozarsky, K. F., Wilson, J. M. (1993). Gene therapy: adenovirus vectors. Curr Opin Genet Dev, 3, pp. 499-503.

Laham, R. J., Sellke, F. W., Edelman, E. R., Pearlman, J. D., Ware, J. A., Brown, D. L., Gold, J. P., Simons, M. (1999). Local perivascular delivery of basic fibroblast growth factor in patients undergoing coronary bypass surgery: results of a phase I randomized, double-blind, placebo-controlled trial. Circulation, 100, pp. 1865-71.

Lee, R. J., Springer, M. L., Blanco-Bose, W. E., Shaw, R., Ursell, P. C., Blau, H. M. (2000). VEGF gene delivery to myocardium: deleterious effects of unregulated expression. Circulation, 102, pp. 898-901.

Li, J., Post, M., Volk, R., Gao, Y., Li, M., Metais, C., Sato, K., Tsai, J., Aird, W., Rosenberg, R. D., Hampton, T. G., Sellke, F., Carmeliet, P., Simons, M. (2000). PR39, a peptide regulator of angiogenesis. Nat Med, 6, pp. 49-55.

Lin, H., Parmacek, M. S., Morle, G., Bolling, S., Leiden, J. M. (1990). Expression of recombinant genes in myocardium in vivo after direct injection of DNA. Circulation, 82, pp. 2217-21.

Losordo, D. W., Vale, P. R., Hendel, R. C., Milliken, C. E., Fortuin, F. D., Cummings, N., Schatz, R. A., Asahara, T., Isner, J. M., Kuntz, R. E. (2002). Phase 1/2 placebo-controlled, double-blind, dose-escalating trial of myocardial vascular endothelial growth factor 2 gene transfer by catheter delivery in patients with chronic myocardial ischemia. Circulation, 105, pp. 2012-8.

Luttun, A., Carmeliet, P. (2003). De novo vasculogenesis in the heart. Cardiovasc Res, 58, pp. 378-89.

Lynch, C. M., Hara, P. S., Leonard, J. C., Williams, J. K., Dean, R. H., Geary, R. L. (1997). Adeno-associated virus vectors for vascular gene delivery. Circ Res, 80, pp. 497-505.

Mann, M. J. (2000). Gene therapy for vein grafts. Curr Cardiol Rep, 2, pp. 29-33.

Mukherjee, D. (2004). Current clinical perspectives on myocardial angiogenesis. Mol Cell Biochem, 264, pp. 157-67.

Mukherjee, D., Bhatt, D. L., Roe, M. T., Patel, V., Ellis, S. G. (1999). Direct myocardial revascularization and angiogenesis--how many patients might be eligible? Am J Cardiol, 84, pp. 598-600, A8.

Mukherjee, D., Comella, K., Bhatt, D. L., Roe, M. T., Patel, V., Ellis, S. G. (2001). Clinical outcome of a cohort of patients eligible for therapeutic angiogenesis or transmyocardial revascularization. Am Heart J, 142, pp. 72-4.

Nayak, L., Rosengart, T. K, (2005). Gene therapy for heart failure. Semin Thorac Cardiovasc Surg, 17, pp. 343-7.

Novina, C. D., Roy, A. L. (1996). Core promoters and transcriptional control. Trends Genet, 12, pp. 351-5.

Park, J. E., Chen, H. H., Winer, J., Houck, K. A., Ferrara, N. (1994). Placenta growth factor. Potentiation of vascular endothelial growth factor bioactivity, in vitro and in vivo, and high affinity binding to Flt-1 but not to Flk-1/KDR. J Biol Chem, 269, pp. 25646-54.

Pennisi, E. (2003). Human genome. A low number wins the GeneSweep Pool. Science, 300, p. 1484.

Pislaru, S., Janssens, S. P., Gersh, B. J., Simari, R. D. (2002). Defining gene transfer before expecting gene therapy: putting the horse before the cart. Circulation, 106, pp. 631-6.

Presta, M., Dell'Era, P., Mitola, S., Moroni, E., Ronca, R., Rusnati, M. (2005). Fibroblast growth factor/fibroblast growth factor receptor system in angiogenesis. Cytokine Growth Factor Rev, 16, pp. 159-78.

Rabinowitz, J. E., Samulski, J. (1998). Adeno-associated virus expression systems for gene transfer. Curr Opin Biotechnol, 9, pp. 470-5.

Risau, W. (1997). Mechanisms of angiogenesis. Nature, 386, pp. 671-4.

Risau, W., Flamme, I. (1995). Vasculogenesis. Annu Rev Cell Dev Biol, 11, pp. 73-91.

Schaper, W., Scholz, D. (2003). Factors regulating arteriogenesis. Arterioscler Thromb Vasc Biol, 23, pp. 1143-51.

Schumacher, B., Pecher, P., von Specht, B. U., Stegmann, T. (1998). Induction of neoangiogenesis in ischemic myocardium by human growth factors: first clinical results of a new treatment of coronary heart disease. Circulation, 97, pp. 645-50.

Shyu, K. G., Manor, O., Magner, M., Yancopoulos, G. D., Isner, J. M. (1998). Direct intramuscular injection of plasmid DNA encoding angiopoietin-1 but not angiopoietin-2 augments revascularization in the rabbit ischemic hindlimb. Circulation, 98, pp. 2081-7.

Simons, M., Annex, B. H., Laham, R. J., Kleiman, N., Henry, T., Dauerman, H., Udelson, J. E., Gervino, E. V., Pike, M., Whitehouse, M. J., Moon, T., Chronos, N. A. (2002). Pharmacological treatment of coronary artery disease with recombinant fibroblast growth factor-2: double-blind, randomized, controlled clinical trial. Circulation, 105, pp. 788-93.

Simons, M., Bonow, R. O., Chronos, N. A., Cohen, D. J., Giordano, F. J., Hammond, H. K., Laham, R. J., Li, W., Pike, M., Sellke, F. W., Stegmann, T. J., Udelson, J. E., Rosengart, T. K. (2000). Clinical trials in coronary angiogenesis: issues, problems, consensus: An expert panel summary. Circulation, 102, pp. E73-E86.

Simons, M., Edelman, E. R., DeKeyser, J. L., Langer, R., Rosenberg, R. D. (1992). Antisense c-myb oligonucleotides inhibit intimal arterial smooth muscle cell accumulation in vivo. Nature, 359, pp. 67-70.

Stewart, D. J., Kutryk, M.J.B. (2007). The NORTHERN Trial: A Prospective, Randomized, Double Blind Placebo-Controlled Evaluation of Intramyocardial VEGF165 Plasmid Gene Transfer in Patients with Refractory Angina. Presented at Transcatheter Therapeutics, Washington, D.C. on 10-24-2007.

Takahashi, T., Kalka, C., Masuda, H., Chen, D., Silver, M., Kearney, M., Magner, M., Isner, J. M., Asahara, T. (1999). Ischemia- and cytokine-induced mobilization of bone marrow-derived endothelial progenitor cells for neovascularization. Nat Med, 5, pp. 434-8.

Thom, T., Haase, N., Rosamond, W., Howard, V. J., Rumsfeld, J., Manolio, T., Zheng, Z. J., Flegal, K., O'Donnell, C., Kittner, S., Lloyd-Jones, D., Goff, D. C., Jr., Hong, Y., Adams, R., Friday, G., Furie, K., Gorelick, P., Kissela, B., Marler, J., Meigs, J., Roger, V., Sidney, S., Sorlie, P., Steinberger, J., Wasserthiel-Smoller, S., Wilson, M., Wolf, P. (2006). Heart disease and stroke statistics--2006 update: a report from the American Heart Association Statistics Committee and Stroke Statistics Subcommittee. Circulation, 113, pp. e85-151.

Tirziu, D., Simons, M. (2005). Angiogenesis in the human heart: gene and cell therapy. Angiogenesis, 8, pp. 241-51.

Tsurumi, Y., Takeshita, S., Chen, D., Kearney, M., Rossow, S. T., Passeri, J., Horowitz, J. R., Symes, J. F., Isner, J. M. (1996). Direct intramuscular gene transfer of naked

DNA encoding vascular endothelial growth factor augments collateral development and tissue perfusion. Circulation, 94, pp. 3281-90.

Udelson, J. E., Dilsizian, V., Laham, R. J., Chronos, N., Vansant, J., Blais, M., Galt, J. R., Pike, M., Yoshizawa, C., Simons, M. (2000). Therapeutic angiogenesis with recombinant fibroblast growth factor-2 improves stress and rest myocardial perfusion abnormalities in patients with severe symptomatic chronic coronary artery disease. Circulation, 102, pp. 1605-10.

Unger, E. F., Goncalves, L., Epstein, S. E., Chew, E. Y., Trapnell, C. B., Cannon, R. O., III, Quyyumi, A. A. (2000). Effects of a single intracoronary injection of basic fibroblast growth factor in stable angina pectoris. Am J Cardiol, 85, pp. 1414-9.

Vale, P. R., Losordo, D. W., Milliken, C. E., McDonald, M. C., Gravelin, L. M., Curry, C. M., Esakof, D. D., Maysky, M., Symes, J. F., Isner, J. M. (2001). Randomized, single-blind, placebo-controlled pilot study of catheter-based myocardial gene transfer for therapeutic angiogenesis using left ventricular electromechanical mapping in patients with chronic myocardial ischemia. Circulation, 103, pp. 2138-43.

van der, Z. R., Murohara, T., Luo, Z., Zollmann, F., Passeri, J., Lekutat, C., Isner, J. M. (1997). Vascular endothelial growth factor/vascular permeability factor augments nitric oxide release from quiescent rabbit and human vascular endothelium. Circulation, 95, pp. 1030-7.

Vile, R. G., Tuszynski, A., Castleden, S. (1996). Retroviral vectors. From laboratory tools to molecular medicine. Mol Biotechnol, 5, pp. 139-58.

Walsh, T. P., Grant, G. H. (1997). Computer modelling of the receptor-binding domains of VEGF and PIGF. Protein Eng, 10, pp. 389-98.

Wang, G. L., Jiang, B. H., Rue, E. A., Semenza, G. L. (1995). Hypoxia-inducible factor 1 is a basic-helix-loop-helix-PAS heterodimer regulated by cellular O_2 tension. Proc Natl Acad Sci USA, 92, pp. 5510-4.

Wolff, J. A., Ludtke, J. J., Acsadi, G., Williams, P., Jani, A. (1992). Long-term persistence of plasmid DNA and foreign gene expression in mouse muscle. Hum Mol Genet, 1, pp. 363-9.

Yancopoulos, G. D., Davis, S., Gale, N. W., Rudge, J. S., Wiegand, S. J., Holash, J. (2000). Vascular-specific growth factors and blood vessel formation. Nature, 407, pp. 242-8.

10.9 Glossary of Terms

AAV - Adeno-associated viruses

Beta blocker - A class of drugs that block beta-adrenergic substances such as adrenaline in the "sympathetic" portion of the autonomic nervous system.

CAD - Coronary artery disease

Calcium channel blockers - A drug that blocks the entry of calcium into the muscle cells of the heart and the arteries. By blocking the entry of calcium, calcium channel blocker decrease the contraction of the heart and widen the arteries.

Cardiomyocyte - The muscle cells of heart muscle tissue.

Cardiomyopathy - A disease or disorder of the heart muscle.

Chemokines - Small proteins secreted by cells that have the ability to attract white blood cells.

EGR-1 - Early growth response protein

FGF - Fibroblast growth factor

GM-CSG - Granulocyte-macrophage colony-stimulating factor

HGF - Hepatocyte growth factor

HIF-1 - Hypoxia-inducible factor-1

Hyperplasia - An abnormal increase in the number of cells in an organ or a tissue with consequent enlargement.

MCP-1 - Monocyte chemoattractant protein-1

PDGF - Placenta-derived growth factor

PIGF - Placenta growth factor

PR39 - Peptide regulator 39

Ranolazine - A medication used for treatment of angina. The mechanism of action is believed to be due to selective ion channel inhibition.

Troponin - A structural protein that is integral to muscle contraction in skeletal and cardiac muscle.

VEGF - Vascular endothelial growth factor

10.10 Review Questions

Q10.1 The leading cause of death in the Western world is:
A. congestive heart failure
B. stroke
C. coronary artery disease
D. cancer

Q10.2 Therapeutic angiogenesis attempts in humans have predominantly used germline gene therapy in the past. True or false?

Q10.3 Arteriogenesis produces fully developed arteries. True or false?

Q10.4 In human trial the following genes were most frequently used:
1. VEGF
2. BRCA
3. FGF
4. MLH-1

A. 1 is correct
B. 2 is correct
C. 4 is correct
D. 1 and 3 are correct
E. 1-4 are correct

Q10.5 Gene products cannot be administered without a viral vehicle.
True or false?

Q10.6 Modes of gene delivery to the heart muscle include:
1. Intravenous
2. Intra-myocardial
3. Intra-coronary

A. 1 is correct
B. 2 is correct
C. 3 is correct
D. 2 and 3 are correct
E. 1-3 are correct

Q10.7 "Off-target" angiogenesis in animals has been not been
documented cause:
A. neoplasms
B. retinopathy
C. accelerated atherosclerosis
D. none of the above

Q10.8 "Off-target" angiogenesis in humans has been documented to
cause:
A. neoplasms
B. retinopathy
C. accelerated atherosclerosis
D. none of the above

Q10.9 Human gene therapy trials to date have shown a significant
mortality benefit compared to placebo. True or false?

Chapter 11

Stem Cell Transplantation Therapy for Heart Disease

Wangde Dai, M.D.[1] and Robert A. Kloner, M.D., Ph.D.[1]

[1] The Heart Institute at Good Samaritan Hospital, Keck School of Medicine Univ. of Southern California, 1225 Wilshire Blvd., Los Angeles, CA 90017 Tel. : 213-977-4050; Fax. : 213-977-4107; EM: wangdedai@yahoo.com; EM: rkloner@goodsam.org

11.1 Introduction

The heart is composed primarily of cardiac muscle that serves as a pump to propel blood through the vasculature of the human body. The cardiac muscle receives an abundant blood supply through the coronary arteries. Occlusion of a coronary artery can restrict the blood supply to the myocardium, and result in injury of these muscle cells (cardiomyocytes) and eventual cardiomyocyte death; this process is termed myocardial infarction (heart attack). Because cardiomyocytes are primarily final differentiated cells without the ability to adequately regenerate, loss of cardiomyocytes after myocardial infarction is replaced by fibrosis, and followed by a scar formation. Over time the myocardial infarct thins and dilates, as does the noninfarcted tissue, leading to left ventricular remodeling, and finally resulting in heart failure. Although pharmacotherapy of myocardial infarction and consequent heart failure has improved quality of life, hemodynamics and survival in clinical practice, the benefits are limited due to the fact that current drug treatments fail to address the underlying scarring and cell loss. Current option to cure this inevitable ventricular remodeling and heart failure is heart transplantation. However, heart transplantation is limited to a small patient collective because of a lack of donor organs. Thus, alternative therapeutic strategies are needed to cure the ischemically injured failing heart which lacks contractile myocardium, functional vasculature, and electrical integrity.

In the last decade, accumulated experimental data have suggested that cell transplantation therapy is a promising approach to repair the damaged heart after myocardial infarction and to prevent post-myocardial infarction left ventricular remodelling. The aim of cell transplantation therapy is to replace the scar tissue with new contractile cardiomyocytes and functional vasculature. Transplanted fetal and neonatal cardiomyocyte donor cells have been shown to truly replace infarcted heart muscle (Figs. 11.1, 2), increase the thickness of the infarct wall (Figs. 11.1, 2), and improve left ventricular stroke volume and ejection fraction in a rat model of myocardial infarction (Muller-Ehmsen et al., 2002). Moreover, these engrafted fetal and neonatal cardiomyocyte donor cells have been demonstrated to integrate structurally and functionally into the host heart myocardium (Soonpaa et al., 1994). However, the clinical application of fetal and neonatal cardiomyocytes for cardiac regeneration is limited due to their ethical restrictions and insufficient numbers of donor cells. Therefore, there is a need to seek other potential sources of cells that may be applicable for cardiac regeneration.

In recent years, stem cells have been proposed to be a novel cell source for cardiovascular regeneration. The working hypothesis of stem cell transplantation therapy for the injured failing heart is described in Fig. 11.3. This chapter will cover the current state of stem cell therapy in the field of cardiac regenerative medicine.

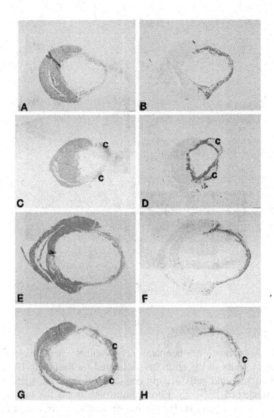

Figure 11.1. A through H, Low-power view of transmural slices of left ventricles stained with hematoxylin and eosin (left column) or picrosirius red (right column). A and B are from a control heart that received medium injection. Note thin free wall of left ventricle composed primarily of collagen (right half of the circular ventricular wall). C and D are from a cell transplant heart. Note two discrete lumps of myocardial cells (c) within the scar that increase wall thickness at the site of the cells. E and F are from a control heart that received medium. Again, note that the free left ventricular wall is thin and composed of collagen. G and H are from a heart that received cell injections into the scar. Note discrete lumps of cells (c) within the scar. Note improved wall thickness. (Originally published as color picture in Muller-Ehmsen et. al, (2002). Reprinted with permission).

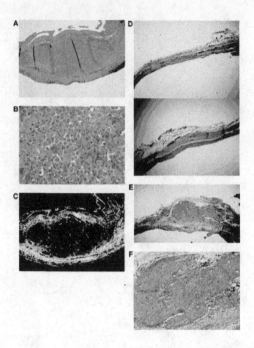

Figure 11.2. A. Appearance of neonatal cell implant (hematoxylin and eosin, x4 objective) within 24 hours of injection into infarcted rat that died. Plane of myocardial infarct scar is disrupted, and cells occupy central portion of the scar, resulting in what appears to be a thickened LV wall. Endocardium is toward the top and epicardium is toward the bottom of the figure. B. Higher-power view of cells within the first 24 hours of transplantation shows a round, immature appearance and large nuclei (original magnification x40). C. Polarized light microscopy of picrosirius red–stained section from the same infarct as in A. Note collagen of scar (white areas) along endocardial and epicardial surfaces of ventricle. Neonatal cell implants are devoid of collagen and appear as dark zones in the center of the ventricular wall. Infarct scar has been bulked up by cell implants (original magnification x4). D. Infarct scar at 6 months of 2 untreated (media only) rats. In both cases, infarcts are composed of collagen and are transmural, thin, and devoid of myocytes. Visceral pericardium appears thickened in bottom panel of D (hematoxylin and eosin, x4 objective). E. Transplanted neonatal cardiomyocytes survived in the infarct and form a bulky muscle patch within the 6-month-old infarct scar. Cell implant is a discrete lump of cells found in the midmyocardium and subepicardium of the scar. We did not observe similar structures in media-treated hearts (hematoxylin and eosin, x4 objective). F. Magnification of transplant from E. Implanted cells formed a discrete lump of cells. There is some degree of myofiber disarray (hematoxylin and eosin, x4 objective). (Originally published as color picture in Muller-Ehmsen et al. (2002). Reprinted with permission.).

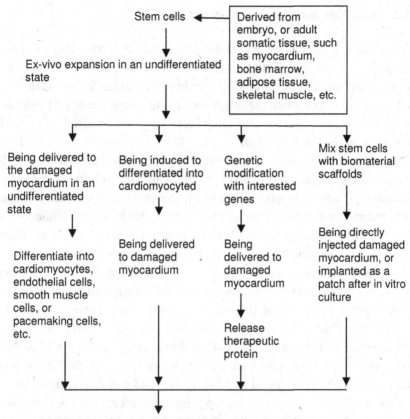

Figure 11.3. Working hypothesis of stem cell transplantation therapy for failing heart. Stem cells derived from various sources are expanded ex-vivo with or without further modification. Then the stem cells are transplanted into the failing heart to form new cardiomyocytes, or new blood vessels, or release paracrine factors to improve cardiac function.

11.2　Definition and Sources of Stem Cells

Stem cells are defined as undifferentiated cells that have the ability to self-renew and to differentiate into different cell types that make up the body. Stem cells can be divided into embryonic stem cells and adult stem cells according to their tissue origination. Embryonic stem (ES) cells are derived from the embryo, and adult stem cells are isolated from adult somatic tissue. Adult stem cells were traditionally believed to differentiate into progeny only within tissue lineage boundaries. But in recent years, adult stem cells have demonstrated plasticity in some laboratories, which means they have the potential ability to differentiate into mature cell phenotypes different from their original lineage in response to microenvironmental cues (termed transdifferentiation). Stem cells can also be divided into totipotent stem cells, pluripotent stem cells, multipotent stem cells and unipotent stem cells according to the number of cell types into which they can differentiate. Totipotent stem cells can form trophoblastic cells of the placenta and all fully differentiated cells of the body. Pluripotent stem cells have the potential to differentiate into cell types of all three germ layers (ectoderm, mesoderm and endoderm), but cannot form the placenta and their supporting structures. Multipotent stem cells are usually found in adult tissue, and can differentiate into a limited number (≥ 2) of cell types appropriate to their location. Unipotent stem cells have the least potential for differentiation, and can only differentiate into one special type of cell. Some popular stem cells used experimentally in cardiovascular regeneration are introduced below.

11.2.1　*Embryonic stem cells*

Embryonic stem cells are isolated from the blastocyst stage of the mammalian embryo. At the blastocyst stage (5 days after fertilization), the embryo is composed of an outer cell layer and an inner cluster of cells. The outer cell layer becomes the trophectoderm that gives rise to the placenta and other supporting tissues. The inner cluster of cells, termed inner cell mass, develops into all tissues of the body and nontrophoblast structures that support the embryo. The inner cell mass of the blastocyst is isolated by selective removal of the outer cell layer using specific antibodies (termed immunosurgery) (Solter and Knowles, 1975), or by mechanical isolation (Bongso, 1994). Compared with immunosurgery, mechanical isolation has the advantage that there is no contact of blastocysts with animal antibodies, but mechanical isolation does carry a risk that not all of the trophectoderm cells may be removed. The overgrowth of residual trophectoderm cells may inhibit the growth of the inner cell mass. The isolated inner cell mass is then plated on a feeder layer (a layer of non-dividing cells, such as lethally irradiated mouse fibroblasts, that provide essential nutrients to cultured ES cells and release cytokines to maintain EC cells in an undifferentiated state) to form colonies. The colonies are mechanically isolated and replated. The procedure is repeated to finally form homogenous colonies. The colony of interest is passaged and expanded to establish an embryonic stem cell line. There are many human ES cell lines available for scientific research [http://stemcells.nih.gov/research/registry/DefaultPage.htm], and there are 23 ES cell lines that have proven viable and have met the NIH criteria to be eligible for federally-sponsored human ES cell research.

Human ES cell-derived cardiomyocytes have the structural and functional properties of early-stage cardiomyocytes (He et al., 2003). In theory, human ES cells can potentially provide an unlimited supply of cardiomyocytes for cell therapy procedures aimed at regenerating functional myocardium. However, there are still many hurdles to be overcome before cardiomyocytes derived from human ES cells are utilized in clinical medicine. Human ES cell-derived cardiac cells may be a mixture of various cell types (such as atrial, immature and mature ventricular cardiomyocytes) (He et al., 2003). Thus, purity of human ES cell-derived cardiac cells is important. Dolnikov et al. (2005) observed that the excitation-contraction coupling properties of the human embryonic stem cell-derived cardiomyocytes differed from the adult myocardium, and suggested that genetic manipulation of the immature cardiomyocytes toward the adult myocardium was needed to mimic the excitation-contraction coupling properties of the adult heart. Many of these human ES cell lines have been derived or grown using mouse embryonic fibroblasts, animal serum or serum replacement containing animal ingredients as part of the feeder preparation. Because feeder cells may be derived from animals or are bathed in ingredients derived from animals, the feeder layers may contain animal pathogens, limiting the medical application of certain human ES cell lines. Therefore, for clinical cell therapy, it is necessary to establish defined conditions for derivation and growth of human ES cells. Other problems include their immunogenicity, teratogenic potential, ethical, and social and political issues.

Recently, two teams of scientists (Takahashi et al., 2007; Yu et al., 2007) independently reported that ordinary human skin cells can be turned into pluripotent stem cells by a "direct reprogramming" technique that adds a cocktail of four genetic factors into human skin cells. From the genetic modified human skin cells, the two teams have been able to isolate cells with the same characteristics as those derived from human embryos. In theory, these newly minted stem cells could be used as a new cell source of donor cardiac cells. These cells would be able to bypass the ethical issues on human embryonic stem cells and eliminate the possibility of rejection.

11.2.2 *Resident cardiac stem cells*

The adult mammalian heart has been considered to be a postmitotic organ without regenerative capacity. However, this notion has been challenged by the accumulated evidence of the existence of resident stem cells within the adult heart (Nadal-Ginard, et al., 2003). The function of the resident stem cells is to maintain tissue homeostasis. Cardiac stem cells can be isolated from myocardial biopsies and expanded ex vivo, and differentiated into cardiomyocytes or vascular lineages (Oh et al., 2003). Transplanted cardiac stem cells may develop into cardiomyocytes or vascular cells. Intramyocardial injection of growth factors can stimulate resident cardiac stem cells to help restore the damaged tissue within the myocardium (Linke et al., 2005). Better understanding of the regulation of cardiac stem cell proliferation and differentiation through growth factor-receptor systems may make the resident cardiac stem cell one of the most appropriate cell sources for future cardiac regeneration.

11.2.3 *Bone marrow-derived stem cells*

Bone marrow cells can be obtained by bone marrow aspiration and expanded in vitro for autologous transplantation. The adult bone marrow contains differentiated and undifferentiated cells. Differentiated cells include stromal cells, vascular cells, adipocytes and osteoblasts. Undifferentiated cells are composed of hematopoietic stem cells, mesenchymal stem cells, and endothelial progenitor cells. These three purified subsets of cells, as well as a mixed population of bone marrow cells, have been used for myocardial regeneration.

Bone marrow hematopoietic stem cells have the capacity to self-renew, form clones, and differentiate into mature blood cell types. The surface markers of hematopoietic stem cells which have been used for isolation vary among species. The hematopoietic stem cells retain developmental plasticity and have the potential to differentiate across boundaries of lineage and tissue. Whether hematopoietic stem cells can transdifferentiate into cardiac muscle cells remains controversial. Reports from some laboratories demonstrated that hematopoietic stem cells can transdifferentiate into smooth muscle cells, endothelial cells, and cardiac muscle cells (Fernandez-Aviles et al., 2004; Yoon et al., 2005); as well as induce endogenous neovascularization and cardiomyogenesis (Yoon et al., 2005). In contrast, Murry et al. (2004) injected haematopoietic stem cells labeled with enhanced green fluorescent protein directly into normal and injured adult mouse hearts, and did not observe that they transdifferentiated into cardiomyocytes by immunohistochemistry. These results indicate that haematopoietic stem cells do not transdifferentiate into cardiac myocytes in myocardial infarcts, and raise a cautionary note for their utilization in infarct repair.

Bone marrow mesenchymal stem cells are a subset of the unfractionated mononuclear cells within the bone marrow, and are characterized by nonhematopoietic multipotent stem cells (Fernandez-Aviles et al., 2004; Yoon et al., 2005). Although the immunophenotype of mesenchymal stem cells has been partially determined, they cannot be distinguished solely by antigen expression. In order to identify mesenchymal stem cells, functional assays demonstrating their multipotent growth and differentiation behavior are necessary (Colter et al., 2000). The mesenchymal stem cells make up only 0.001~0.01% of the unfractionated bone marrow cell population. After plating, mesenchymal stem cells adhere quickly to the culture dish, and form visible colonies at 1 week (Pittenger and Martin, 2004). Mesenchymal stem cells can be induced to differentiate into multiple phenotypes in the presence of growth factors and cytokines (Pittenger et al., 1999). In the presence of 5-aza-cytidine, mesenchymal stem cells differentiated into cardiomyocytes which beat spontaneously and synchronously, and responded to isoproterenol and β_1-blocking agents (Makino et al., 1999). Thus, mesenchymal stem cells are a potential cell source for cardiac regeneration.

Endothelial progenitor cells have the capacity to proliferate, migrate, and differentiate into mature endothelial cells. Endothelial progenitor cells have been detected not only in the bone marrow, but they also have been isolated from peripheral blood (Asahara et al., 1997) and human umbilical cord blood (Nieda et al., 1997). The majority of endothelial progenitor cells reside in the bone marrow. About 0.01% of the peripheral circulating mononuclear cells are composed of endothelial progenitor cells under normal physiological conditions (Rafii et al., 2002). The mobilization of endothelial progenitor cells from bone marrow into the peripheral circulation can be enhanced by endogenous stimuli or exogenous cytokine therapy. Tissue ischemia, such as acute myocardial infarction can mobilize the endothelial progenitor cells as one of the endogenous stimuli. Exogenous cytokines, such as vascular endothelial growth factor, angiopoietin-1, fibroblast growth factor, stromal cell-derived growth factor-1, granulocyte-macrophage colony-stimulating factor, have been shown to promote the mobilization of endothelial progenitor cells. Isolated endothelial progenitor cells have been successfully expanded and formed an endothelial cell-like phenotype in vitro, and have been shown to incorporate into capillaries in vivo (Asahara et al., 1997). Although the expression of CD34, CD133, vascular endothelial growth factor receptor-2 have been used as markers to identify the endothelial progenitor cells, the unique markers for the lineage and exact phenotype of endothelial progenitor cells requires further characterization (Szmitko et al., 2003).

11.2.4 *Human umbilical cord blood*

Umbilical cord blood is usually discarded after delivery. Umbilical cord blood contains a large number of progenitor cells, which can be easily extracted and cryopreserved. Establishment of HLA-type stem cell banks can offer HLA-identical allogeneic cells for transplantation to avoid an immune rejection response. Because the T cells of umbilical cord blood are relatively immature, the risk of graft-versus-host is relatively low (de La Selle et al., 1996).

Compared with adult peripheral blood or bone marrow-derived stem cells, umbilical cord blood-derived stem cells are easier to isolate, and have the capacity to form a greater number of colonies. They also have a higher cell-cycle rate and a longer telomere length (Melo et al.). Transplantation of cord blood-derived EPCs into the ischemic limb muscles of non-immunocompetent rats augmented reparative neovascularization and improved blood flow recovery (Murohara et al., 2000).

11.2.5 *Adipose tissue derived stem cells*

As a mesodermally-derived organ, adipose tissue, also known as fat tissue, contains microvascular endothelial cells, smooth muscle cells and stem cells (Zuk et al., 2001). Adipose-derived adult stem cells are multipotent and can differentiate into various cell phenotypes in vitro (Aust et al., 2004). Adipose tissue-derived mesenchymal stem cells triggered angiogenesis through paracrine pathways and differentiated into cardiomyocytes after transplantation into the scarred myocardium of rats (Miyahara et al., 2006). Thus, adipose tissue-derived mesenchymal stem cells may be a potential cell source strategy for cardiac tissue regeneration.

11.2.6 *Muscle-derived stem cells*

Skeletal muscle is a convenient source of stem cells. Stem cells can be isolated from skeletal muscle biopsies and expanded ex vivo. There are two kinds of stem cells in skeletal muscle: muscle-derived stem cells (MDSCs) and satellite cells. MDSCs are self-renewing and multipotential cells, and are considered to be distinct from satellite cells (Deasy and Huard, 2002). The MDSCs are derived from the interstitial spaces or connective tissue of the skeletal muscle, while the satellite cells are located beneath the basal lamina of mature muscular fibers. The satellite cells are also capable of self-renewal and myogenic lineage differentiation. Compared with the satellite cells, MDSCs have a broader range of differentiation capabilities, and may be a precursor of the satellite cell. Both MDSCs and satellite cells are able to differentiate into a myogenic cell type (Alessandri et al., 2004), and have the potential for cardiac repair. The advantages of skeletal myoblasts are that they are autologous and resistant to ischemia.

11.2.7 *Side population cells*

Side population cells represent a tissue-specific progenitor cell population characterized by an intrinsic capacity to efflux Hoechst dye through an ATP-binding cassette transporter. These side population cells were initially isolated from bone marrow by fluorescence-activated cell sorting (FACS) (Goodell et al., 1996). Side population cells also exist in other tissues, such as skeletal muscle and heart. Side population cells are multipotent stem cells, and can be used for cardiac repair. Jackson et al. (2001) demonstrated that bone marrow derived-side population cells migrated into ischemic cardiac muscle and differentiated into cardiomyocytes and endothelial cells in a mouse ischemia/reperfusion model. Pfister et al. (2005) isolated side population cells from cardiac tissue, and observed that these cells were capable of functional differentiation into cardiomyocytes in vitro.

11.3 Undifferentiated and Differentiated Culture of Stem Cells

In order to replace myocardium damaged by a heart attack, a large number of cardiomyocytes are needed for transplantation. An ideal approach is to isolate and produce a large number of stem cells in an undifferentiated state in vitro, and induce them to differentiate into cardiomyocytes before transplantation.

The conditions for isolation and culture of stem cells differ for different stem cell types. Many culture systems, such as plating ES cells on a feeder layer, are able to maintain stem cells in an undifferentiated state during culture expansion. However, these available culture systems may contain animal feeder cells, animal serum or albumin purified from animals, and have the potential risk of cross-transfer of animal pathogens in clinical therapeutic application. Thus, challenges in expansion of undifferentiated stem cells for clinical applications include the removal of feeder layers and non-defined components in the culture medium. In order to eliminate animal materials to make a pathogen-free culture system for clinical application, it is necessary to establish defined culture conditions to support stem cell growth. Development of pathogen-free culture systems depends upon deeper understanding of signaling pathways and molecular mechanisms in the maintenance of the undifferentiated state of stem cells (Rao and Stice, 2004).

Although undifferentiated adult stem cells have been transplanted to repair injured myocardium and have been reported to differentiate spontaneously into cardiac cells in vivo within the recipient heart, the efficacy of cardiomyogenic lineage differentiation was low, and the stem cells tended to spontaneously differentiate into multiple lineages after transplantation in vivo (Odorico et al., 2001). Moreover, undifferentiated adult stem cells may differentiate into an undesired tissue type that could impair the heart function after transplantation into the heart (Wang et al., 2001). In the case of ES cells, the potential to form teratomas after transplantation in vivo is another major consideration. Thus, directing cardiomyogenic differentiation of stem cells in vitro prior to transplantation will be necessary. There are many techniques that could be possibly employed to direct cardiomyogenic differentiation of stem cells (for review, see Heng et al., 2004a; Heng et al., 2004b). Understanding the molecular regulation of stem cell differentiation will provide a foundation for strategies to direct the differentiation of stem cells to clinically relevant cell types.

11.4 Enrichment of Stem Cell-Derived Cardiomyocytes

There is a potential risk to form teratomas within the recipient heart if the transplanted stem cell-derived cardiomyocytes contain undifferentiated stem cells. It has been shown that the ES cells generate teratomas after transplantation into post-natal animals (Wobus et al., 1984). Thus, it is necessary to eliminate undifferentiated cells to avoid teratoma formation after transplantation for clinical application. Many methods, such as Percoll density centrifugation (Xu et al., 2002), genetic manipulation (Klug et al., 1996), green fluorescent protein expression plus fluorescence-activated cell sorting (Muller et al., 2000), have been developed to enrich differentiated cardiomyocytes. On the other hand, clinical application of stem cell-derived cardiomyocyte transplantation for cardiac regeneration requires a large number of donor cells. Thus, methods for scalable production of stem cell-derived cardiomyocytes are in need of development (Zandstra et al., 2003).

11.5 Potential Application of Stem Cell Therapy for Heart Diseases

The failing heart lacks adequate contractile myocardium, functional vasculature, and electrical integrity. Currently, stem cell transplantation therapy has been used to replace lost cardiomyocytes, generate new blood vessels, and prevent cardiac arrhymias. Many encouraging preclinical experimental results have been reported (Dai et al., 2007; Matsumoto et al., 2005; Orlic et al., 2001; Potapova et al., 2004; Shyu et al., 2006; Tang et al., 2005).

11.5.1 *Replacement of lost cardiomyocytes*

Cardiac cell loss caused by ischemic necrosis of a myocardial infarction results in scar formation, and ultimately heart failure. Replacement of dead cells with viable cells is a possible strategy to overcome this loss of muscle cells. Stem cells have been applied to regenerate damaged tissues because of their plasticity. Studies from various laboratories have demonstrated that stem cell therapy improves cardiac function after myocardial infarction (Dai et al., 2005 b). Orlic et al. (2001) transplanted adult bone marrow derived hematopoietic stem cells into myocardial infarction in mice. They observed that newly formed myocardium occupied 68% of the infarcted portion of the ventricle at 9 days after bone marrow cell transplantation, and the cardiac function was improved. This study suggested that locally delivered bone marrow cells can generate de novo myocardium. Recently, our research group demonstrated that transplanted hESC-derived cardiomyocytes survived and formed sizeable grafts within the nude rat heart subjected to ischemia/reperfusion at 4 weeks after transplantation and matured toward an adult cardiomyocyte (Dai et al., 2007). These data suggest that stem cell transplantation is a promising approach to repair the damaged myocardium.

In our recent study (Dai et al., 2005 a), we injected allogeneic MSCs into the scar of a 1-week-old myocardial infarction in Fischer rats, and demonstrated that grafted MSCs survived in the infarcted myocardium as long as 6 months. The transplanted MSCs did not express muscle-specific markers at 2 weeks, but expressed some muscle markers at 3 months, and further expression of muscle markers had occurred by 6 months (Figs. 11.4-11.7). Grafted MSCs did not result in visible replacement of scar with sheets of muscle cells (Fig. 11.8), and did not increase the scar thickness (Fig. 11.8) and prevent LV remodeling at either 4 weeks or 6 months after treatment. The global LV function was improved at 4 weeks; however, the benefit was lost at 6 months. The fact that function was improved at 4 weeks without thickening of the infarct scar with muscle suggested that a paracrine effect of transplanted MSCs played a role in the improvement of cardiac function. Paracrine effect refers to a cell-to-cell communication that is mediated by the action of regulatory molecules (such as cytokines, growth factors) produced by adjacent cells. The paracrine hypothesis is also supported by the recent studies of Dr Dzau's group (Gnecchi et al., 2006; Mirotsou et al., 2007). Thus, an improvement in cardiac function does not necessarily mean that the injected stem cells have differentiated into an adult cardiomyocyte phenotype. The mechanisms of beneficial effects of stem cell therapy need to be clarified in future studies.

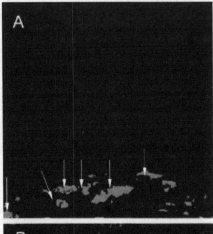

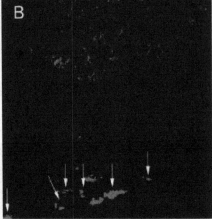

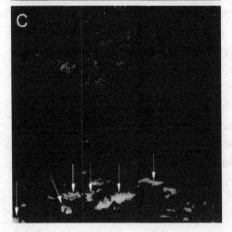

Figure 11.4. Confocal microscopy of fluorescent immunohistochemical staining of DiI-labeled cells in infarcted myocardium for α-actinin at 6 months. A. DiI-labeled MSCs indicated by white arrows. B. Sections were stained with antibody to muscle marker α-actinin. White arrows point to MSC transplant. Fluorescent cells at the top of the panel represent native rat cardiomyocytes that also stain positive for muscle markers. C. Merged image of A and B shows DiI-labeled MSCs express α-actinin indicated by white arrows. Original magnification x400. (Originally published as color picture in Dai et al. (2005a). Reprinted with permission.).

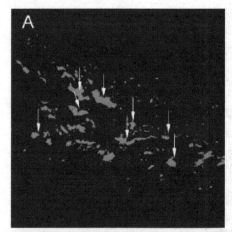

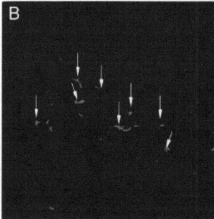

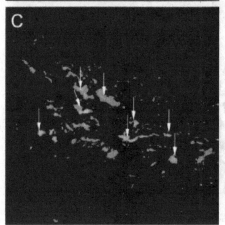

Figure 11.5. Confocal microscopy of fluorescent immunohistochemical staining of DiI-labeled cells in infarcted myocardium for MF-20 at 6 months. A. DiI-labeled MSCs indicated white arrows. B. Sections were stained with antibody to muscle marker MF-20. White arrows point to MSC transplant. C. Merged image of A and B shows DiI-labeled MSCs express MF-20 indicated by white arrows. Original magnification x400. (Originally published as color picture in Dai et al. (2005a). Reprinted with permission.).

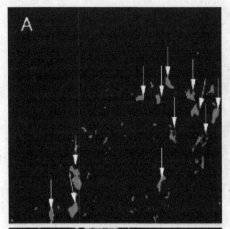

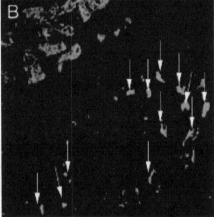

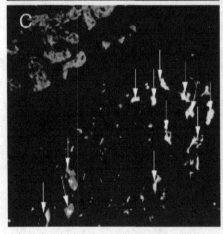

Figure 11.6. Confocal microscopy of fluorescent immunohistochemical staining of DiI-labeled cells in infarcted myocardium for phospholamban at 6 months. A. DiI-labeled MSCs indicated by white arrows. B. Sections were stained with antibody to muscle marker phospholamban. White arrows point to MSC transplant. C. Merged image of A and B shows DiI-labeled MSCs express phospholamban indicated by white arrows. Original magnification x400. (Originally published as color picture in Dai et al. (2005a). Reprinted with permission.).

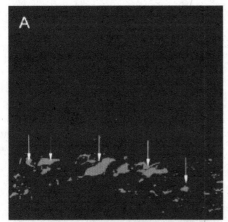

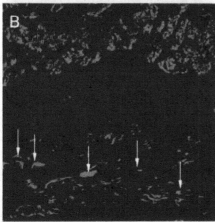

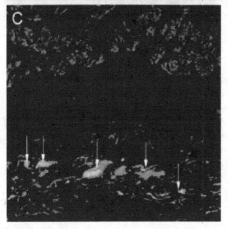

Figure 11.7. Confocal microscopy of fluorescent immunohistochemical staining of DiI-labeled cells in infarcted myocardium for tropomyosin at 6 months. A. DiI-labeled MSCs indicated by white arrows. B. Sections were stained with antibody to muscle marker tropomyosin. White arrows point to MSC transplant. C. Merged image of A and B shows DiI-labeled MSCs express tropomyosin indicated by white arrows. Original magnification x400. (Originally published as color picture in Dai et al. (2005a). Reprinted with permission.).

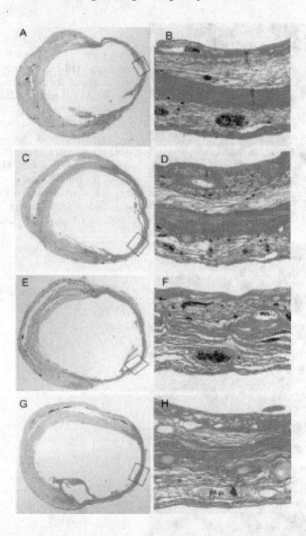

Figure 11.8. Representative picrosirius red stained sections of myocardial infarction show thin-walled, transmural collagenous scars (seen on the right-hand side of panels A, C , E and G as dark colored tissue). No grafts appearing to "bulk-up" the infarcted wall with new cardiac muscle were observed. **A** (4 weeks) and **E** (6 months) represent the heart after saline treatment; **C** (4 weeks) and **G** (6 months) represent the heart after MSC treatment. **B**, **D**, **F** and **H** are the higher magnification (×100) of the boxed area in the picture **A**, **C**, **E** and **G**, respectively. (Originally published as color picture in Dai et al. (2005a). Reprinted with permission.).

11.5.2 *Therapeutic neovascularization*

Myocardial regeneration requires the formation of new blood vessels to supply oxygen and nutrients to facilitate the survival of transplanted cells. The development of the vascular system involves vasculogenesis, angiogenesis and arteriogenesis. Vasculogenesis is the in situ blood vessel formation from hemangioblasts during embryonic development. Vasculogenesis is now proposed to occur in adults as well. Angiogenesis refers to the sprouting of new capillary vessels from the already present primitive vasculature. Arteriogenesis is the remodeling of the existing arterioles to form collateral vessels. A functional new vasculature requires resistance arterioles to supply blood and a capillary network to delivery oxygen.

Cell transplantation may serve as a novel strategy to promote the formation of natural bypasses or collaterals within the ischemic tissue. Transplanted stem cells can differentiate into endothelial cells and smooth muscle cells to incorporate into a vascular structure, or release pro-angiogenic factors to effectively stimulate angiogenesis (for review, see Losordo and Dimmeler, 2004). Tang et al. (2005) transplanted autologous MSCs into myocardial infarctions in rats, and detected that the angiogenic factors basic fibroblast growth factor and vascular endothelial growth factor, as well as stem cell homing factor increased in the MSC-treated hearts. This phenomenon was accompanied by increased angiogenesis and cytoprotection, and improved left ventricular contractility. Shyu et al. (2006) demonstrated that human bone marrow-derived mesenchymal stem cell transplantation was better at increasing capillary density than angiogenic growth factor gene therapy (angiopoietin-1 or vascular endothelial growth factor) in a mouse myocardial infarction model.

Genetically modulated stem cells carrying exogenous genes encoding for angiogenic factors have been used for therapeutic angiogenesis. Matsumoto et al (2005) transfected the VEGF165 gene into MSCs of Lewis rats using an adenoviral vector, and injected the VEGF-transfected cells into syngeneic rat hearts 1 hour after left coronary artery occlusion. The capillary density of the infarcted region, alpha-smooth muscle actin-positive cells and LV function were significantly increased. Cell transplantation with gene therapy could be a useful therapy for angiogenesis in infarcted heart.

11.5.3 *Prevention of cardiac arrhythmias*

In normal hearts the cardiac impulse is initiated in a group of cells (termed pacemaking cells) that can spontaneously depolarize at a constant rate in the sinoatrial node. The electrical impulses of the pacemaking cells propagate through the atria to the atrioventricular node, and then through the specialized His-Purkinje system to trigger cardiac contraction. Tissue loss or dysfunction at critical sites in the cardiac conduction system may result in cardiac arrhythmias. Cardiac arrhythmias include abnormally low heart rates (bradyarrhythmias), abnormally fast beating rates (tachyarrhythmias), and various uncoordinated beating. Currently, antiarrhythmic strategies include pharmacotherapy, focal injury (surgery or catheter ablation), and implantable devices (pacemakers or implantable cardiac defibrillators). Recently, with the development of molecular and cell biology, as well as new tissue engineering technologies, a novel strategy, cell therapy, has been proposed to replace or modify the diseased pacemaking cells or cardiac conduction system to treat cardiac arrhythmias.

Cell therapy can replace the diseased cells of the conduction system. One of the possible cell sources is human ES cell lines. ES cells can differentiate into different subtypes of cardiomyocytes in vitro, including pacemaking, atrial, ventricular, and Purkinje-like phenotypes (He et al., 2003). ES cell-derived cells have a stable pacemaker activity and electrical propagation, and can respond to adrenergic and cholinergic stimuli. Kehat et al. (2004) demonstrated that human ES cell-derived cardiomyocytes formed structural and electromechanical connections with cultured rat cardiomyocytes in a coculture system. Moreover, in an in vivo study in a model of swine with complete atrioventricular block, transplanted human ES cell-derived cardiomyocytes paced the hearts assessed by detailed three-dimensional electrophysiological mapping and histopathological examination. These results suggest that human ES cell-derived cardiomyocytes have the potential to act as a rate-responsive biological pacemaker.

Adult stem cells or autologous myocardial cells from biopsies can also be used as pacemaking cells through in vitro genetic modification. The considerable methods include selective increase of the cellular response to adrenergic stimulation (Edelberg et al., 1998), reduction of the inward diastolic rectifying current (Miake et al., 2003), and increase in the inward depolarizing current (Qu et al., 2003).

Stem cells can act as a gene delivery system to create cardiac pacemakers. The hypothesis is that the stem cells that are genetically modified with a cardiac pacemaker gene can generate inward current that may spread to the coupled myocytes via gap junctions after transplantation within the heart. The coupled host myocytes will be driven to threshold to function as a cardiac pacemaker. Potapova et al. (2004) transfected human mesenchymal stem cells with a cardiac pacemaker gene, mHCN2, that generated an inward current necessary for cardiac excitation. The mHCN2-transfected human mesenchymal stem cells were able to generate a depolarizing current, but were not excitable themselves due to lacking other currents that were required to generate an action potential. The in vitro and in vivo results showed that the mHCN2-transfected human mesenchymal stem cells influenced the beating of coupled cardiac myocytes. These results suggested that human mesenchymal stem cells might act as a gene delivery system to create cardiac pacemakers.

Although it is possible to obtain cells with similar electrophysiological properties to pacemaker cells, and some animal studies show that cell therapy for replacement of diseased pacemaking cells is promising, cell therapy as a biological solution for rhythm disorders still requires extensive investigation before it is applicable to routine clinical medicine.

11.6 Combination of Stem Cell and Gene Therapy

The stem cell can serve as a platform for gene therapy. Selected cells can be genetically manipulated ex vivo to serve as a vehicle for delivering the recombinant proteins of interest. In recent years, genetic modification of stem cells with therapeutic genes before transplantation has been suggested as a new treatment strategy for heart diseases. Although proangiogenic cytokines and cardio-protective gene therapy have been used as strategies for protection, rescue, and repair of ischemic myocardium, direct gene transfer within the myocardium has some disadvantages. One of the limitations of this approach is that some of the available vectors cannot infect non-dividing cardiac cells, and some have very low transfection efficiency. Cell-based gene therapy may overcome some of the disadvantages of direct gene transfer. Transfer efficiency may be maximized in vitro because cultured cells are dividing, and the transduced cells can be selected in vitro.

Constitutive high-level expression of the transfected genes may be associated with some side effects, such as hemangiomas (Schwarz et al., 2000) and generation of tumors (Meuillet et al., 2003). Thus, the growth of the genetically manipulated stem cells will need controls to prevent abnormal growth. A suicide gene system can be used to control the growth of the transplanted cells with overexpressed gene. A suicide gene system is composed of thymidine kinase gene of Herpes Simplex Virus (TK) and Ganciclovir (GCV). Cells transfected with TK can be killed by GCV (Miyagawa et al., 2006). Cell-based gene therapy using the TK-GCV suicide gene system is promising for delivering target genes and conrolling their expression in vivo.

On the other hand, selected expression of proteins by genetic manipulation may improve the survival and function of grafted stem cells. Overexpression of the prosurvival gene Akt1 (encoding the Akt protein, which is a general mediator of survival signals for cell survival) (Mangi et al., 2003) and heme oxygenase-1 (HO-1) plasmid (Tang et al., 2005) have been demonstrated to improve survival of grafted genetically engineered mesenchymal stem cells within the ischemic myocardium of the rat myocardial infarction model. Yau et al. (2005) demonstrated that multimodal cell-based gene therapy may maximize the benefits of cell transplantation. In this study, rat bone marrow cells were transfected with vascular endothelial growth factor (VEGF), insulin-like growth factor I (IGF-I) separately, or VEGF plus IGF-I, and then transplanted into 3-week old myocardial infarction in rats. Transplantation of bone marrow cells with VEGF plus IGF-I reduced cell apoptosis of the graft, and improved cell survival and LV function at 2 and 4 weeks after transplantation.

11.7 Stem Cell Delivery Approaches

In order to repair the damaged myocardium, the stem cells have to be delivered to the injured site. Many strategies have been developed for cell delivery to the infarcted heart. Ex-vivo expanded stem cells can be injected directly into the cardiac muscle. In contrast, they can be injected into the systemic vasculature with the idea that the stem cells can "home" to injured myocardium. Bone marrow stem cells can be mobilized and "home" to the myocardial infarction area. Intrinsic cardiac stem cells can be stimulated to proliferation and differentiate into cardiomyocytes in the ischemic heart. With the advancement of developmental biology, cardiac muscle cell biology, and material science, tissue engineering scientists are creating functional three dimensions cardiac tissue for the replacement of damaged myocardium.

Direct injection of stem cells into infarcted myocardium can be performed during open-heart surgery, by minimally invasive thoracoscopic procedures or percutaneously by injecting cells via a catheter. Catheter injection includes catheter-based needle injection from the left ventricular cavity, ultrasound-directed intramyocardial injection through the coronary sinus or the great cardiac vein, and injection of cells via an intracoronary route.

Stem cell "homing" through the systemic vasculature is another approach for cell delivery. Stem cell homing is a multistep process within ischemic tissue, including adhesion of the cells to the endothelium, transmigration through the blood vessel wall and migration within the target tissue. The site of introducing stem cells into the circulatory system includes intravenous injection, intracoronary injection, intra- aortic root administration and retrograde venous infusion. A disadvantage of these techniques is that the cells may have the potential to cause embolization if they are too big or clump into aggregates, or if very large quantities of cells are infused. The homing process is complicated and its mechanisms remain unclear. Better understanding of the mechanisms of homing might help to enhance local homing signals or increase the ability of stem cells to respond to the stimulation after myocardial infarction, or adhere to the tissue areas in need of new cells.

Enhancing mobilization of bone marrow stem cells may serve as an alternative delivery approach. Bone marrow stem cells are spontaneously mobilized after myocardial infarction, and this naturally occurring process might contribute to the process of recovery following myocardial infarction (Leone et al., 2005). A number of cytokines and drugs, such as granulocyte colony-stimulating factor (G-CSF), and statins, have been used for stem cell mobilization. Many studies have reported that mobilized stem cells can regenerate myocardium, forming myocytes, capillaries and arterioles (Kawada et al., 2004; Ohtsuka et al., 2004). However, in a recent study by Sesti et al. (2005), G-CSF and stem cell factor (SCF) mobilized hematopoietic progenitor cells from bone marrow into the circulation, and improved left ventricular functional reserve but not resting LV function. G-CSF did not benefit LV remodeling, nor did it replace the scar with new muscle cells. The results suggested that the combination of G-CSF and SCF improve left ventricular function by enhancing the functional reserve of the heart, not by replacing muscle.

The heart may contain intrinsic cardiac stem cells that help to regenerate myocardium after infarction (Dawn et al., 2005). Linke et al. (2005) recently reported that intramyocardial injection of a hepatocyte growth factor (HGF) and an insulin-like growth factor 1 (IGF-1) can stimulate resident cardiac progenitor cells to form myocytes and coronary vessels within the infarct, and result in a marked recovery of contractile performance of the infarcted heart. The authors suggested that activating the growth reserve of the myocardium might be an approach to repair the damaged myocardium after ischemic injury.

Biomaterial scaffolds have been used as an adjunct to transplanted stem cells. The three dimensional engineered cardiac tissue can be generated in vitro by combination of stem cells and biomaterial scaffolds, and be subsequently implanted in vivo. Another approach is injecting the mixture of cells and a scaffold into the myocardium to create in situ engineered cardiac tissue (Leor et al., 2006). Liu et al.

(2004) seeded autologous porcine mesenchymal stem cells within a fibrin matrix patch and applied this patch to myocardial infarction in a swine model. The transplanted cells differentiated into both endothelial cells and cells with myocyte-like properties. Magnetic resonance imaging data indicated a significant increase of left ventricular systolic wall thickening fraction in the infarct zone. The patch-based autologous stem cell procedure may serve as a therapeutic modality for myocardial repair. Christman et al. (2004) injected skeletal myoblasts embedded in fibrin glue into the infarcted area in rats. Fibrin glue increased cell transplant survival, decreased infarct size, and increased blood flow to ischemic myocardium. The results suggest that fibrin glue may have potential as a biomaterial scaffold to improve cellular cardiomyoplasty treatment of myocardial infarction.

11.8 Clinical Trials of Stem Cell Therapy for Heart Disease

A variety of stem cells have been used for cardiac repair in animal studies. Although embryonic stem cells are pluripotent stem cells, and are able to differentiate into cardiomyocytes which display structural and functional properties of early-stage cardiomyocytes, their utilization in clinical practice is far away because of many unresolved problems such as ethical and legal issues, tumorigenicity and immuno-rejection.

Compared with ES cells, adult stem cells present fewer risks. Adult stem cells, especially bone marrow cells and skeletal muscle satellite cells, are easier to obtain from autologous tissue, and to expand ex vivo. Currently, bone marrow cells and skeletal muscle satellite cells have been used for clinical trials of cell therapy for myocardial regeneration. Recently, several groups have reported the results of randomized, controlled clinical trials which investigated the effect of bone marrow cells on ventricular function after a myocardial infarction (Assmus et al., 2006; Lunde et al., 2006; Meyer et al., 2006; Schachinger et al., 2006). The clinical trial results are mixed. The available clinical trial results have not yet clearly answered the question of whether stem cell therapy is or is not a promising therapeutic strategy for routine clinical practice.

11.9 Potential Problems of Stem Cell Therapy and Possible Prevention

The transplanted cells might cause arrhythmias in the recipient heart after cell transplantation therapy. Some studies suggest that stem cells have proarrhythmic potential (Zandstra et al., 2003). For example, cultured mouse embryonic stem cell-derived cardiomyocytes showed characteristics of arrhythmogenicity, including heterogeneity of their action potential morphology, with reduced maximum upstroke velocities and prolonged action potential durations and high proclivity toward triggered arrhythmias (Zandstra et al., 2003). Skeletal myoblast transplantations were observed to increase the risk of malignant ventricular arrhythmias in human clinical trials (Smits et al., 2003). The pathogenesis of cell transplant-associated arrhythmias remains poorly understood. The possible mechanisms may be due to proarrhythmic potential of the stem cells themselves or the disruption of electrical signals around these cells when they have not formed normal gap junctions with host cells. It will be necessary to develop methods to prevent cell transplant-associated arrhythmias.

The plasticity of adult stem cells continues to be uncertain. For example, Orlic et al. (2001) injected murine hematopoietic stem cells into the contracting wall bordering the infarct in mice. The transplanted cells transdifferentiated into cardiomyocytes and blood vessels at 9 days after transplantation. In contrast, Murry et al. (2004) reported that haematopoietic stem cells did not transdifferentiation into cardiomyocytes at 1-4 weeks after transplantation into normal and injured adult mouse hearts. The fusion of transplanted stem cells with host cardiomyocyte may also challenge the existence of stem cell transdifferentiation (Wurmser and Gage, 2002).

The low survival rate of the grafted cells after transplantation is one of the major limitations for cell therapy in the heart. Many factors may influence the fate of the transplanted cells. The cells may be damaged during injection. Some cells escape into the systemic circulation through the vascular system of the heart (Dow et al., 2005). The retention of injected cells in myocardium is extremely low. The hypoxic environment of the damaged myocardium in poorly vascularized areas of the heart can induce apoptosis or necrosis. The inflammatory response or the soluble factors released by the surrounding host cells are also able to affect the cell survival rate. A dose-effect relationship between the cell survival rate and the functional outcome of cell therapy has been observed (Tambara et al., 2003). Thus, it is important to develop strategies for enhancing transplanted cell survival. Approaches to improve the graft blood supply include revascularization of the ischemic area through coronary artery bypass surgery or an interventional procedure, co-injection of angiogenic growth factors, genetically engineering the transplanted cells with genes encoding growth factors. Another approach to limit cell loss from the injection site and to protect the cells from harmful environmental factors is embedding the cells in bio-absorbable materials (Christman et al., 2004).

Immunological rejection is a potential barrier for the use of allogeneic stem cells in human clinical therapy that needs to be solved. Nuclear transfer techniques may provide an unlimited supply of histocompatible ES cells (therapeutic cloning) (Lanza et al., 2004). Stem cell banks may be another alternative approach.

11.10 Summary

Stem cell transplantation provides a novel and promising approach to treat cardiovascular disease. Despite the exciting advances described, there are still many unaddressed biological and technical problems that remain to be solved. Major questions include: what is the optimal cell source, how to produce large quantities of undifferentiated stem cells, as well as their large-scale differentiation, how to keep the cells in the desired location of transplantation, and how to aid in appropriate electro-physiologic connections with the host cells. While some clinical trials suggest that bone marrow cell therapy may improve cardiac function in ischemic heart disease, other studies are negative or only show a transient benefit. Nevertheless, this new field of research promises to produce many exciting findings in the future that will greatly benefit mankind.

11.11 References

Alessandri, G., Pagano, S., Bez, A., Benetti, A., Pozzi, S., Iannolo, G., Baronio, M., Invernici, G., Caruso, A., Muneretto, C., Bisleri, G. and Parati, E. (2004). Isolation and culture of human muscle-derived stem cells able to differentiate into myogenic and neurogenic cell lineages. *Lancet*, 364(9448), pp. 1872-1883.

Alhadlaq, A. and Mao, JJ. (2004). Mesenchymal stem cells: isolation and therapeutics. *Stem Cells Dev*, 13, pp. 436-448.

Asahara, T., Murohara, T., Sullivan, A., Silver, M., van der Zee, R., Li, T., Witzenbichler, B., Schatteman, G. and Isner, JM. (1997). Isolation of putative progenitor endothelial cells for angiogenesis. *Science*, 275(5302), pp. 964-967.

Assmus, B., Honold, J., Schachinger, V., Britten, MB., Fischer-Rasokat, U., Lehmann, R., Teupe, C., Pistorius, K., Martin, H., Abolmaali, ND., Tonn, T., Dimmeler, S. and Zeiher, AM. (2006). Transcoronary transplantation of progenitor cells after myocardial infarction. *N Engl J Med*, 355(12), pp. 1222-1232.

Aust, L., Devlin, B., Foster, SJ., Halvorsen, YD., Hicok, K., du Laney, T., Sen, A., Willingmyre, GD. and Gimble, JM. (2004). Yield of human adipose-derived adult stem cells from liposuction aspirates. *Cytotherapy*, 6(1), pp. 7-14.

Bongso, A., Fong, CY., Ng, SC. and Ratnam, S. (1994). Isolation and culture of inner cell mass cells from human blastocysts. *Hum Reprod*, 9(11), pp. 2110-2117.

Christman, KL., Vardanian, AJ., Fang, Q., Sievers, RE., Fok, HH. and Lee, RJ. (2004). Injectable fibrin scaffold improves cell transplant survival, reduces infarct expansion, and induces neovasculature formation in ischemic myocardium. *J Am Coll Cardiol*, 44(3), pp. 654-660.

Colter, DC., Class, R., DiGirolamo, CM. and Prockop, DJ. (2000). Rapid expansion of recycling stem cells in cultures of plastic-adherent cells from human bone marrow. *Proc Natl Acad Sci U S A*, 97(7), pp. 3213-3218.

Dai, W., Field, LJ., Rubart, M., Reuter, S., Hale, SL., Zweigerdt, R., Graichen, RE., Kay, GL., Jyrala, AJ., Colman, A., Davidson, BP., Pera, M. and Kloner RA. (2007). Survival and maturation of human embryonic stem cell-derived cardiomyocytes in rat hearts. *J Mol Cell Cardiol*, 43(4), pp. 504-516.

Dai, W., Hale, SL., Martin, BJ., Kuang, JQ., Dow, JS., Wold, LE. and Kloner, RA. (2005a). Allogeneic mesenchymal stem cell transplantation in postinfarcted rat myocardium: short- and long-term effects. *Circulation*, 112(2), pp. 214-223.

Dai, W., Hale, SL. and Kloner, RA. (2005b). Stem cell transplantation for the treatment of myocardial infarction. *Transpl Immunol*, 15(2), pp. 91-97.

Dawn, B., Stein, AB. and Urbanek, K. (2005). Cardiac stem cells delivered intravascularly traverse the vessel barrier, regenerate infarcted myocardium, and improve cardiac function. *Proc Natl Acad Sci U S A*, 102(10), pp. 3766-3771.

de La Selle, V., Gluckman, E. and Bruley-Rosset, M. (1996). Newborn blood can engraft adult mice without inducing graft-versus-host disease across non H-2 antigens. *Blood*, 87(9), pp. 3977-3983.

Deasy, BM. and Huard, J. (2002). Gene therapy and tissue engineering based on muscle-derived stem cells. *Curr Opin Mol Ther*, 4(4), pp. 382-389.

Dolnikov, K., Shilkrut, M., Zeevi-Levin, N., Danon, A., Gerecht-Nir, S., Itskovitz-Eldor, J. and Binah, O. (2005). Functional properties of human embryonic stem cell-derived cardiomyocytes. *Ann N Y Acad Sci*, 1047, pp. 66-75.

Dow, J., Simkhovich, BZ., Kedes, L. and Kloner, RA. (2005). Washout of transplanted cells from the heart: a potential new hurdle for cell transplantation therapy. *Cardiovasc Res*, 67(2), pp. 301-307.

Edelberg, JM., Aird, WC. and Rosenberg, RD. (1998). Enhancement of murine cardiac chronotropy by the molecular transfer of the human beta2 adrenergic receptor cDNA. J Clin Invest, 101, pp. 337-343.

Fernandez-Aviles, F., San Roman, JA., Garcia-Frade, J., Fernandez, ME., Penarrubia, MJ., de la Fuente, L., Gomez-Bueno, M., Cantalapiedra, A., Fernandez, J., Gutierrez, O., Sanchez, PL., Hernandez, C., Sanz, R., Garcia-Sancho, J. and Sanchez, A. (2004). Experimental and clinical regenerative capability of human bone marrow cells after myocardial infarction. *Circ Res*, 95(7), pp. 742-748.

Gnecchi, M., He, H., Noiseux, N., Liang, OD., Zhang, L., Morello, F., Mu, H., Melo, LG., Pratt, RE., Ingwall, JS. and Dzau VJ. (2006). Evidence supporting paracrine hypothesis for Akt-modified mesenchymal stem cell-mediated cardiac protection and functional improvement. *FASEB J*, 20(6), pp. 661-669.

Goodell, MA., Brose, K., Paradis, G., Conner, AS. and Mulligan, RC. (1996). Isolation and functional properties of murine hematopoietic stem cells that are replicating in vivo. *J Exp Med*, 183, pp. 1797-1806.

He, JQ., Ma, Y., Lee, Y., Thomson, JA. and Kamp, TJ. (2003). Human embryonic stem cells develop into multiple types of cardiac myocytes: action potential characterization. *Circ Res*, 93(1), pp. 32-39.

Heng, BC., Cao, T., Haider, HK., Wang, DZ., Sim, EK. and Ng, SC. (2004a) An overview and synopsis of techniques for directing stem cell differentiation in vitro. *Cell Tissue Res*, 315(3), pp. 291-303.

Heng, BC., Haider, HKh., Sim, EK., Cao, T. and Ng, SC. (2004b). Strategies for directing the differentiation of stem cells into the cardiomyogenic lineage in vitro. *Cardiovasc Res*, 62(1), pp. 34-42.

Jackson, KA., Majka, SM., Wang, H., Pocius, J., Hartley, CJ., Majesky, MW., Entman, ML., Michael, LH., Hirschi, KK. and Goodell, MA. (2001). Regeneration of ischemic cardiac muscle and vascular endothelium by adult stem cells. *J Clin Invest*, 107(11), pp. 1395-1402.

Kawada, H., Fujita, J. and Kinjo, K. (2004). Nonhematopoietic mesenchymal stem cells can be mobilized and differentiate into cardiomyocytes after myocardial infarction. *Blood*, 104(12), pp. 3581-3587.

Kehat, I., Khimovich, L., Caspi, O., Gepstein, A., Shofti, R., Arbel, G., Huber, I., Satin, J., Itskovitz-Eldor, J. and Gepstein, L. (2004). Electromechanical integration of cardiomyocytes derived from human embryonic stem cells. *Nat Biotechnol*, 22(10), pp. 1282-1289.

Klug, MG., Soonpaa, MH., Koh, GY. and Field LJ. (1996). Genetically selected cardiomyocytes from differentiating embronic stem cells form stable intracardiac grafts. *J Clin Invest*, 98(1), pp. 216-224.

Lanza, R., Moore, MA., Wakayama, T., Perry, AC., Shieh, JH., Hendrikx, J., Leri, A., Chimenti, S., Monsen, A., Nurzynska, D., West, MD., Kajstura, J. and Anversa, P. (2004). Regeneration of the infarcted heart with stem cells derived by nuclear transplantation. *Circ Res*, 94(6), pp. 820-827.

Leone, AM., Rutella, S. and Bonanno, G. (2005). Mobilization of bone marrow-derived stem cells after myocardial infarction and left ventricular function. *Eur Heart J*, 26(12), pp. 1196-1204.

Leor, J., Landa, N. and Cohen, S. (2006). Renovation of the injured heart with myocardial tissue engineering. *Expert Rev Cardiovasc Ther*, 4(2), pp. 239-352.

Linke, A., Muller, P. and Nurzynska, D. (2005). Stem cells in the dog heart are self-renewing, clonogenic, and multipotent and regenerate infarcted myocardium, improving cardiac function. *Proc Natl Acad Sci U S A*, 102(25), pp. 8966-8971.

Liu, J., Hu, Q. and Wang, Z. (2004). Autologous stem cell transplantation for myocardial repair. *Am J Physiol Heart Circ Physiol*, 287(2), pp. H501-11.

Losordo, DW. and Dimmeler, S. (2004). Therapeutic angiogenesis and vasculogenesis for ischemic disease: part II: cell-based therapies. *Circulation*, 109(22), pp. 2692-2697.

Lunde, K., Solheim, S., Aakhus, S., Arnesen, H., Abdelnoor, M., Egeland, T., Endresen, K., Ilebekk, A., Mangschau, A., Fjeld, JG., Smith, HJ., Taraldsrud, E., Grogaard, HK., Bjornerheim, R., Brekke, M., Mulle, C., Hopp, E., Ragnarsson, A., Brinchmann, JE. and Forfang, K. (2006). Intracoronary injection of mononuclear bone marrow cells in acute myocardial infarction. *N Engl J Med*, 355(12), pp. 1199-1209.

Makino, S., Fukuda, K., Miyoshi, S., Konishi, F., Kodama, H., Pan, J., Sano, M., Takahashi, T., Hori, S., Abe, H., Hata, J., Umezawa, A. and Ogawa, S. (1999). Cardiomyocytes can be generated from marrow stromal cells in vitro. *J Clin Invest*, 103(5), pp. 697-705.

Mangi, AA., Noiseux, N., Kong, D., He, H., Rezvani, M., Ingwall, JS. and Dzau, VJ. (2003). Mesenchymal stem cells modified with Akt prevent remodeling and restore performance of infarcted hearts. *Nat Med*, 9(9), pp. 1195-1201.

Matsumoto, R., Omura, T., Yoshiyama, M., Hayashi, T., Inamoto, S., Koh, KR., Ohta, K., Izumi, Y., Nakamura, Y., Akioka, K., Kitaura, Y., Takeuchi, K. and Yoshikawa, J. (2005). Vascular endothelial growth factor-expressing mesenchymal stem cell transplantation for the treatment of acute myocardial infarction. *Arterioscler Thromb Vasc Biol*, 25(6), pp. 1168-1173.

Mayani, H. and Lansdorp, PM. (1994). Thy-1 expression is linked to functional properties of primitive hematopoietic progenitor cells from human umbilical cord blood. *Blood*, 83(9), pp. 2410-2417.

Meuillet, EJ., Mahadevan, D., Vankayalapati, H., Berggren, M., Williams, R., Coon, A., Kozikowski, AP. and Powis G. (2003). Specific inhibition of the Akt1 pleckstrin homology domain by D-3-deoxy-phosphatidyl-myo-inositol analogues. *Mol Cancer Ther*, 2(4), pp. 389-399.

Meyer, GP., Wollert, KC., Lotz, J., Steffens, J., Lippolt, P., Fichtner, S., Hecker, H., Schaefer, A., Arseniev, L., Hertenstein, B., Ganser, A. and Drexler, H. (2006). Intracoronary bone marrow cell transfer after myocardial infarction: eighteen months' follow-up data from the randomized, controlled BOOST (BOne marrOw transfer to enhance ST-elevation infarct regeneration) trial. *Circulation*, 113(10), pp. 1287-1294.

Miake, J., Marban, E. and Nuss, HB. (2003). Functional role of inward rectifier current in heart probed by Kir2.1 overexpression and dominant-negative suppression. *J Clin Invest*, 111(10), pp. 1529-1536.

Mirotsou, M., Zhang, Z., Deb, A., Zhang, L., Gnecchi, M., Noiseux, N., Mu, H., Pachori, A. and Dzau V. (2007). Secreted frizzled related protein 2 (Sfrp2) is the key Akt-mesenchymal stem cell-released paracrine factor mediating myocardial survival and repair. *Proc Natl Acad Sci U S A*, 104(5), pp. 1643-1648.

Miyagawa, S., Sawa, Y., Fukuda, K., Hisaka, Y., Taketani, S., Memon, IA. and Matsuda, H. (2006). Angiogenic gene cell therapy using suicide gene system regulates the effect of angiogenesis in infarcted rat heart. *Transplantation*, 81(6), pp. 902-907.

Miyahara, Y., Nagaya, N., Kataoka, M. Yanagawa, B., Tanaka, K., Hao, H., Ishino, K., Ishida, H., Shimizu, T., Kangawa, K., Sano, S., Okano, T., Kitamura, S. and Mori, H. (2006). Monolayered mesenchymal stem cells repair scarred myocardium after myocardial infarction. *Nat Med*,12(4), pp. 459-465.

Muller, M., Fleischmann, BK. and Selbert, S. (2000). Selection of ventricular-like cardiomyocytes from ES cells in vitro. *FASEB J*. 14(15), pp. 2540-2548.

Muller-Ehmsen, J., Peterson, KL., Kedes, L., Whittaker, P., Dow, JS., Long, TI., Laird, PW. and Kloner RA. (2002). Rebuilding a damaged heart: long-term survival of transplanted neonatal rat cardiomyocytes after myocardial infarction and effect on cardiac function. *Circulation*,105(14), pp. 1720-1726.

Murohara, T., Ikeda, H., Duan, J., Shintani, S., Sasaki, K., Eguchi, H., Onitsuka, I., Matsui, K. and Imaizumi T. (2000). Transplanted cord blood-derived endothelial precursor cells augment postnatal neovascularization. *J Clin Invest*, 105(11), pp. 1527-1536.

Murry, CE., Soonpaa, MH., Reinecke, H., Nakajima, H., Nakajima, HO., Rubart, M., Pasumarthi, KB., Virag, JI., Bartelmez, SH., Poppa, V., Bradford, G., Dowell, JD., Williams, DA. and Field, LJ. (2004). Haematopoietic stem cells do not transdifferentiate into cardiac myocytes in myocardial infarcts. *Nature*, 428(6983), pp. 664-668.

Nadal-Ginard, B., Kajstura, J., Leri, A. and Anversa, P. (2003). Myocyte death, growth, and regeneration in cardiac hypertrophy and failure. *Circ Res*, 92(2), pp. 139-150.

Nieda, M., Nicol, A., Denning-Kendall, P., Sweetenham, J., Bradley, B. and Hows, J. (1997). Endothelial cell precursors are normal components of human umbilical cord blood. *Br J Haematol*, 98(3), pp. 775-777.

Odorico, JS., Kaufman, DS. and Thomson JA. (2001). Multilineage differentiation from human embryonic stem cell lines. *Stem Cells*, 19(3), pp. 193-204.

Oh, H., Bradfute, SB., Gallardo, TD., Nakamura, T., Gaussin, V., Mishina, Y., Pocius, J., Michael, LH., Behringer, RR., Garry, DJ., Entman, ML. and Schneider, MD. (2003). Cardiac progenitor cells from adult myocardium: homing, differentiation, and fusion after infarction. *Proc Natl Acad Sci U S A*, 100(21), pp. 12313-12318.

Ohtsuka, M., Takano, H. and Zou, Y. (2004). Cytokine therapy prevents left ventricular remodeling and dysfunction after myocardial infarction through neovascularization. *FASEB J*, 18(7), pp. 851-853.

Orlic, D., Kajstura, J., Chimenti, S., Jakoniuk, I., Anderson, SM., Li, B., Pickel, J., McKay, R., Nadal-Ginard, B., Bodine, DM., Leri, A. and Anversa, P. (2001). Bone marrow cells regenerate infarcted myocardium. *Nature*, 410(6829), pp. 701-705.

Pfister, O., Mouquet, F., Jain, M., Summer, R., Helmes, M., Fine, A., Colucci, WS. and Liao, R. (2005). CD31- but Not CD31+ cardiac side population cells exhibit functional cardiomyogenic differentiation. *Circ Res*, 97(1), pp. 52-561.

Pittenger, MF. and Martin, BJ. (2004). Mesenchymal stem cells and their potential as cardiac therapeutics. *Circ Res*, 95, pp. 9-20.

Pittenger, MF., Mackay, AM., Beck, SC., Jaiswal, RK., Douglas, R., Mosca, JD., Moorman, MA., Simonetti, DW., Craig, S. and Marshak, DR. (1999). Multilineage potential of adult human mesenchymal stem cells. *Science*, 284(5411), pp. 143-147.

Potapova, I., Plotnikov, A., Lu, Z., Danilo, P Jr., Valiunas, V., Qu, J., Doronin, S., Zuckerman, J., Shlapakova, IN., Gao, J., Pan, Z., Herron, AJ., Robinson, RB., Brink, PR., Rosen, MR. and Cohen IS. (2004). Human mesenchymal stem cells as a gene delivery system to create cardiac pacemakers. *Circ Res*, 94(7), pp. 952-959.

Qu, J., Plotnikov, AN., Danilo, P Jr., Shlapakova, I., Cohen, IS., Robinson, RB. and Rosen, MR. (2003). Expression and function of a biological pacemaker in canine heart. *Circulation*, 107(8), pp. 1106-1109.

Rafii, S., Heissig, B. and Hattori K. (2002). Efficient mobilization and recruitment of marrow-derived endothelial and hematopoietic stem cells by adenoviral vectors expressing angiogenic factors. *Gene Ther*, 9(10), pp. 631-641.

Rao, RR. and Stice, SL. (2004). Gene expression profiling of embryonic stem cells leads to greater understanding of pluripotency and early developmental events. *Biol Reprod*, 71(6), pp. 1772-1778.

Schachinger, V., Erbs, S., Elsasser, A., Haberbosch, W., Hambrecht, R., Holschermann, H., Yu, J., Corti, R., Mathey, DG., Hamm, CW., Suselbeck, T., Assmus, B., Tonn, T., Dimmeler, S. and Zeiher, AM. (2006). Intracoronary bone marrow-derived progenitor cells in acute myocardial infarction. *N Engl J Med*, 355(12), pp. 1210-1221.

Schwarz, ER., Speakman, MT., Patterson, M., Hale, SS., Isner, JM., Kedes, LH. and Kloner, RA. (2000). Evaluation of the effects of intramyocardial injection of DNA expressing vascular endothelial growth factor (VEGF) in a myocardial infarction model in the rat--angiogenesis and angioma formation. *J Am Coll Cardiol*, 35(5), pp. 1323-1330.

Sesti, C., Hale, SL., Lutzko, C. and Kloner, RA. (2005). Granulocyte Colony-Stimulating Factor and Stem Cell Factor Improve Contractile Reserve of the Infarcted Left Ventricle Independent of Restoring Muscle Mass. *J Am Coll Cardiol*, 46(9), pp. 1662-1669.

Shyu, KG., Wang, BW., Hung, HF., Chang, CC. and Shih, DT. (2006). Mesenchymal stem cells are superior to angiogenic growth factor genes for improving myocardial performance in the mouse model of acute myocardial infarction. *J Biomed Sci*, 13(1), pp. 47-58.

Smits, PC., van Geuns. RJ., Poldermans, D., Bountioukos, M., Onderwater, EE., Lee, CH., Maat, AP. and Serruys, PW. (2003). Catheter-based intramyocardial injection of autologous skeletal myoblasts as a primary treatment of ischemic heart failure: clinical experience with six-month follow-up. *J Am Coll Cardiol*, 42(12), pp. 2063-2069.

Solter, D. and Knowles BB. (1975). Immunosurgery of mouse blastocyst. *Proc Natl Acad Sci USA*, 72, pp. 5099-5102.

Soonpaa, MH., Koh, GY., Klug, MG. and Field, LJ. (1994). Formation of nascent intercalated disks between grafted fetal cardiomyocytes and host myocardium. *Science*, 264(5155), pp. 98-101.

Szmitko, PE., Fedak, PW., Weisel, RD., Stewart, DJ., Kutryk, MJ. and Verma, S. (2003). Endothelial progenitor cells: new hope for a broken heart. *Circulation*, 107(24), pp. 3093-3100.

Takahashi, K., Tanabe, K., Ohnuki, M., Narita, M., Ichisaka, T., Tomoda, K. and Yamanaka, S. (2007). Induction of pluripotent stem cells from adult human fibroblasts by defined factors. *Cell*, 31(5), pp. 861-872.

Tambara, K., Sakakibara, Y., Sakaguchi, G., Lu, F., Premaratne, GU., Lin, X., Nishimura, K. and Komeda, M. (2003). Transplanted skeletal myoblasts can fully replace the infarcted myocardium when they survive in the host in large numbers. *Circulation*, 108 Suppl 1, pp. II-259 - II-263.

Tang, YL., Tang, Y., Zhang, YC., Qian, K., Shen, L. and Phillips, MI. (2005). Improved graft mesenchymal stem cell survival in ischemic heart with a hypoxia-regulated heme oxygenase-1 vector. *J Am Coll Cardiol*, 46(7), pp. 1339-1350.

Tang, YL., Zhao, Q., Qin, X., Shen, L., Cheng, L., Ge, J. and Phillips, MI. (2005). Paracrine action enhances the effects of autologous mesenchymal stem cell transplantation on vascular regeneration in rat model of myocardial infarction. *Ann Thorac Surg*, 80(1), pp. 229-236.

Wang, JS., Shum-Tim, D., Chedrawy, E. and Chiu, RC. (2001). The coronary delivery of marrow stromal cells for myocardial regeneration: pathophysiologic and therapeutic implications. *J Thorac Cardiovasc Surg,*,122(4), pp. 699-705.

Wobus, AM., Holzhausen, H., Jakel, P. and Schoneich, J. (1984). Characterization of a pluripotent stem cell line derived from a mouse embryo. *Exp Cell Res*, 152(1), pp. 212-219.

Wurmser, AE. and Gage, FH. (2002). Stem cells: cell fusion causes confusion. *Nature*, 416(6880), pp. 485-487.

Xu, C., Police, S., Rao, N. and Carpenter, MK. (2002). Characterization and enrichment of cardiomyocytes derived from human embryonic stem cells. *Circ Res*, 91(6), pp. 501-508.

Yau, TM., Kim, C., Li, G., Zhang, Y., Weisel, RD. and Li, RK. (2005). Maximizing ventricular function with multimodal cell-based gene therapy. *Circulation*, 112(9 Suppl), pp. I-123 - I-128.

Yoon, YS., Wecker, A., Heyd, L., Park, JS., Tkebuchava, T., Kusano, K., Hanley, A., Scadova, H., Qin, G., Cha, DH., Johnson, KL., Aikawa, R., Asahara, T. and Losordo, DW. (2005). Clonally expanded novel multipotent stem cells from human bone marrow regenerate myocardium after myocardial infarction. *J Clin Invest*, 115(2), pp. 326-338.

Yu, J., Vodyanik, MA., Smuga-Otto, K., Antosiewicz-Bourget, J., Frane, JL., Tian, S., Nie, J., Jonsdottir, GA., Ruotti, V., Stewart, R., Slukvin, II. and Thomson, JA. (2007). Induced Pluripotent Stem Cell Lines Derived from Human Somatic Cells. *Science*, 318, pp. 1879-1880.

Zandstra, PW., Bauwens, C. and Yin, T. (2003). Scalable production of embryonic stem cell-derived cardiomyocytes. *Tissue Eng*, 9(4), pp. 767-778.

Zhang, YM., Hartzell, C., Narlow, M. and Dudley, SC Jr. (2002). Stem cell-derived cardiomyocytes demonstrate arrhythmic potential. *Circulation*, 106(10), pp. 1294-9.

Zuk, PA., Zhu, M., Mizuno, H., Huang, J., Futrell, JW., Katz, AJ., Benhaim, P., Lorenz, HP. and Hedrick, MH. (2001). Multilineage cells from human adipose tissue: implications for cell-based therapies. *Tissue Eng*, 7(2), pp. 211-228.

11.12 Glossary of Terms

Adipocyte - a connective tissue cell within the fat tissue, also named fat cell.

Adipose tissue - derived stem cell: stem cells are isolated from adipose tissue.

Adult stem cell - stem cells are isolated from the tissue of a physically fully grown and mature individual.

Autologus - in transplantation, referring to a graft in which the donor and recipient tissue is derived from the same individual, or to blood that the donor has previously donated and receives back, usually during surgery.

Blastocysts - the modified blastula stage of mammalian embryos, consisting of the inner cell mass and a thin trophoblast layer enclosing the blastocele.

Bone marrow - derived stem cell: stem cells are isolated from bone marrow tissue.

Cardiomyocyte - A heart muscle cell.

Cytokine: any of numerous hormonelike, low-molecular-weight proteins, secreted by various cells types, which regulate the intensity and duration of immune response and mediate cell-cell communication.

Embryonic stem cell - stem cells are isolated from the inner cell mass of the blastocyst stage of the mammalian embryo.

Embryo: in humans, the developing organism from conception until approximately the end of the second month; developmental stages from this time to birth are commonly designated as fetal. An organism in the early stages of development.

Hematopoietic stem cell - stem cells pertaining to or related to the formation of blood cells.

Pluripotent stem cell - cells that may still differentiate into various specialized types of tissue elements.

Mesenchymal stem cell - stem cells that can develop into connective tissue, skeletal tissue, and the circulatory and lymphatic system. Mesenchymal stem cells are derived from adult organs, such as bone marrow.

Mitosis - the usual process of somatic reproduction of cells consisting of a sequence of modifications of the nucleus that results in the formation of two daughter cells with exactly the same chromosome and nuclear DNA content as the original cell.

Muscle-derived stem cell - stem cells are isolated from skeletal muscle.

Multipotent - the ability of a cell to differentiate into two or more than two types of cells.

Osteoblasts - a bone-forming cell that is derived from mesenchymal osteoprogenitor cells and forms an osseous matrix in which it becomes enclosed as an osteocyte.

Stem cell - Stem cells are defined as undifferentiated cells that have the ability to self-renew and the potential to differentiate into various cell types that make up the body. Stem cells can be isolated from embryo, or various adult somatic tissues.

Totipotent stem cell - stem cells that can form trophoblastic cells of the placenta and all fully differentiated cells of the body.

Transdifferentiation - stem cells derived from adult somatic tissue can develop into mature cell phenotypes different from their original lineage in response to microenvironmental cues and this phenomenon is termed transdifferentiation. For example, hematopoietic stem cells from bone marrow turning into cardiac muscle cells would be termed transdifferentiation.

Unipotent – referring to those cells that produce a single type of daughter cell.

11.13 Review Questions

Q11.1 What is a myocardial infarction?

Q11.2 What is a stem cell?

Q11.3 Which of the following is (are) correct regarding the definition of embryonic stem cell?

A. Embryonic stem cells are isolated from the blastocyst stage of the mammalian embryo.

B. Embryonic stem cells are isolated from adult somatic tissue.

C. Embryonic stem cells are derived from the inner cluster of cells in the embryo.

D. Embryonic stem cells are derived from the outer cell layer of the embryo.

Q11.4 Mechanisms of improvement of cardiac function by cell transplantation therapy after myocardial infarction remain unknown. Which of the following may be involved (there can be more than one answer)?

A. Replacement of lost cardiac cells with new cardiomyocytes (muscle cells).

B. Formation of new blood vessel cells.

C. Use of cells to replace the electrical (conduction) system of the heart.

D. Prevention of left ventricular remodeling.

Q11.5 What is the transdifferentiation of stem cells?

Q11.6 What are the potential approaches to deliver ex-vivo expanded stem cells into the injured heart?

Q11.7 What is "homing" of stem cells?

Q11.8 Which kind of cells has been currently used for clinical trials of stem cell therapy for heart disease?

A. Bone marrow derived cells.

B. Embryonic stem cells.

C. Skeletal muscle satellite cells.

D. Adipose tissue derived cells.

VI

JOINTS

Chapter 12

Total Knee Replacement

W. Thomas Gutowski, M.D.[1]

[1] Princeton Orthopaedic Associates
325 Princeton Ave., Princeton, NJ 08540
PH: 609-924-8131; FX: 609-924-8532; EM: tridoc6950@aol.com

12.1 Introduction

12.1.1 *Overview*

According to the American Academy of Orthopaedic Surgeons, approximately 300,000 knee replacement operations are performed annually in the United States. In the coming years, this is likely to increase significantly. Most recent projections (Fig. 12.1) regarding primary total knee replacements suggest that by the year 2030, the number of primary knee arthroplasties will grow to 3.48 million procedures annually (growth of 673 percent). If these numbers are correct, the number of orthopaedic surgeons that will need to be trained to successfully complete these procedures must go up significantly. Additionally, the Medicare and private insurance dollars allocated to cover this burgeoning joint replacement demand must also increase. Unfortunately, to my knowledge, there is no major effort underway to carefully study these projections and thus increase the number of surgeons and dollars to provide for this dramatic increase.

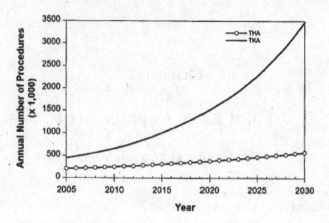

Figure 12.1. Projected number of primary total hip arthroplasty (THA) and total knee arthroplasty (TKA) procedures in the United States from 2005 to 2030. (Kurtz et al., 2007)

Through a combination of improved surgical techniques and better implants, total knee arthroplasty is considered one of the most important and successful advances of the 20th Century. Although a significant portion of the increasing number of total knee replacements is related to the burgeoning number of seniors, younger people – who are no longer willing to live with their arthritis – are also fueling the growth in knee replacement surgery.

12.1.2 *Indications*

As the knee gradually becomes more arthritic, patients begin seeking treatment for their painful and/or deformed joint. Initially, treatment such as nonsteroidal anti-inflammatory medication (i.e., ibuprofen), light bracing (i.e., neoprene/elastic knee sleeve), physical therapy, and activity modification are employed. Glucosamine sulfate, chondroitin, MSN, and other over-the-counter products may be attempted. It is at this point that x-rays are oftentimes done which may reveal joint space narrowing (Fig. 12.2), and the doctor may recommend an MRI scan. Should the MRI reveal a concomitant torn meniscus (cartilage), then an arthroscopic procedure aimed at removing and/or repairing the torn cartilage might be suggested.

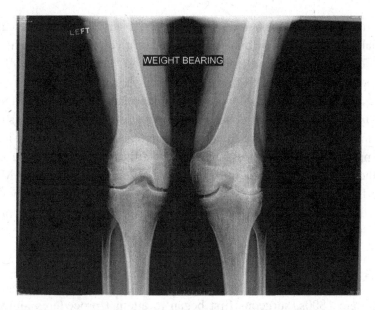

Figure 12.2. Weightbearing x-rays of knees demonstrating marked narrowing of the lateral compartment (outer portion) of the right knee (right image). There is complete obliteration of the outer joint space with bone articulating on bone (see arrows). On the inner aspect of this same knee, and in the image on the left-hand side, note the normal maintenance of the joint space between the femur and the tibia.

Despite this type of treatment, however, arthritis gradually worsens and – it is at this point that intraarticular injections of a local anesthetic (i.e., lidocaine), a steroid (i.e., cortisone), or hyaluronic acid (known as viscosupplementation) may be tried. With this later treatment, a series of joint injections are administered which serve to lubricate and enhance the arthritic cartilage function. In properly selected patients with moderate osteoarthritis, viscosupplementation therapy has been reported to secure complete or near-complete relief in pain in 39-56% of cases (Rosier and O'Keefe, 2000). If successful, it can be repeated in 9-15 months until it is no longer effective. If the MRI scan shows no evidence of torn cartilage or other correctible pathology – and merely shows a advancing osteoarthritis – then arthroscopic surgery has not proven effective (Kirkley et al., 2008).

Once conservative measures are no longer effective and pain with associated swelling and deformity progress, more complex surgical procedures can be considered. Occasionally, a surgical procedure called a tibial osteotomy can be done on the knee of a younger patient who has significant deformity and arthritis localized to just one section of the knee joint. In this complex operation, which used to be done much more frequently before the advent of joint replacement surgery, a wedge of bone is removed from the upper portion of the tibia and the bone is then bent into this void in order to create an angular change in the leg itself. This procedure removes pressure from the arthritic segment of the knee and then shifts the pressure to a more normal section of the knee. Much more frequently, however, when the arthritis is end-stage and involves more extensive aspects of the joint, knee replacement is the appropriate surgical procedure.

12.1.3 *History*

In the late 1800s, surgeons first began to attempt procedures aimed at replacing damaged knee joints. Unfortunately, these procedures failed miserably. In the early 1950s, prostheses designed as simple hinges (Fig. 12.3) made of more biocompatible materials were first attempted. The two moving components were linked, however, in a constrained way. This constraint placed far too much stress on the attachment points of the prosthesis to the bone, and most of these prostheses failed. It wasn't

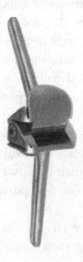

Figure 12.3. Complete metal-on-metal fixed-bearing hinge knee developed in the early 1950s by Dr. Walldius in Sweden. Because of its metal articulation and mechanically-linked components, it rapidly failed.

until the mid 1960s that surgeons learned to unlink the femoral and tibial components (unconstrained total knee) that the moderate era of total knee replacement surgery began.

The human knee is an immensely complex joint that continues to confound investigators even today. In its simplest form, it is a hinge that can normally bend between 0° and 150°. Flexion is its most important function, but the joint also rotates (spins around a vertical axis by about 15°) and translates (moves forward and backward between 10-15mm) as it bends (Fig. 12.4).

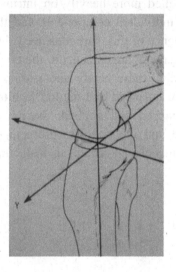

Figure 12.4. Picture showing three arcs of motion occurring in the knee joint.

In designing a knee replacement, it is vitally important to recognize the complexity of knee kinematics so that the mechanical total knee replacement can mirror the natural knee. The first total knee replacements designed in the 1950s did not rotate or translate. They moved as simple hinges and were considered constrained prostheses. Constraint is defined as limitation between two bodies linked by a joint. In simple terms, the constrained hinged prosthesis had two stems – one of which was inserted into the femur and the other down into the tibia. The early prosthesis moved in a single flexion axis, despite the fact that the normal knee wanted to move in three axes simultaneously. The consequence of this constraint mismatch was that huge forces were applied to the attachment of the prosthesis at the bone, and consequentially, the cemented prosthesis rapidly lost its bony fixation and became loose. It was not that the hinge itself failed, but rather – because the knee could not rotate or translate – the stresses on the mechanical knee were directly transferred to bone which became overwhelmed and caused the prosthesis to loosen with subsequent pain.

By the late 1960s, researchers recognized the need to mimic the mechanics of the normal knee and began designing prostheses with less constraint. These new knees produced significantly less strain on the cemented bone-attachment points and relied more heavily on intrinsic stability produced by the shape of the individual components and the retained natural ligaments. As a consequence of this, surgeons needed to pay significantly more attention to the ligament attachments to the bone, as these ligaments were required to "hold" these newly unconstrained knee prostheses together in a much more balanced and natural fashion. If the ligaments were not properly balanced and aligned, the newly unconstrained knees would be unstable and the opposite problem of a constrained hinge would occur – namely, mechanical instability (Figs. 12.5a, b).

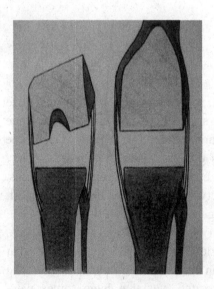

Figure 12.5a. Picture on right showing well-balanced collateral ligaments, while the picture on the left shows that one ligament is excessively long (stretched) resulting in joint space imbalance.

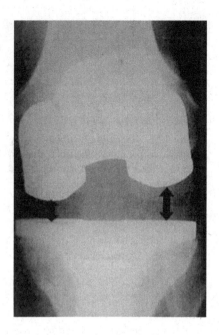

Figure 12.5b. X-ray picture demonstrating the asymmetrical joint space created by failure to properly balance ligaments resulting in potential instability. In a well-balanced and properly done total knee replacement, the components will appear parallel to one another as a consequence of the surgeon making proper bony cuts and carefully balancing the ligaments. Here, an x-ray picture demonstrates an asymmetrical joint space created by failure to properly balance the ligaments resulting in lateral liftoff (elongated arrow) resulting in potential instability.

And so began the modern era of total knee replacement surgery – respecting the need to use relatively unconstrained ligament "friendly" prostheses which would mimic the natural knee. The consequence of this was prostheses which placed significantly less stress on the bony attachment points and hence, promoted better motion, durability, and longevity of the prostheses.

12.1.4 *Anatomy*

Once it was realized that for proper knee replacement function all three axes of motion need to be taken into account, a great deal of research centered on how best to mechanically achieve this goal. The key to achieving satisfactory performance centered around a new appreciation for properly balancing the patient's own ligaments at surgery so that the knee would be snug when straightened fully (extended) as well as when the knee was flexed (bent). Instruments were developed which accurately reflected the alignment of the leg and permitted the surgeon to make precise bone cuts (Fig. 12.6).

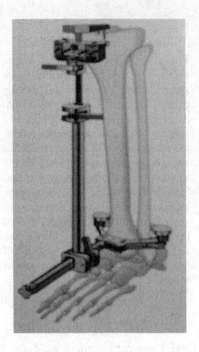

Figure 12.6. Example of tibial cutting guide placed parallel to the tibial shaft in order to make a precise 90° cut across the upper tibia.

There are four basic ligaments within the knee: the medial and lateral collateral ligaments, which sit on the inner and outer side of the bone, and – the two crossing ligaments in the center of the knee, referred to as the anterior and posterior cruciate ligaments. Additionally, two quarter moon-shaped "bumper pad" like cartilage pads sit on the inner and outer aspect of the knee and are referred to as the medial and lateral menisci. They serve to cushion and protect the two moving bones as well as providing some intrinsic support (Fig. 12.7). In order to achieve optimal function of the knee replacement, the two collateral ligaments must be retained and carefully balanced in the operating room. Oftentimes, the knee is deformed and angled. This creates a situation in which one of the collateral ligaments is too tight and the other ligament is overly stretched or elongated. Obviously, a well done total knee replacement must restore the correct alignment of the new knee through proper bone cuts (the deformed angulation must be brought back to neutral). Once this is done, though, the surgeon must address the

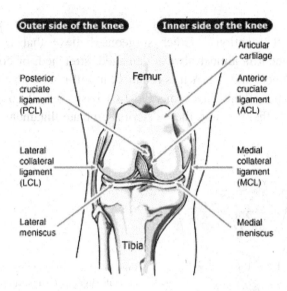

Figure 12.7. Drawing which shows the four major ligaments of the knee as well as the menisci.

unbalanced ligaments – namely lengthening the contracted or shorter ligament and/or tightening the stretched or excessively lax ligament. These considerations changed the total knee operation from merely completing a series of bone cuts to one in which lengthening and tightening the pivotal collateral ligaments throughout the normal arc of knee motion must be accurately achieved. Additionally, the two central ligaments (cruciate ligaments) also had to be addressed, as they help control rotation and translation. The vast majority of contemporary total knee replacement designs removes the anterior cruciate ligament and compensate for its loss by specific design characteristics in the prosthesis. In regard to the posterior cruciate ligament, though, certain surgical designs remove the posterior cruciate ligament and substitute a cam and post in the center of the knee to take its place (Fig. 12.8), while other prostheses are designed to retain and utilize the posterior cruciate ligament (Fig. 12.9). As just stated, almost all contemporary total knee replacements remove the anterior cruciate ligment. The issue regarding the posterior cruciate ligament continues to be a controversial one for orthopaedic surgeons today. Some surgeons feel that retaining the posterior cruciate ligament allows for better guided motion and perhaps better function. Other surgeons believe that the posterior cruciate ligament is almost always damaged, stretched, or contracted in the arthritic knee, and that if it is retained, it will not be able to function normally. Thus, there have emerged two basic schools of thought in regard to whether or not the posterior cruciate ligament should be retained.

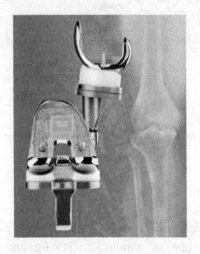

Figure 12.8. Picture of the posterior cruciate ligament substituting total knee replacement design.

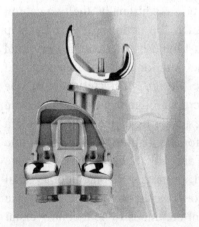

Figure 12.9. Picture of posterior cruciate ligament retaining total knee design.

In the United States today, there is no absolute direction as to which technique is better, but it does appear that there is a gradual shift to more surgeons embracing the posterior cruciate ligament substituting prosthesis (i.e., removing the posterior cruciate ligament and using prosthetic mechanics) as opposed to retaining the posterior cruciate ligament. Several studies appear to show that those prosthetic designs which substitute for the posterior cruciate ligament may perform somewhat better regarding improved range of motion and better stair-climbing mechanics (Hirsch et al., 1995).

12.1.5 *Prosthetic materials*

Besides issues of constraint and laxity, another important issue in joint replacement surgery involves the potential for wear of the components – or that tendency of a bearing surface to abrade, fatigue, or delaminate much like a rubber tire gradually wears out. All contemporary knee replacements use a combination of metal and plastic. The ability to withstand wear involves the toughness of these surfaces. Additionally, the amount of contact surface which abrades or rubs, - the ability of surfaces to withstand millions of cycling of motion, - the impact of microscopic debris on these surfaces, - and the level of stress or activity which the surfaces must endure (i.e., jogging, tennis, obesity) are all issues which need to be carefully understood when designing a contemporary knee prosthesis. After much research, most orthopaedic components employ chromium cobalt metal on the femoral side (Fig. 12.10a) and titanium on the tibial base plate (Fig. 12.10b) with a polyethylene-molded plastic insert placed between these two metal components. The plastic polyethylene insert essentially functions like the cartilage in the natural knee – providing a smooth, contoured, gliding surface between the two hard metal replacement surfaces (Fig. 12.10c). Additionally, a small plastic polyethylene button is typically cemented to the back side of the patella (kneecap) so it, too, can glide on the metal femoral component (Fig. 12.10d).

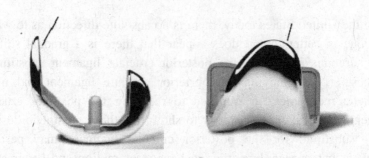

Figure 12.10a. Picture of femoral component.

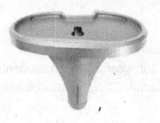

Figure 12.10b. Picture of tibial component.

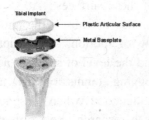

Figure 12.10c. Picture of polyethylene articular surface which locks into the tibial component.

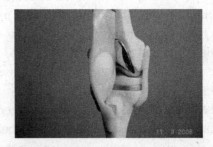

Figure 12.10d. Model of a total knee replacement in which the patellar tendon and its associated patella (right) has been tipped 90° to its normal position in order to visualize the patellar prosthetic "button" (left) cemented onto the patella bone (bone not visible as it is covered with the new patellar component).

12.1.5.1 *Polyethylene*

In the past, the polyethylene molded component – placed between the two metal sections – wore out rather rapidly and thus impacted the ability of these prostheses to perform reliably over many years (Fig. 12.11).

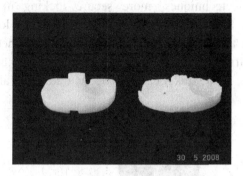

Figure 12.11. Picture of a new tibial component (left) next to a markedly worn component which was removed from a patient after eight years of use.

Factors that adversely affect tibial polyethylene inserts include:
- poor production quality,
- oxidation of the polyethylene,
- application of abnormally-high focal stresses due to poor prosthetic design,
- obesity,
- excessive activity,
- improper surgical implant technique,
- improper sterilization techniques, etc. (Blunn et al., 1997; Conditt et al., 2000).

Excessive constraint also placed high stresses and friction on the plastic. As the polyethylene deteriorated, small microscopic debris particles were shed which had a highly toxic effect on the adjacent bone. It produced an inflammatory reaction in the bone, causing it to slowly dissolve (osteolysis), and with this, the metal knee components became loose. Over the last few years, however, wear rates of the plastic polyethylene have improved significantly as a consequence of manufacturing processes to improve plastic toughness as well as better implant design and implantation techniques. A process called "crosslinking" in which the polyethlene is radiated and heated in order to quench free radicals has helped to prevent plastic oxidation and subsequent early polyethylene failure (Fig. 12.12). Similarly, better surgical implant techniques, more secure locking mechanisms (the manner in which the tibial polyethylene plastic is locked onto the cemented metal tibial base plate), and improved prosthetic design have resulted in significantly improved polyethylene wear (Rand et al., 2003; Muratoglu et al., 2001; Baker et al., 2003; Muratoglu et al., 2003; Collier et al., 1991).

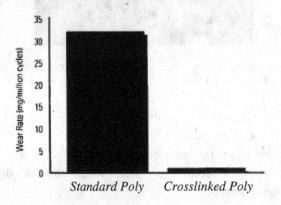

Figure 12.12. Typical simulator findings whereby standard polyethylene is seen to wear significantly faster (left) compared to crosslinked polyethylene (right) after approximately five million wear cycles. (Courtesy of Zimmer.)

12.2 Surgical Technique and Design Considerations

12.2.1 *Surgical technique*

The goal of every properly performed total knee replacement is to restore the joint to its correct alignment which means making a bowed leg or knocked-knee deformity straight again. To do this properly, the surgeon requires calibrated instruments which take rigid reference from the normal bone so that bone cuts can be made accurately and reproducibly (Fig. 12.13). In addition, as mentioned previously, a better understanding and respect for ligament balancing is essential. Recent improvements such as minimally-invasive surgical techniques which employ methods that attempt to minimize muscle and tendon injury during surgery have also helped.

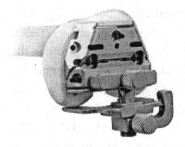

Figure 12.13. An example of a femoral cutting jig rigidly applied to the end of the femur with saw capture cutting slots which precisely hold the cutting blade when preparing the femur for its properly sized implant.

Although the effects of these minimally-invasive techniques can be quite helpful, it is still important to recognize that the same basic surgical tenants must occur (alignment, soft tissue balance, good cement technique, etc.) simply through smaller and less extensive incisions and dissections (Heim et al., 1996; Dalury and Jiranek, 1999; White et al., 1999). Obviously, with smaller incisions, the surgeon cannot "see" as much as in the past, and the potential for misaligning components is very real. For this reason, excellent surgical training, well-calibrated smaller instruments, and proper technique are essential. Newer technologies which involve computer-assisted navigation and other emerging technologies may further this effort. While most people believe that computer navigation can help the surgeon tremendously, its track record to date has been inconsistent and its performance has lagged. It is not that the computer can't perform adequately – but rather, the ability of the computer to accurately register where the bones are in space and thus tell the surgeon to make completely reliable bone cuts has been inconsistent. These computer navigation technologies are improving and in the future should be able to produce more consistent results.

12.2.2 *Unique design considerations – mobile-bearing versus fixed-bearing*

In the past 20 years, two schools of thought have emerged regarding the tibial component portion of a total knee replacement procedure. In one design, the metal tibial tray is rigidly attached (usually with cement) to the tibia bone, and the polyethylene spacer is then locked onto this tray (Fig. 12.14). This results in some limited tibial constraint (the tibia base and its plastic insert are fixed rigidly to the tibia bone) and is referred to as a fixed-bearing tibial component. In the other design, the polyethylene tibial portion has a cylindrical extension on its undersurface which drops down into a similar-shaped hole in the metal tibial tray which is fixed to the bone. This is referred to as a mobile-bearing knee (D'Lima et al., 2001; Haas et al., 2002; Ranawat et al., 2004). The polyethylene component is free to rotate around the cylindrical post and thereby potentially reduce certain stresses on the total knee compared to the fixed-bearing component (Fig. 12.15). While the theoretical advantage of a mobile-bearing component occurs by decreasing constraint, it also creates a potential for instability if the operation is not done correctly and also has the potential for greater polyethylene wear as the polyethylene rotates about the post on the metal tray itself (Fig. 12.16). Rarely, as alluded to above, the tibial plastic can rotate too far, and the total knee becomes painful and occasionally disjointed. Additionally, when range of motion following fixed-bearing versus mobile-bearing components were compared, the range of motion appeared slightly better in the fixed-bearing components than in the mobile-bearing (Dennis et al., 1998). Notwithstanding much of this data, it does appear that from a clinical perspective, whether or not the surgeon chooses a mobile-bearing or a fixed-bearing component – the outcomes tend to be quite good if the design mechanics of the component are respected, the quality of the polyethylene is good, the ligaments are properly balanced, and the components are properly implanted by the surgeon.

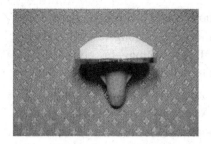

Figure 12.14. Example of a fixed-bearing tibial component in which the tibial polyethylene is locked onto the tibial base plate.

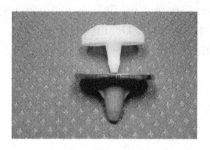

Figure 12.15. Example of a mobile-bearing knee replacement in which the tibial polyethylene has a conical post which slides down into the metal tibial tray and allows the polyethylene to rotate on the base plate.

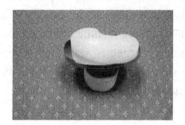 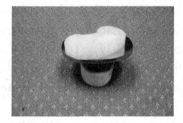

Figure 12.16. Example of a mobile-bearing knee replacement (two perspectives) in which the tibial component is free to rotate about the tibial base plate.

12.2.3 *Posterior cruciate-retaining versus posterior cruciate-sacrificing total knee replacement*

As described previously, two other schools of thought have emerged regarding how the posterior cruciate ligament should be managed in joint replacement surgery. By retaining the posterior cruciate ligament, some surgeons believe that the knee will move more naturally, maintaining better mechanics. Unfortunately, in the case of longstanding arthritis and deformity, the posterior cruciate ligament may be contracted or deformed, and thus – when retained – is unbalanced. This can cause a loss of motion, difficulty with pain, trouble with stair-climbing, and hence, produce a poor clinical result. As a consequence of this, another school of surgeons believes that the posterior cruciate ligament can be safely removed and substituted with a post and cam built into the prosthesis, which more consistently and correctly mimics the normal posterior cruciate ligament and thus produces fewer problems and better results (Bertin et al., 2002; Dennis et al., 2001; Dennis et al., 2003; Dennis et al., 2004; Dennis et al., 2003). While both schools of thought have their detractors and proponents, it appears that the number of surgeons preferring posterior cruciate substituting operation is gradually increasing in this country.

12.2.4 *Cement versus noncement*

Traditionally, total knee replacements were always secured to the bone by utilizing bone cement. Unfortunately, like any static bond, this interface may fail and result in the component losing its attachment to the bone (Fig. 12.17). To avoid this problem, surgeons designed knee components in which the metallic surface was coated with a bio-friendly porous surface into which the bone could actually grow (porous coating). While this design has met with some good success, the bone has not always successfully grown into the components and thus, despite the surgeon's best attempts to secure biologic fixation, the component remains unfixed – and thus painful. As a consequence of this, the majority of surgeons in this country prefer to use cement when attaching the tibial base tray to the tibial bone itself.

On the femoral side, these same issues also pertain, and surgeons may choose to cement or not cement the femoral component based on a host of issues such as the quality of bone, the implant design, and the particular surgeon's training or expertise.

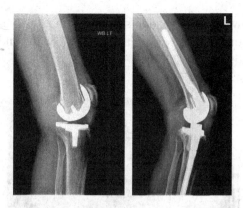

Figure 12.17. X-ray of a mechanically-loose cemented total knee replacement. Note the gap between the anterior femoral component and its underlying bone with a piece of loose cement interposed (left). On the right, the x-ray showing the extensive revision that was necessary to rectify this problem.

12.2.5 *Unicompartmental versus total knee replacement*

The anatomical knee can be thought of as being composed of three distinct parts – a medial compartment (the inner side), a lateral compartment (the outer side), and the patellofemoral space (knee cap portion). When a person's arthritis affects two or three of these compartments simultaneously, then a total knee replacement is required to solve the problem. Conversely, if the arthritis affects only one side or compartment (as is often the case years following an open meniscectomy) – and the other two compartments of the knee are essentially normal – then the patient may be a candidate for a partial knee replacement (Fig. 12.18). During this operation, only the single diseased compartment is replaced. The remaining two compartments – comprised of mostly normal cartilage tissue – can be preserved and hence the knee should function in a more natural way – as only a single compartment has been replaced (Fig. 12.19a). Unfortunately, most people's arthritis involves more than one compartment and hence, the vast majority of arthroplasties done are total knee replacements in which all three compartments are replaced (Figs. 12.19b, c). In the United States today, between 5-10% of knee arthroplasties are unicompartmental arthroplasties. With current surgical techniques and well-designed components, recent data suggest greater than 90% survival at 11-year follow-up in 41 patients younger than 60 years of age who had unicompartmental knee replacements (Svard and Price, 2001; Romanowski and Repicci, 2002).

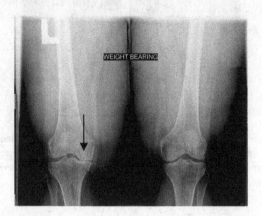

Figure 12.18. X-ray demonstrating joint space narrowing (arrow) on the inner (medial) aspect of the left knee, while the x-ray to the right shows symmetrical joint spaces between the femur and tibia on both the inner and outer compartments.

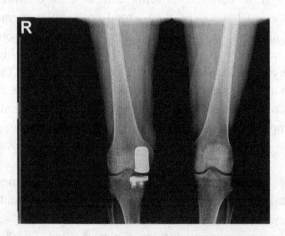

Figure 12.19a. X-ray demonstrating a unicompartmental knee replacement of the inner (medial) aspect of the knee. The "gap" between the two metal components is filled with the polyethylene-bearing surface which locks onto the tibial tray and is not visible with regular x-ray.

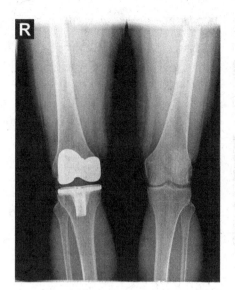
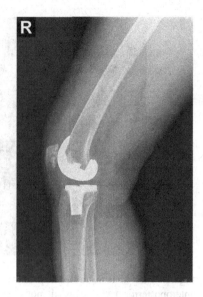

Figures 12.19b, c. Anteroposterior (AP) and lateral x-rays of total knee replacement.

12.2.6 *Patellofemoral arthroplasty*

A somewhat less frequent area of <u>localized</u> osteoarthritis involves deterioration in the patellofemoral joint (knee cap part of the joint). Isolated patellofemoral osteoarthritis may occur in up to 11% of men and 24% of women older than 55 years old (Merchant, 2004; Smith et al., 2002). Oftentimes, through a combination of activity modification, various medications, exercise, and bracing, symptoms can be managed. Unfortunately, there are times when the arthritic deterioration becomes so severe that patellofemoral arthroplasty (replacing the kneecap joint alone) can be considered (Figs. 12.20a, b) (Lonner, 2004).

Isolated patellofemoral arthroplasty is by far the least common arthroplasty done today. In the last several years, improved component design has significantly diminished the complications associated with this procedure, and with further refinements in component design we can expect better long-term patient outcomes which may then result in an increasing percentage of patellofemoral arthroplasties in the future.

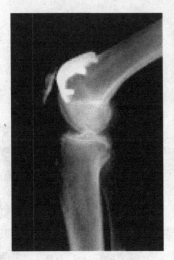 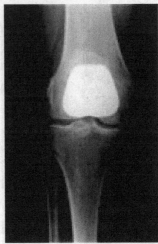

Figures 12.20a, b. X-ray of a patellofemoral arthroplasty (replacement). Lateral and anteroposterior (AP) x-ray demonstrating the front (anterior) portion of the femur replaced by a trapezoidal-shaped metal component and, although not seen on this x-rays, the patella has been replaced with a small plastic button.

12.2.7 *Minimally-invasive total knee arthroplasty*

Prior to 2000, the majority of total knee replacement surgeries were done with incisions ranging between 25-30cm. Typically, the quadriceps was incised and the patella (kneecap) inverted. This resulted in a significantly slower recovery, more scar, and the potential for diminished long-term quadriceps function (Mahoney et al., 2002; Silva et al., 2003). As a consequence of this, surgeons began working with smaller incisions which were significantly more tissue friendly (i.e., "quad sparing") (Fig. 12.21). In completing a minimally-invasive total knee replacement, however, it is important to recognize that the surgeon will see less, and hence the potential for misplacing the components is very real. Notwithstanding this, current clinical results in large series of patients in which the procedure has been done correctly showed reduced recovery time, lessened pain, and more rapid return to work. The incisions vary between 7-10cm. It is unclear whether a long-term advantage – such as an improved arc of motion or better quadriceps strength – can be expected with minimally-invasive knee surgery compared to traditional incision knee replacement surgery (Tria and Coon, 2003; Haas et al., 2004; Hozack et al., 2004).

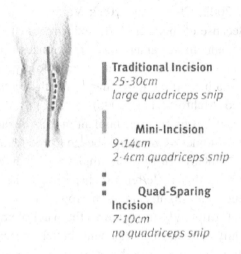

Figure 12.21. Picture of a traditional long total knee replacement scar (left), a minimally-invasive total knee replacement (middle), and a complete quadriceps total knee replacement scar (right) incision.

12.2.8 *Gender-specific total knee arthroplasty*

It has long been recognized that there are different anatomical characteristics which typically distinguish the male versus the female knee (Fig. 12.22). These issues involve the shape and angular change in

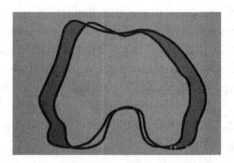

Figure 12.22. Male (dark) to female (light) comparison using three-dimensional CT scan data from over 800 cadaveric femurs.

the patellofemoral joint as well as a difference in the height versus width of the end of the femur. Additionally, anatomical differences have also been noted in different populations (Woodland and Francis, 1992; Csintalan et al., 2002; Chin et al., 2002; Vaidya et al., 2000; Mahfouz et al., 2006). Because of this, scientists and surgeons recognized that by taking into account these anatomical differences in their specific populations – and designing implants more closely resembling their natural anatomy – a potential improvement in both function and outcome might be achieved (Mahfouz et al., 2006).

In the early part of this century, implant makers began looking at this issue and the Zimmer Company began production of "Gender Solutions™ NexGen® High-Flexion Implant" which was deliberately designed to address this male/female disparity. The gender type of femoral component is slightly more narrow, thinner in profile, and shaped somewhat differently in regard to the patellofemoral joint. This results in a slightly less bulky component, better kneecap tracking, and hence potentially better motion in the majority of female patients. Other implant makers are also actively involved in optimizing components to address this issue.

12.2.9 *Outcomes*

Long-term studies currently report ten-year survivorship of total knee replacements in the 95% range. Additional studies looking at between 15- and 20-year survivorship still show numbers in the 90%+ range (Buechel, 2002; Hofmann et al., 2001; Back et al., 2001). A number of factors, however, can have a negative impact on survivorship, such as poor implant design (Forster, 2003; Furnes et al., 2002), patient comorbidity such as diabetes (Meding et al., 2003; Shrader et al., 2003), obesity, and excessive postoperative activity level (Lavernia et al., 2001). As a consequence of this, while patients are encouraged to remain physically active following their total knee replacements, they are advised to refrain from certain activities which could pose risk to long-term survivorship (Table 12.1).

Table 12.1. Recommended activities following total knee replacement.

Recommended activities following total knee replacement (Healy, 2000; Kuster, 2000)		
Low-load activities	*Moderate-level activities performed on a recreational level*	*Discouraged high-impact activities to be avoided post total knee replacement*
Walking	Skiing	Running/jogging
Swimming	Hiking	Basketball
Bike riding	Doubles tennis	Gymnastics
Light weight training	Aerobics	Football
Dancing	Bowling	Lacrosse
Golf, etc.	Horseback riding, etc.	Singles tennis, etc.

12.3 Computer-Assisted Technology/Robotics

12.3.1 *Background*

Currently, computer-assisted navigation technology is available in our operating rooms to assist a surgeon in making more accurate bony cuts and doing a better job at balancing ligaments. Unfortunately, the ability of the computer to consistently and reproducibly "understand" the exact position, alignment, and anatomy of the joint in space has been problematic. In order to get this technology to work correctly, the bone and joint need to be accurately registered in the computer so that the computer can precisely recognize the positions of the bones in space and thus correctly orient the surgeon to make proper bone cuts and ligament releases. This technology is only as good as the information secured by the computer during this registration process. The difficulty with accurately registering the patient's anatomy has led to some inconsistency in precisely and reproducibly "telling" the surgeon how to cut and how much ligament to release (Saragaglia et al., 2001; Sparmann et al., 2003; Stulberg et al., 2002). The field of computer-assisted surgery continues to mature, and more consistent and reliable results can be expected in the future.

12.3.2 *Robotic technology in orthopaedics (Bargar, 2003)*

Unlike computer-<u>assisted</u> surgery in which the surgeon still manually makes the cuts and/or releases – robotic surgery involves cutting tools which are directly connected to an automated machine which follows a predefined trajectory. The surgeon may supervise or observe what the robot is doing, but it is the mechanical robotic device making the cut – not the surgeon's hands. Hybrid robots are being developed involving a semi-active role of the machine so that the surgeon does partake – to a degree – in the cuts or releases. These systems are still in their infancy, although in the future they could play a more active role in knee replacement surgery.

12.4 Other Considerations

12.4.1 *Revision knee replacement surgery*

One of the largest burdens faced by the orthopaedic community – in the future – will be the increasing number of revision knee replacements. The need for this surgery is a consequence of either the knee wearing out, or becoming loose, painful, or infected. As more and more primary knee replacements are done on younger and more active patients, the demand for revision surgery will clearly grow. These revision procedures are typically more complex, expensive, time consuming, and riskier than the patient's initial procedure (Fig. 12.23) (Coyte, 1999). Oftentimes, the revision is necessary for an infection which may require multiple surgical procedures as well as months of antibiotics to resolve. The quality of the host bone when the revision procedure is done is never as good as it was at the time of the original procedure. Additionally, patients are typically older and have more medical comorbidities. The collective consequence of this is that revision knee surgery is much more complex and will place a much greater burden on our healthcare system in the future. Typically, the results are never as good or long-lasting as the original procedure.

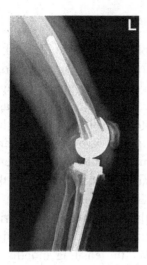

Figure 12.23. Lateral x-ray of the revision knee replacement done for the loose femoral component which was shown in Fig. 12.16.

12.4.2 *Surgical risks*

Once the patient and surgeon agree that a knee replacement should be done, a thorough discussion regarding potential risks should occur. The major risks of knee replacement surgery include anesthetic issues (spinal versus epidural versus general anesthesia), blood clot in leg veins (thrombophlebitis) or lungs (pulmonary embolism) (Clagett et al., 1998), infection, knee stiffness, damage to adjacent structures (such as nerves or arteries), and perisurgical events such as stroke or heart attack. With improved anesthetic techniques – oftentimes which avoid general anesthesia and rather rely on regional anesthesia – risks have diminished and outcomes have improved (Rodgers et al., 2000). Additionally, utilizing thromboembolic prophylaxis – whereby patients are administered various treatments to prevent clots including elastic stockings, pneumatic compression stockings, blood thinners (Colwell, 1999), and rapid out-of-bed mobilization, etc., have reduced this risk. By using prophylactic antibiotics, infection rates of less than 1% are reported in most major institutions (Peersman et al., 2001). All of these issues, as well as others, need to be thoroughly discussed and understood before surgery.

12.4.3 *Future considerations: biological solutions*

A great deal of research now centers on technologies which could heal or replace damaged cartilage with new healthy articular cartilage. At birth, all of our joints are lined with pristine, smooth articular hyaline cartilage. As a consequence of injury, disease, genetics, aging, etc., this cartilage becomes pitted, eroded, and irregular in osteoarthritis. Because this cartilage does not have its own good blood supply, regrowing or getting damaged cartilage to heal is still an extremely challenging problem. Currently we can take healthy segments of articular cartilage from the knee (as a biopsy) and get these cells to reproduce in a Petrie dish. Unfortunately, when we attempt to replant this new cartilage material over a very broad and uncontained surface (as happens with extensive osteoarthritis), the cells may survive, but over the ensuing months of wear – the new cartilage material delaminates from the bone, much like an orange peel coming off an orange. Conversely, if the arthritic defect in the joint is isolated and small – much like a pothole–then the sidewalls of the damaged articular cartilage lesion serve as a buttress to the transplanted cartilage material and indeed, we can get these cells to grow and survive. A great deal of future research needs to be devoted to these issues so that ultimately we can secure a biological solution to the damaged arthritic knee as opposed to the current mechanical (metal and plastic) solutions. These technological advances may also require some manipulation of the genome as we attempt to alter and change the body's ability to heal cartilage damage. Unfortunately, these biotechnologies are still years off in helping patients with advanced tricompartmental knee osteoarthritis – and total knee replacement will remain the mainstay of advanced arthritis treatment for years to come.

12.4.4 *Note to people considering undergoing a total knee replacement*

It has been said that knowledge is power – the ability to better understand and comprehend an issue in order to confidently make a good decision. Hopefully, this chapter – and the book in general – can aid patients in better understanding their body. If you are considering undergoing a total knee replacement, though, there are several additional issues which you may wish to consider.

Physical conditioning of your body and leg both before and after surgery is vital to a successful outcome. Despite excellent prosthetic design and surgical skills, muscular training and conditioning through physical therapy is mandatory. Ideally, six weeks before surgery you should begin a program of progressive quadriceps muscle strengthening, as well as general lower extremity strengthening in preparation for your surgery. Cardiovascular conditioning (such as stationary bike riding or swimming) is also helpful.

When selecting your surgeon, Board certification in orthopaedic surgery should be a prerequisite standard in your selection process. Your surgeon should also be open to discussing the issues reviewed in this chapter. Additionally, it has been shown that surgeons who perform this type of total knee replacement surgery – frequently – often have better outcomes than those who do the operation only occasionally (Katz et al, 2004. As a rough rule, surgeons who do more than 20-25 cases per year – at a minimum – generally seem to have better patient outcomes than those that do less than this number. It is not unreasonable to ask your surgeon about his knee replacement case load.

Lastly, try not to put too much pressure on yourself to heal too quickly. Despite the advances discussed in this chapter, the knee still needs to biologically heal. This means that the soft tissues have to mend while coping with the fact that you will be walking on the leg – and moving the joint. This obviously produces inflammation, pain, and swelling, but these issues can be managed and moderated during your recovery. Remember, as your knee became progressively arthritic, your joint became stiff and the surrounding muscles increasingly weak. After your joint replacement, the new joint may take some time to gradually regain its motion and strength. You should understand that your recovery will more likely unfold over months as opposed to weeks.

12.5 Summary

In the past 35 years, a knee replacement operation initially designed as a
simple hinge has evolved into an extremely complex and reproducible
procedure taking into account three simultaneous axes of motion and
many of the complexities and nuances of the natural knee.
Contemporary prostheses are designed to mimic a knee's normal
kinematics as much as possible so that it feels and acts naturally.
Improvements in materials, design, anatomical understandings, careful
ligament balancing, and a respect for the soft tissue envelope have
proven tremendously successful at improving knee replacement
outcomes. The number of people who can now benefit from this
technology is increasing, and this operation will become evermore
popular. Future developments including computer-assisted navigation,
better implant design and materials, biologics (cartilage transplantation
technologies), and other emerging technologies will further improve
outcome and longevity.

12.6 References

Back, D. L., Cannon, S. R., Hilton, A., Bankes, M. J., and Briggs, T. W. (2001). The
Kinemax total knee arthroplasty: Nine years' experience. *J. Bone Joint Surg. [Br]*
83, pp. 359-363.

Baker, D., Bellare, A., Pruitt, L. (2003). The effects of degree of crosslinking on the
fatigue crack initiation and propagation resistance of orthopedic grade polyethlene.
J. Biomed Mater Res. 66, pp. 146-154.

Bargar, W. (2003). Robotic hip surgery and current development with the Robodoc
system. In: Stiehl, J. B., Konermann, W. H., Haaker, R. G. (eds). *Navigation and
robotics in total joint and spine surgery.* Springer-Verlag, Berlin, Heidelberg, New
York, Tokyo. pp. 119-121.

Bertin, K. C., Komistek, R. D., Dennis, D. A., Hoff, W. A., Anderson, W. A., Langer, T.
(2002). In vivo determination of posterior femoral rollback for subjects having a
NexGen posterior cruciate-retaining total knee arthroplasty. *J. Arthroplasty* 17,
pp. 1040-1048.

Blunn, G. W., Joshi, A. B., Minns, R. J., Lidgren, L., Lilley, P., Ryd, L., Engelbrecht, E.,
Walker, P. S. (1997). Wear in retrieved condylar knee arthroplasties. *J. Arthroplasty*
12, pp. 281-290.

Buechel, F. F. (2002). Long-term follow-up after mobile-bearing total knee replacement.
Clin. Orthop. Relat. Res. 404, pp. 40-50.

Callaghan, J. J., Insall, J. N., Greenwald, A. S., Dennis, D. A., Komistek, R. D., et al. (2000). Mobile-bearing knee replacement. *J. Bone Joint Surg. [Am]* 82, pp. 1020-1041.

Chin, K. R., Dalury, D. F., Zurakowski, D., Scott, R. D. (2002). Intraoperative measurements of male and female distal femurs during primary total knee arthroplasty. *J. Knee Surg.* 15(4), pp. 213-217.

Clagett, G. P., Anderson, F. A. Jr., Geerts, W., et al. (1998). Prevention of venous thromboembolism. *Chest* 114[Suppl 5], pp. 531S-560S.

Collier, J. P., et al. (1991). Analysis of the failure of 122 polyethylene inserts from uncemented tibial knee components. *Clin. Orthop.* 273, pp. 232-242.

Colwell, C. W. Jr., Collis, D. K., Paulson, R., et al. (1999). Comparison of enoxaparin and warfarin for the prevention of venous thromboembolic disease after total hip arthroplasty: Evaluation during hospitalization and three months after discharge. *J. Bone Joint Surg. [Am]* 81, pp. 932-940.

Conditt, M., Stein, J., Noble, P. (2000). Backside polyethylene wear in modular tibial inserts. *46th Annual Meeting Orthopaedic Research Society* p. 197.

Coyte, P. C., Hawker, G., Croxford, R., Wright, J. G. (1999). Rates of revision knee replacement in Ontario, Canada. *J. Bone Joint Surg. [Am]* 81, pp. 773-782.

Csintalan, R. P., Schulz, M. M., Woo, J., McMahon, P. J., Lee, T. Q. (2002). Gender differences in patellofemoral joint biomechanics. *Clin. Orthop. Relat. Res.* 402, pp. 260-269.

D'Lima, D. D., Trice, M., Urquhart, A. G., Colwell, C. W. Jr. (2001). Tibiofemoral conformity and kinematics of rotating-bearing knee prostheses. *Clin. Orthop.* 386, pp. 235-242.

Dalury, D. F., Jiranek, W. A. (1999). A comparison of the midvastus and paramedian approaches for total knee arthroplasty. *J. Arthroplasty* 14, pp. 33-37.

Dennis, D. A., Komistek, R. D., Stiehl, J. B., Walker, S. A., Dennis, K. (1998). Range of motion following total knee arthroplasty: The effect of implant design and weightbearing conditions. *J. Arthroplasty* 13, pp. 748-752.

Dennis, D. A., Komistek, R. D. (2003). Evaluation of range of motion after PFC Sigma posterior stabilized rotating platform total knee arthroplasty. Internal Report at the Rocky Mountain Musculoskeletal Research Laboratory.

Dennis, D. A., Komistek, R. D., Cheal, E. J., Walker, S. A., Stiehl, J. B. (2001). In vivo femoral condylar lift-off in total knee arthroplasty. *J. Bone Joint Surg. [Br]* 83, pp. 33-39.

Dennis, D. A., Komistek, R. D., Mahfouz, M. R., Haas, B. D., Stiehl, J. B. (2003). Multicenter determination of in vivo kinematics after total knee arthroplasty. *Clin. Orthop. Relat. Res.* 416, pp. 37-57.

Dennis, D. A., Komistek, R. D., Mahfouz, M. R., Walker, S. A., Tucker, A. (2004). A multicenter analysis of axial femorotibial rotation after total knee arthroplasty. *Clin. Orthop. Relat. Res.* 428, pp. 180-189.

Dennis, D. A., Komistek, R. D., Mahfouz, M. (2003). In vivo fluoroscopic analysis of fixed-bearing total knee replacements. *Clin. Orthop. Relat. Res.* 410, pp. 114-130.

Forster, M. C. (2003). Survival analysis of primary cemented total knee arthroplasty: Which designs last? *J. Arthroplasty* 18, pp. 265-270.

Furnes, O., Espehaug, B., Lie, S. A., Vollset, S. E., Engesaeter, L. B., Havelin, L. I. (2002). Early failures among 7,174 primary total knee replacements: A follow-up study from the Norwegian Arthroplasty Register 1994-2000. *Acta Orthop. Scan* 73, pp. 117-129.

Gluck, T., Arch,. Klin. (1891). *Clin.* 41, p. 186.

Haas, S., Cook, S., Beksac, B. (2004). Minimally-invasive total knee replacement through a mini-midvastus approach: A comparative study. *Clin. Orthop. Relat. Res.* 428, pp. 68-73.

Haas, B. D., Dennis, D. A., Komistek, R. D., Brumley, J. T., Hammill, C. (2001). Range of motion of posterior-cruciate-substituting total knee replacements: The effect of bearing mobility. *J. Bone Joint Surg. [Am]* 83[Suppl 2], pp. 51-55.

Haas, B. D., Komistek, R. D., Stiehl, J. B., Anderson, D. T., Northcut, E. J. (2002). Kinematic comparison of posterior cruciate sacrifice versus substitution in a mobile-bearing total knee arthroplasty. *J. Arthroplasty* 17, pp. 685-692.

Healy, W. L., Iorio, R., Lemos, M. J. (2000). Athletic activity after total knee arthroplasty. *Clin. Orthop.* 380, pp. 65-71.

Heim, C. M., et al. (1996). Factors influencing the longevity of UHMWPE tibial components. *AAOS Instructional Course Lectures* 45, pp. 303-314.

Hirsch, H. S., Lotke, P. A., Morrison, L. D. (1995). The posterior cruciate ligament in total knee replacement surgery: Save, sacrifice, or substitute? *Clin. Orthop.* 309, pp. 64-68.

Hofmann, A. A., Evanich, J. D., Ferguson, R., et al. (2001). Ten- to 14-year clinical follow-up of the cementless Natural Knee system. *Clin. Orthop. Relat. Res.* 388, pp. 85-94.

Hozack, W. J., Krismer, M., Nogler, M., et al. (eds). (2004). *Minimally Invasive Total Joint Arthroplasty*. New York, NY, Springer-Verlag.

Jazrawi, L. M., et al. (2000). The accuracy of computer tomography for determining femoral and tibial total knee arthroplasty component rotation. *J. Arthroplasty* 15, pp. 761-766.

Katz, J. N., Barrett, J., Mahomed, N. N., Baron, J. A., Wright, R. J., Losina, E. (2004). Association between hospital and surgeon procedure volume and the outcomes of total knee replacement. *J. Bone Joint Surg. [Am]* 86A, 9, pp. 1909-1916.

Katz, J. N., Mahomed, N. N., Baron, J. A., Barrett, J. A., Fossel, A. H., Creel, A. H., Wright, J., Wright, E. A., Losina, E. (2007). Association of hospital and surgeon procedures volume with patient-centered outcomes of total knee replacement in a population-based cohort of patients age 65 years and older. *Arthritis Rheum.* 56(2), pp. 568-574.

Kirkley, A., Birmingham, T. B., Litchfield, R. B., Griffin J. R., et al. (2008). A randomized trial of arthroscopic surgery for osteoarthritis of the knee. *NE Jour. Med.* 359, pp. 1097-1107.

Kurtz, S., Ong, K., Lau, E., et al. (2007). Projections of primary and revision hip and knee arthroplasty in the United States from 2005 to 2030. *J. Bone Joint Surg. Am* 89, pp. 780-785.

Kuster, M. S., Spalinger, E., Blanksby, B. A., Gatchter, A. (2000). Endurance sports after total knee replacement: A biomechanical investigation. *Med. Sci. Sports Exerc.* pp. 721-724.

Lavernia, C. J., Sierra, R. J., Hungerford, D. S., Krackow, K. (2001). Activity level and wear in total knee arthroplasty. *J. Arthroplasty* 4, pp. 446-453.

Lonner, J. H. (2004). Patellofemoral arthroplasty: Pros, cons, design considerations. *Clin. Orthop. Relat. Res.* 428, pp. 158-165.

Mahfouz, M., Booth, R. Jr., Argenson, J., Merkl, B. C., Abdel Fatah, E. E., Kuhn, M. J. (2006). Analysis of variation of adult femora using sex-specific statistical atlases. Presented at Computer Methods in Biomechanics and Biomedical Engineering Conference.

Mahoney, O. M., McClung, C. D., dela Rosa, M. A., Schmalzried, T. P. (2002). The effect of total knee arthroplasty design on extensor mechanism function. *J. Arthroplasty* 17, pp. 416-421.

Meding, J. B., Reddleman, K., Keathing, M. E., et al. (2003). Total knee replacement in patients with diabetes mellitus. *Clin. Orthop. Relat. Res.* 417, pp. 208-216.

Merchant, A. C. (2004). Early results with a total patellofemoral joint replacement arthroplasty prosthesis. *J. Arthroplasty* 19, pp. 829-836.

Muratoglu, O. K., Bragdon, C. R., O'Connor, D. O., Jasty, M., Harris, W. H. (2001). A novel method of cross-linking ultra-high-molecular-weight polyethylene to improve wear, reduce oxidation, and retain mechanical properties. Recipient of the 1999 HAP Paul Award. *J. Arthroplasty* 16, pp. 149-160.

Muratoglu, O. K., Mark, A., Vittetoe, D. A., Harris, W. H., Rubash, H. E. (2003). No abstract polyethylene damage in total knees and use of highly crosslinked polyethylene. *J. Bone Joint Surg. [Am]* 85, pp. S7-S13.

Oakshott, R., Komistek, R. D., Anderson, D. T., Haas, B. D., Dennis, D. A. (2000). In vivo passive vs. weightbearing knee kinematics for subjects implanted with a mobile bearing that can freely translate and rotate. Internal report at Rocky Mountain Musculoskeletal Research Laboratory.

Parentis, M. A., Rumi, M. N., Deol, G. S., et al. (1999). A comparison of the vastus splitting and median parapatellar approaches in total knee arthroplasty. *Clin. Orthop.* 367, pp. 107-116.

Peersman, G., Laskin, R., Davis, J., Peterson, M. (2001). Infection in total knee replacement: A retrospective review of 6489 total knee replacements. *Clin. Orthop. Relat. Res.* 392, pp. 15-23.

Pennington, D. W., Swienckowski, J. J., Lutes, W. B., Drake, G. N. (2003). Unicompartmental knee arthroplasty in patients sixty years of age or younger. *J. Bone Joint Surg. [Am]* 85(A), pp. 1968-1973.

Ranawat, C. S., Komistek, R. D., Rodriguez, J. A., Dennis, D. A., Anderle, M. (2004). In vivo kinematics for fixed and mobile-bearing posterior stabilized knee prostheses. *Clin. Orthop.* 419, pp. 1-7.

Rand, J. A., Trousdale, R. T., Ilstrup, D. M., Harmsen, W. S. (2003). Factors affecting the durability of primary total knee prostheses. *J. Bone Joint Surg. [Am]* 85, pp. 259-265.

Rodgers, A., Walker, N., Schug, S., et al. (2000). Reduction of postoperative mortality and morbidity with epidural or spinal anaesthesia: Results from overview of randomised trials. *BMJ* 321(7275), p. 1493.

Romanowski, M. R., Repicci, J. A. (2002). Minimally-invasive unicondylar arthroplasty: 8-year follow-up. *J. Knee Surg.* 15, pp. 17-22.

Rosier, R. M., O'Keefe, R. J. (2000). Hyduronic acid therapy. *Instructional Course Lecture* 49, pp. 495-502.

Saragaglia, D., et al. (2001). Computer-assisted knee arthroplasty: Comparison with a conventional procedure. Results of 50 cases in a prospective randomized study. *Rev. Chir. Orthop. Reparatrice Appar. Mot.* 87, pp. 18-28.

Shrader, M. W., Morrey, B. F. (2003). Primary TKA in patients with lymphedema. *Clin. Orthop. Relat. Res.* 416, pp. 22-26.

Silva, M., Shepherd, E., Jackson, W., Pratt, J., McClung, C., Schmalzried, T. (2003). Knee strength after total knee arthroplasty. *J. Arthroplasty* 18, pp. 605-611.

Smith, A. M., Peckett, W. R. C., Butler-Manuel, P. A., Venu, K. M., d'Arey, J. C. (2002). Treatment of patellofemoral arthritis using the Lubinus patellofemoral arthroplasty: A retrospective review. *Knee* 9, pp. 27-30.

Sparmann, M., et al. (2003). Positioning of total knee arthroplasty with and without navigation support. A prospective, randomised study. *J. Bone Joint Surg. [Br]* 85, pp. 830-835.

Stiehl, J. B., Dennis, D. A., Komistek, R. D., Keblish, P. (2000). In vivo comparison of posterior cruciate retaining and sacrificing mobile-bearing total knee arthroplasty. *Am. J. Knee Surg.* 13, pp. 13-18.

Stiehl, J. B., Dennis, D. A., Komistek, R. D., Keblish, P. A. (1997). In vivo kinematic analysis of a mobile-bearing total knee prosthesis. *Clin. Orthop.* 345, pp. 60-66.

Stulberg, S. D., et al. (2002). Computer-assisted navigation in total knee replacement: Results of an initial experience in thirty-five patients. *J. Bone Joint Surg. [Am]* 84, pp. 90-98.

Svard, U. C., Price, A. J. (2001). Oxford medial unicompartmental knee arthroplasty: A survival analysis of an independent series. *J. Bone Joint Surg. [Br]* 83, pp. 191-194.

Tria, A., Coon, T. (2003). MIS TKA quad sparing approach. *Clin. Orthop. Relat. Res.* 416, pp.185-190.

Vaidya, S. V., Ranawat, C. S., Aroojis, A., Laud, N. S. (2000). Anthropometric measurements to design total knee prostheses for the Indian population. *J. Arthroplasty* 15(1), pp. 79-85.

Van Ham, G., et al. (1998). Machining and accuracy studies for a tibial knee implant using a force-controlled robot. *Comput. Aided Surg.* 3, pp. 123-133.

Victor, J., et al. (2004). Image-based computer-assisted total knee arthroplasty leads to lower variability in coronal alignment. *Clin. Orthop.* 428, pp. 131-139.

White, R. E., Allman, J. K., Trauger, J. A., et al. (1999). Clinical comparison of the midvastus and medial parapatellar surgical approaches. *Clin. Orthop.* 367, pp. 117-122.

Woodland, L. H., Francis, R. S. (1992). Parameters and comparisons of the quadriceps angle of college-aged men and women in the supine and standing positions. *Amer. J. Sports Med.* 20(2), pp. 208-211.

12.7 Review Questions

Q12.1 Total knee replacement surgery is becoming evermore popular because:

    A. insurance pays for it.

    B. it can be done arthroscopically.

    C. surgical techniques, implants, and outcomes have improved significantly over the last 30 years.

    D. results have improved so much that you can now run marathons with a total knee replacement.

Q12.2 When deciding to undergo a unicompartmental (partial) knee replacement, only one compartment of the knee can be arthritic (True/False).

Q12.3 A well-done contemporary total knee replacement, if properly cared for, should last between 15-20 years in approximately:

    A. 50% of the cases.

    B. 75% of the cases.

    C. forever.

    D. > 90% of the cases.

Q12.4 When considering undergoing a total knee replacement, significant operative risks include:

    A. blood clots.

    B. infection.

    C. anesthetic issues.

    D. damage to an adjacent structure such as a blood vessel or nerve.

    E. All of the above.

Q12.5 Recommended activities following a total knee replacement (select 3):

    A. swimming.

    B. basketball.

    C. doubles tennis.

    D. singles tennis.

    E. bowling

VII

MASTERS ATHLETE

Chapter 13

Medical Advances in Treating the Masters Athlete

Anthony Luke, M.D., M.P.H.[1] and Marc R. Safran, M.D.[2]

[1] Depts. of Orthopaedics and Family and Community Medicine
Univ. of California at San Francisco, 500 Parnassus Ave., MU-320W
San Francisco, CA 94143-0728
PH: 415-353-7586; FX: 415-353-9675; EM: LukeA@orthosurg.ucsf.edu

[2] Stanford University Medical Center, 300 Pasteur Dr., Edwards R-105
Stanford, CA 94305-5341
PH: 650-736-7600; FX: 650-498-7186; EM: safranm@orthosurg.ucsf.edu

13.1 Introduction

"The doctor of the future will give no medicine, but will interest his patients in the care of human frame, and in the cause and prevention of disease." - T. A. Edison

Over the next few decades, the aging population will continue to increase as a proportion of society. With this change in demographics and the continued urgency that people remain active during their entire lives, a new phenomenon in sports medicine has been developing. "Boomeritis" refers to the complex of conditions that arise as bone, cartilage, muscle and tendon degenerate while we age. Osteoarthritis, tendinosis, osteoporosis, and chondromalaciae are a few of the medical conditions that contribute to "boomeritis". In 2004, the direct and indirect medical costs associated with all forms of arthritis was estimated to exceeded $86 billion (Liu et al., 2004). Unfortunately, the idea of a "cure" for these problems remains an elusive goal. Investigating the cellular effects of aging can help understand the physiologic changes, the pathologic processes and directions for treatment in the hopes of finding a possible "cure" for problems in the older athlete.

With each decade, a larger proportion of the population is living longer. In 1900, the over-65 age group represented only 4% of the population of the United States. By 1988, they accounted for 12.4%, and is projected to account for 22% by the year 2030 (Elders, 2000). There is a need for these individuals to continue to maintain a very active lifestyle. On the other hand, more and more individuals are participating in athletic activity into their later years. It is estimated that more than 68% of people older than 55 years of age will have osteoarthritis based on radiographic evidence (Elders, 2000). It has been estimated that approximately one in 6 individuals have arthritis, which corresponds to 43 million individuals, most of them being older than 45 years (Elders, 2000). This will increase to approximately 59.4 million persons by the year 2020 (Elders, 2000).

In this chapter, we will discuss the physiology of the Masters athlete and the natural history of degenerative changes that inevitably occur. We discuss the physiologic changes that occur during aging as well as the pathophysiology associated with degenerative changes in the body. We will use the knee joint as a model for physiologic aging and pathologic problems, since the knee has been studied in depth and knee osteoarthritis is such a heavy burden of disease. We review standard treatment options available for osteoarthritis of the knee. Subsequently, we explore the advances that are being made in trying to heal and preserve cartilage so that osteoarthritis might be prevented before it can progress. New treatments are being investigated in the fields of gene therapy and tissue engineering, which use stem cells and growth factors to induce healing. It is difficult to summarize the vast amount of research which is being undertaken in the field of molecular genetics. Nevertheless, we aim to provide an overview of major areas of advancement in Orthopaedics in addressing problems in the Masters athlete.

13.2 The Masters Athlete

Age is a relative concept, as some athletes are physiologically younger than their chronological age. By definition, the Masters athlete are individuals who participate in organized Masters sports competition after the age of 50 (Jokl et al., 2004). Managing the older athlete requires understanding their activity level and their personal exercise goals. Exercise is clearly safe for most individuals including the elderly. There are several benefits for exercise in the older population, and very few contraindications exist. It is recommended that an age-specific pre-participation physical exam be carried out, especially for individuals starting a new exercise program.

Moderate exercise improves bone density, improves function in osteoarthritis, and is vital for patients with coronary artery disease (Kavanagh and Shephard, 1977). Several studies have demonstrated that the Masters athlete can build, maintain, and increase strength with appropriate strength training programs, even when they have not been previously engaged in the program (Galloway and Jokl, 2000). It is recommended that seniors participate in 30 to 50 minutes of aerobic exercise at least 3 times a week (Galloway and Jokl, 2000).

13.2.1 *Physiologic changes with aging and sports*

Several physiologic changes occur with aging that affect strength and metabolism which can result in performance changes (Powell, 2005). Strength changes include decrease in muscle mass. Aging results in changes in fiber type, with a shift towards a higher percentage of type I fibers. Lexell et al. (1988) showed that after age 25, a loss in the number of type 1 (slow-twitch) and type 2 fibers (fast-twitch fibers) occurs equally among fiber types as well as a reduction in these size of fibers. Secondly, the type 2 fibers lose more cross-sectional area than the type 1 fibers, which also occurs with aging (Lexell et al., 1988). Several studies have demonstrated that Masters athlete can still build, maintain, and increase strength with appropriate strength training programs, even during a short interval of training (Galloway and Jokl, 2000).

Neuromuscular changes also occur with aging. By approximately age 60, individuals lose spinal motor neurons and motor units. While muscle atrophy is attenuated by resistance training with aging, it is unclear whether resistance training can reduce the loss of spinal motor neurons, motor units, and muscle fiber number (Booth et al., 1994).

Endurance changes can result in decreased athletic performance, including a decrease in maximum heart rate, and decrease in VO_2 max. Maximal oxygen consumption (VO_2 max), which is an index of maximal cardiovascular (CV) function, has been estimated to decline approximately 5 to 15% per decade after the age of 25 years old (Heath et al., 1981). Fortunately, the age-related decrease in VO_2 max of Masters athletes who continue to engage in regular vigorous endurance exercise training experience about one-half the rate of decline compared with age-matched individuals who live a sedentary lifestyle. Endurance exercise training may also reduce the rate of decline in maximal heart rate that typically occurs as an individual ages (Roger et al., 1990).

With advancing age, musculoskeletal soft tissue changes as well as degenerative diseases can affect an individual's function and mobility, which can lead to pain and physical impairments. One proposal for the continued loss of flexibility with aging involves the development of increased cross links between fibers in muscle and tendon throughout the body. Loss of hip extension is one of the typical problems that can occur which has been associated with falls (Lee et al., 2005). Maintaining an active stretching and flexibility program can help improve range of motion and mobility (DiBenedetto et al., 2005).

13.2.2 *Articular cartilage/osteoarthritis knee model*

To discuss degenerative changes in the Masters athlete we will use the knee as a model. The knee has an articular cartilage surface, which consists of the hard, smooth areas covering bones at the articulating surfaces of the joint. The ultimate stress for articular cartilage (dry) is approximately 5 MPa or 500 N/cm^2, and its friction coefficient is 0.0025, which is the lowest for any solid material (Nigg, 1998). There is a matrix or "solid phase" of cartilage which consists of large hydrophilic proteoglycan molecules and type II collagen that form a tight lattice structure (Ghivizzani and Evans, 2000). Proteoglycans are carbohydrate polymers making up which are major components of the matrix. Water is associated with the matrix and is referred to the "liquid phase", which gives cartilage its resilient mechanical properties and produces a cushioning effect. For example, upon initial loading of a joint, up to 75% of the compressive stress is absorbed by the fluid in the matrix. Under load for greater than 5 minutes, the deformation that occurs in the cartilage takes several minutes to recover (Nigg, 1998). The arrangement of type II collagen restrains the large proteoglycans and limits their ability to swell, providing a pressure that contributes to the stiffness of cartilage enabling it to withstand heavy loads (Fig. 13.1). If the proteoglycans are less compact, they can "imbibe additional water", reducing the stiffness of cartilage (Ghivizzani et al., 2000).

There is a small population of chondrocytes (or cartilage cells) responsible for maintaining and replacing the cartilage. Chondrocytes are continually involved in the degradation, digestion, and synthesis of the matrix (Buckwalter and Mankin, 1998). Proteoglycans can be turned over in days or weeks, while fibrillar collagens are replaced over months or years.

In addition to articular cartilage, the knee specifically has meniscal cartilage structures. The menisci are thick disks of fibrocartilage that are located in the medial and lateral compartments of the knee between the tibia and femur. They are congruently shaped to help support and stabilize the tibia and femur, to absorb and handle load placed on the knee, and to protect the articular cartilage. Almost 85 per cent of the load on the knee is transmitted through the meniscus during knee flexion, while 50 per cent is transmitted through the meniscus during extension (DeHaven and Arnoczky, 1994).

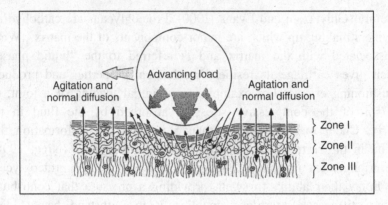

Figure 13.1. Effect of load on articular cartilage. Reprinted from Stanish and Wood (1998), pg. 682, Fig. 6, with permission of Oxford University Press.

13.2.3 *Pathologic changes that occur with aging*

It is normal that as individuals age, degenerative changes occur in certain areas of the body. For examples, degenerative changes develop in the rotator cuff for the shoulder leading to tendon tears. Intervertebral disks and joint surfaces can deteriorate in the lumbar spine leading to degenerative disk disease and osteoarthritis. Similarly, meniscal tears and osteoarthritis can occur in the knee. These conditions are common among the aging population. However, while these degenerative problems may demonstrate changes on imaging studies, they may be symptomatic or clinically silent causing no symptoms.

With age, increased loss of the meniscus results in decreased contact area and increased pressure in the involved compartment (Baratz et al., 1986). Direct blunt trauma or torsional loading can cause acute injury to the joint surface, while repetitive impact or joint malalignment can lead to abnormal loading of the articular cartilage that may gradually lead to eventual injury (Ghivizzani and Evans, 2000). Damage to the joint can fracture the matrix and cause chondrocyte necrosis. Pain and dysfunction may lead to an altered load distribution pattern causing excess stress to surrounding areas of cartilage. The process of mineralization may be activated, which causes thickening of the subchondral bones, and thinning of the articular cartilage leading to early osteoarthritis (Ghivizzani and Evans, 2000). The underlying changes to cells can have permanent effects, which lead to degenerative changes. Apoptosis, also known as programmed cell death, is a cascade of events that occur on a cellular level following trauma. Immobilization due to pain may affect the nutrient flow to the chondrocytes, leading to further chondrocyte death.

During the healing process, the remaining chondrocytes respond through the mediation of cytokines (signalling proteins) and attempt to restore the matrix. Movement and controlled loading of the joint are important to restore adequate nutrition via the circulation of synovial fluid. A fibrin clot with platelet aggregation can occur from bleeding, drawing chondrocyte-like cells to the area. A typical inflammatory response may occur, however, the collagen which is laid down forms a fibrocartilage scar, which has weaker strength and less durability than that of the surrounding matrix. As a result, the area of fibrocartilage may fracture and fragment, leaving exposed bone. Clinically, pressure on exposed bone, which is innervated, can cause pain. Swelling and catching are symptoms due to the irregular surfaces of the joint, while locking and loose body sensations represent bone and cartilage fragments within the knee.

Damage to the articular surface and subchondral bone may lead to osteoarthritis in some athletes. This appears to be particularly more prevalent in athletes with significant malalignment, previous injury or surgery. Also there are genetic predispositions to osteoarthritis that are in the early stages of being understood. Studies on osteoarthritis patients demonstrate genetic predispositions where different inflammatory markers are expressed, which are associated with specific gene configurations as well as poorer physical functioning (Nicklas et al., 2005).

Sports can have both a protective and detrimental impact on future joint health. On one hand, exercise improves muscular strength, loads bones that lead to improved bone mineral density. Osteoporosis is "a skeletal condition characterized by decreased density (mass/volume) of normally mineralized bone" (Glaser and Kaplan, 1997). Bone density decreases with age especially in women after menopause due to the lack of the protective effect of estrogen on bone health. Interestingly, osteoporosis actually has an inverse relationship with osteoarthritis. There are less fragility fractures in individuals with osteoarthritis, which may suggest that patients with osteoarthritis actually have more bone density to resist damage from loading (Dequeker et al., 2003). On the other hand, sports also lead to increase exposure to injury and subsequent development of osteoarthritis. Several studies indicated that there is higher prevalence of osteoarthritis in competitive athletes, most likely due to the higher incidence of knee injuries that occur in active individuals (Deacon et al., 1997; Drawer and Fuller, 2001; Kujala et al., 1995; Thelin et al., 2006).

Table 13.1. Risk factors for degenerative conditions in Masters athletes.

• Age
• Trauma
• Biomechanical abnormalities (malalignment, congenital deformities, acquired disability)
• Obesity
• Compensation loading for other joint injury
• Rheumatologic disease or connective tissue disease
• Genetic predisposition
• Activities: Sports

13.3 Current Management

At the present time, management of osteoarthritis of the knee is directed towards treating symptoms and preventing further deterioration of the knee. As with many degenerative diseases, there is no "cure" for osteoarthritis or the many articular cartilage conditions. The treatments with the best outcomes involve treating end-stage arthritis with joint implant technologies.

13.3.1 *Conservative treatment*

Lifestyle changes are important for reducing degenerative joint disease. For osteoarthritis of the knee, reducing weight and activity modification are cornerstones of management. The goal is to reduce impact across the joint. Changing sports to involve low impact activities such as biking, swimming and exercise machines such as the elliptical trainer can assist in improving overall functional level and reducing daily pain.

Exercise can stimulate body's natural healing response to allow a better repair. Cardiovascular training through endurance exercise can improve the aerobic capacity of muscle, while resistance training can improve central nervous system recruitment of muscle and increase muscle mass (Kirkendall and Garrett, 1998). Load bearing is important to promote proper cell differentiation for healing connective tissues. For example, following cyclic loading in tendon, cells line up better and become more tendon-like though they are still one to two orders lower than normal values. Mechanical load at site of repair influences what type of tissue is formed. It also helps form the proper cross-linking needed for strength after healing. Similarly some tension is also necessary for tissue healing.

13.3.1.1 *Assistive devices*

When osteoarthritis is confined to one area of the knee, such as the medial compartment, braces and orthotics can help improve biomechanical function and loading of the joint. Heel wedges and orthotics can improve medial knee osteoarthritis symptoms by changing the mechanical weight bearing axis and reducing the varus torque during walking (Kerrigan et al., 2002). Knee sleeves have been described to provide warmth and improve neuromuscular properioception. A more substantial device, the custom unloader brace, is designed to off-load an arthritic area of the knee usually the medial or lateral sides of the knee resulting in less symptoms and more functional activity. Patient with medial knee osteoarthritis may benefit significantly from use of a knee brace in addition to standard medical treatment. The unloader brace provided more effective relief for pain and function than a neoprene sleeve after 6 months, with a difference in quality of life reported (Kirkley et al., 1999). Though the braces can only make minor adjustments with angular realignment, the braces have been shown to load share and reduce the stresses especially in the medial compartment or weight-bearing portion of the knee (Pollo and Jackson, 2006; Pollo et al., 2002). As a last resort, a cane or walking stick can mechanically unload the affected lower extremity when used in the opposite hand, again leading to improve function and mobility.

13.3.1.2 *Medications*

Medieations such as Acetaminophen, Non-steroidal anti-inflammatory drugs (NSAIDs) and other arthritis medications are aimed mainly to decrease symptoms of pain and work by affecting the mediators of inflammation and pain pathways. Choice of medications are determined by the severity of the condition, the potency of the medications and the side effect profile of the drug. For examples, NSAIDs have effects on the gastrointestinal wall, the kidney and platelets. The risk of gastrointestinal complications is 3 to 10 times higher in users of nonspecific NSAIDs vs nonusers. Risk factors for NSAID associated gastrointestinal ulcers are: advanced age, history of previous ulcer, concomitant corticosteroids or anticoagulants, high doses of NSAID, serious systemic disorders, smoking and alcohol consumption (Wolfe et al., 1999). The newer class of cyclo-oxygenase – 2 inhibitors differ from NSAIDs, by reducing concerns about bleeding and gastrointestinal side effects since they were more specific for inhibiting inflammatory effects. However, their initial promise was reduced as the drugs in that class have demonstrated increased heart attack rates, especially at maximum drug doses, where it has as high as five times the risk (Bresalier et al., 2005). Only one drug from that class (Celecoxib) remains on the market, since it has not been shown to have the same cardiovascular risks at the prescribed doses (Adapt Research Groups, 2006).

13.3.1.3 *Supplements*

Glucosamine Sulfate and Chondroitin Sulfate are nutritional supplements which has been marketted for treatment of articular cartilage and arthritic conditions. Sales of glucosamine and chondroitin totalled $730 Million in 2004 (Hui et al., 2005). The mechanism of action is unclear. Both molecules are glycosaminoglycans that are building blocks for cartilage. Some randomized controlled studies have demonstrated less progression of osteoarthritis on X-rays over 3 years (Reginster et al., 2001; Pavelka et al., 2002), while most positive studies demonstrate improved short-term pain scores (Richy et al., 2003). A recent study named the GAIT Trial randomized 1583 patients with symptomatic osteoarthritis of the knees to the following treatment groups: 1500 mg of glucosamine daily; 1200 mg of chondroitin sulfate daily; or both; 200 mg of celecoxib daily; or Placebo RCT for 24 weeks (Clegg et al., 2006). The effect of glucosamine and/or chondroitin was not significantly improved among patients with varying degrees of osteoarthritis, except in patients with moderate-to-severe pain at baseline, in whom combined therapy was better than placebo (79.2 percent vs. 54.3 percent, $P = 0.002$) (Clegg et al., 2006).

13.3.1.4 *Viscosupplementation*

Synovial fluid, which normally exists in the knee, has smaller molecular weight and poorer viscous qualities in patients with osteoarthritis. The use of intra-articular injections of high elastoviscous solutions of hyaluronans or its derivatives have been indicated for treatment of knee osteoarthritis since the late 1990's. Hyaluronic acid which is a component of synovial fluid, is manufactured from rooster comb cells or cultured bacteria. In the United States, it is considered a medical device rather than a medication by the Federal Drug Administration.

The viscoelasticity of synovial fluid depends on: (1) Molecular weight, (2) concentration, and (3) molecular interaction of hyaluronan. The suspected mechanism of action involves stimulating the joint's synovium to produce intrinsic synovial fluid of higher molecular weight with increased quantity of hyaluronic acid, leading to improved viscous properties.   Patients receiving injections report decreased pain scores. Though the mechanism of pain relief is uncertain, it is suspected to be from decreased levels cytokines, specifically, Interleukin 1, prostaglandin E2, and matrix metallo-proteins (MMP) (Altman and Moskowitz, 1998), and decreased free radical production.

The ideal patient for viscosupplementation is someone who has mild osteoarthritis, where other conservative treatments do not provide adequate relief.   Hyaluronic acid injections had a pooled mean improvement in pain symptoms of 7.9% (4.1% to 11.7% 95 C.I.'s) over phosphate buffered saline (PBS) injections which served as placebo (Wang et al., 2004).   A second similar review found that 63 studies reported improvements from baseline on the order of 11-54% for pain and 9-15% for function at 5-13 weeks, which demonstrate more prolonged effects than corticosteroids. The concerns for the papers published are that they are often poor quality and may have publication bias for positive results (Bellamy et al., 2006a, b).   Two to four percent of patients experience some side effects following viscosupplementation (Lussier et al., 1996), typically a local sterile, intra-articular effusion which appears often within 2 days.   There are no reported cases of infection from contamination.

13.3.2 *Surgical options*

13.3.2.1 *Arthroscopy*

Arthroscopy has been one of the most significant advances in sports medicine.   It enables minimally invasive surgery to be performed for both diagnostic and therapeutic purposes.   Because of arthroscopy, surgical time and anesthesia needs are reduced as well as surgical morbidity and complications.   The arthroscope is typically a rigid rod-lens system, transmitting light and images through an array of lenses to a video camera using fiber optic light sources (Cautilli, 1997).   Fiber-optic arthroscopes use fibrils that conduct light and project the image on a video monitor in the operating room (Cautilli, 1997). Fluid irrigation via gravity or a pump system distends the joint and enables the surgeon to visualize through the arthroscope, as small debris and blood are cleared by the inflow and removed by the outflow. A number of specialized tools can now resect, drill, burr, and suture within the joint though small incisions referred to as portals.

Arthroscopy for knee osteoarthritis usually involves debridement of loose, scaly, desquamating articular cartilage fragments or mobile flaps or degenerative tears of meniscal cartilage. Abrasion arthroplasty or "Microfracture" is a common treatment at the present time for articular cartilage lesions which have poor healing capacity. By drilling holes through the cartilage into the subchondral bone, bleeding occurs allowing mesenchymal stem cells to come from the healthy bone into the cartilage repair site. This leads to the development of a fibrocartilage surface which allows some protection for the underlying bone. Unfortunately, the fibrocartilage can degenerate within 5 years so these procedures are temporizing measures and not usually recommended for osteoarthritis.

The effectiveness of arthscopic surgery for knee osteoarthritis has been called into question. In a landmark paper, Moseley et al. (2002) demonstrated that arthroscopic debridement, arthroscopic lavage and placebo surgery had no difference after 2 years of follow up. There were concerns with the study including that there were participants with varying severities of arthritis. However, the use of arthroscopy for osteoarthritis has decreased unless patients have mechanical symptoms for which removal of internal derangements in the knee are appropriate. The procedure may also postpone more significant surgery, and allow individuals to await newer techniques and technology to develop.

13.3.2.2 *Realignment surgery*

For severe stages of osteoarthritis, more significant surgical procedures are required. If the arthritis is worst in one compartment due to the malalignment, performing an osteotomy with the goal of redistributing the mechanical forces away from the arthritic compartment to areas of more normal cartilage can succeed in providing relief. A surgical cut is made through either the tibia or the femur with either a wedge of bone removed (closing wedge osteotomy) or the bone is distracted to the appropriate angle (opening wedge osteotomy) to realign the mechanical axis to the desired area of the joint (Fig. 13.2). The advantages of such a procedure over a knee replacement surgery are that the individual's own bone is preserved, the individual can often return to a higher level of activity, and it avoids the complications of the knee replacement. The disadvantages are that the general level of symptom improvement is not as good as implant surgery. The procedure is technically difficult and there is a small chance of delayed union or even non-union of the healing surgery site.

A "High tibial osteotomy (HTO)" is best done on a young, active patient with severe medial knee osteoarthritis. The results of the HTO demonstrate good to excellent results between 73% to 95% at 5 years; 45% to 80% at 10 years and 30% to 46% at 20 years post operative. The distal femoral osteotomy is often preferred, cutting the femur as opposed to the tibia, for lateral compartment osteoarthritis of the knee. The results are good to excellent in 90% of patients at 5 years, which drops to 71% after 8 years. Unfortunately, this procedure has a high rate of non union healing between 4 to 19%.

13.3.2.3 *Arthroplasty surgery*

Arthroplasty is the branch of Orthopaedics involved in replacement of the joints where the weight bearing surfaces are replaced with an implant. These implants most commonly have a metal-on polyethylene design, though various ceramic, metal, and polyethylene alternatives have been used (Jazrawi et al., 1998). For example, an alternative option for a patient with osteoarthritis in one compartment of the knee is a unicondylar knee replacement. This replaces only half of the articulating surface of the knee with a metal implant. The benefits of unicondylar knee replacement are that they are minimally invasive and provide more reliable pain relief than the osteotomy surgeries. Patients can resume weight bearing more quickly since they have an implant and do not need to wait for the bone to heal in the same way as an osteotomy. The surgery is not as involved as the total knee replacement, which is often the next step for definitive care, should the patient continue to have problems. The unicondylar replacement is consider in the younger

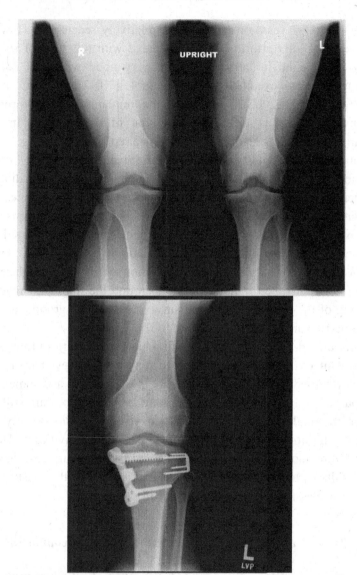

Figure 13.2. (Left) X-ray showing a Left knee medial compartment osteochondral defect with early osteoarthritis. (Right) X-ray demonstrating a high tibial osteotomy to protect medial compartment osteoarthritis. The opening wedge technique realigns the knee to shift the weight from away from the medial aspect of the knee.

patients 40 to 60 years of age who are relatively sedentary. However, patellofemoral joint arthritis cannot be aided with this type of surgery. Results of unicondylar arthroplasty are very good with 87% to 98% reporting good to excellent results as far as 10 years from surgery (Archibeck et al., 2002). However, the implants are still prone to polyethylene wear, as well as progression of osteoarthritis in other compartments, usually leading to a total knee replacement.

Total knee arthroplasty is the most definitive treatment at the present for osteoarthritis in the knee, as well as other joints including the shoulder, hip and ankle. The goal is to replace all the joint surfaces. The advantages include excellent, reliable pain relief. A meta-analysis of 11 series patients who underwent knee replacement surgery reported 93% good to excellent results with a complications rate of 11%. Of the complications, four percent required revision of the knee replacement and 21% demonstrated radiolucent lines around the implant, suggesting loosening of the hardware. Overall survivorship in the group was 90 to 95% at more than 10 to 15 years.

After a total knee arthroplasty, individuals may return to low impact sports. Out of 159 patients 65% who played sports even up to their surgery, returned to their sports, including bowling, golf and some tennis (Bradbury et al., 1998). Because the long term outcomes are still a bit unclear, the total knee arthroplasty is reserved for physiologically older patients, who do not wish to return to impact type activities. Though there is some morbidity associated replacing the joint surfaces, there are good results with overall improvements, making knee arthroplasty one of the most successful surgeries in orthopaedics to date.

13.4 Advances and Future Management of Knee Osteoarthritis

Since articular cartilage has a limited capacity to heal or grow in vivo, the goal of future treatments is to restore the normal structure and composition of tissues such as articular cartilage. Instead of treating pain and other symptoms, the ideal goal is to promote adequate healing over the chronically injured area. Rather than replace tissues, investigators are trying to manipulate the bodies intrinsic repair processes at the cellular and molecular level. Most of these techniques are still in the experimental phase and are demonstrating interesting results in vitro and animal studies.

13.4.1 *Tissue engineering*

Tissue engineering aims to reconstitute tissues functionally and structurally by employing seed cells and biodegradable materials to generate various tissues "in vitro" or or "in vivo" (Langer and Vacanti, 1993; Liu et al., 2004; Hunziker, 2001). The concept is to simulate the embryonic or fetal cell or tissue differentiation processes in order to create repair tissue (Hunziker, 2001). The essential components of tissue engineering include matrix scaffolds, stem or precursor cells, and signaling molecules (Fig. 13.3).

There are 4 key requirements of tissue engineering for the optimal treatment for cartilage lesions. A biodegradable scaffold is necessary to anchor, deliver and orient cells. Secondly, reagents or molecular factors provide instructional cues to guide cartilage growth and orientation. Third, the appropriate cells must be present that respond to their environment, continue to grow and ultimately attain similar biomechanical characteristics as normal articular cartilage. Finally, biomechanical stimulation and adequate blood supply must exist to enhance the speed and maturation of the implant. Three biologic strategies for healing cartilage are to introduce: (1) cells alone, (2) cells with matrix scaffolds, or (3) scaffolds alone (Fig. 13.3) (Khademhosseini et al., 2006).

13.4.1.1 *Autologous Chondrocyte Implanation*

An example of the tissue engineering strategy of adding cultured cells into a repair site is autologous chondrocyte implantation. Autologous Chondrocyte Implantation (ACI) involves harvesting articular cartilage from the non-weightbearing areas of the knee. The cartilage cells are then cultured "in vitro" and re-implanted into the area of cartilage loss approximately six weeks after the initial procedure. The use of autologous cells has great advantages in avoiding immunological and ethical issues. However, due to the limited amount of expendable, harvestable cartilage, expansion of the number of cells is required prior to cell implantation. The results do show promise, though further experimental study continues to improve the procedures.

In a series of 46 patients, where the a second arthroscopy was performed to assess the healing of the implanted cells, biopsies showed that approximately 80% of the samples demonstrated hyaline-like repair tissue consisting of Type 2 collagen. The clinical outcome of the patients also correlated with the histology (Peterson et al., 2002). To compare with a common treatment, a prospective randomized controlled trial compared ACI with micro fracture surgery. From 1999 to 2004,

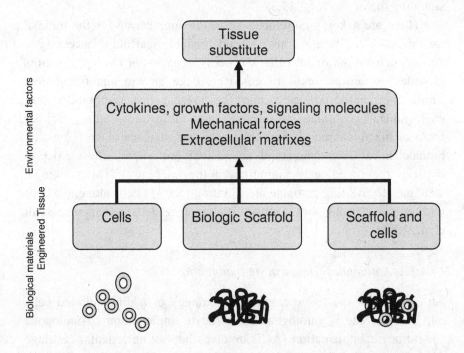

Figure 13.3. Schematic describing biologic strategies to heal cartilage.

eighty patients were followed for 24 months with a biopsy performed at the end of 2 years. The microfracture group had less failures and less reoperations, while the histological quality of the repair tissue was not different in either group. Meanwhile, the patients' Lysholm and visual analog pain scales improved in both groups after two years (Knutsen et al., 2004).

13.4.1.2 *Stem cells*

Stem cells are cells that are able to divide indefinitely. They have the potential to develop into different types of cells, such as muscle, nerve, bone, heart cells, or cartilage. There are several chondroprogenitor cell pools (Table 13.2) that can differentiate into chondrocytes: (1) cells from the cambial layers of the perichondrium and periosteum, (2) adult chondrocytes themselves, (3) bone-marrow stroma cells (which include mesenchymal stem cells) and (4) the synovium. Fat-derived stem cells are another source of potential cells that have been investigated to solve joint related problems.

Chondroprogenitor cells, in particular mesenchymal stem cells (MSCs), are attractive candidates for gene therapy approaches (Caplan, 2000). MSCs are capable of differentiating into multiple cell types specifically osteoblasts, chondroblasts, and adipoblasts and have all have been shown to produce extracellular cartilage matrix. Therefore, they can be particularly useful in situations where both cartilage and bone must be repaired or replaced, such as osteochondral defects from trauma or osteonecrosis. These cells can be readily isolated from bone marrow as well as from a number of different tissues including fat, muscle, bone, synovium, and periosteum. These progenitor cells are easily expanded in tissue culture and can be directed to differentiate into specific cell types by altering their chemical and physical environment.

Table 13.2. Chondroprogenitor cell pools (Hunziker, 2001; Fraser et al., 2006).

	Location	Advantages	Disadvantages
Chondrocytes	Found in articular cartilage	Autogenic and allogenic, can be embedded in collagenous matrix	Long term stability questioned
Perichondrial/periosteal cells	In cambial layer of the perichondrium and periosteum	High proliferative potential and capacity to differentiate into chondrocytes	Short survival period; numerical density declines with time
Bone marrow stromal cells	In bone marrow	Pluripotent mesenchymal stem cells	Numbers decline with time; ability to proliferate and differentiate deteriorate with age
Synovial cells	Synovium of joint	Sustain high proliferative potential and able to differentiate despite age of individual	
Fat derived cells	Adipose tissue	Numerous cells in adipose tissue; low morbidity	

The challenges of using stem cells include the cellular characterization and chondrogenic potency of isolated stem cells (Hui et al., 2005; Richy et al., 2003). Adipose derived stem cells derived from adult humans in vitro have shown chondrogenic nodules while mouse inguinal fat pad derived cells developed the chondrocyte phenotype in vitro (Richy et al., 2003). Purification methods for heterogeneous stem cell populations such as adult tissue derived stem cells have not been well established. The development of a cell-coating technology, known as painting, enables researchers to introduce informational proteins to the outer surface of cells (Caplan, 2005).

13.4.1.3 *Matrix scaffolds*

A matrix is a three dimensional structure which allows cell adhesion and bonding. The matrix provides an acellular extra-cellular scaffold upon which genetically modified cells can be seeded. A matrix can also be introduced without cells for cartilage repair. However, the addition of cartilage growth stimulating factors would be required to promote any potential healing. Important properties of the matrix (Table 13.3) include being biocompatible to avoid unnecessary loss of the cells and biodegradable, so that the construct and cells can remodel. The scaffold should be permeable so that growth factors, cytokines and nutrients can enable cellular growth and produce extracellular matrix within the construct. The scaffold should be mechanically stable, so it can support the cells but also be shaped to match the size and shape of an area of damaged articular cartilage (Kim et al., 2006).

There are four main classes of scaffolds to date (Table 13.4). Matrices can be made from (1) protein-based polymers, such as fibrin or collagen, (2) carbohydrate-based polymers (i.e. Hyaluronan), (3) artificial polymers like Dacron and (4) different polymer combinations (Table 13.1).

Table 13.3. Requirements for the Ideal Scaffold (from Hunziker, 2001, pg. 440).

1) Biocompatible
2) Not cytotoxic
3) Biodegradable
4) Support cells
5) Permeable
6) Mechanically stable
7) Hold cells
8) Reproducible and readily available
9) Versatile for full thickness and partial thickness lesions.

Second generation of biologic 3-D scaffolds made of collagen and hyaluronan are under investigation and are the more popular ones being used in humans. Products which are being used in Europe and other countries include the MACI (Matrix Induced Autologous Chondrocyte Implantation) technique, the Hyalograft technique, and PLA/PGA Fleece techniques. In a fashion similar to ACI, autologous chondrocytes are harvested and cultured. The MACI technique places the cells in a collagen scaffold, while the Hyalograft ® technique places the cells in a hyaluronic acid based scaffold (Kim et al., 2006). The Hyalograft ®

(Fidia, Advanced Biopolymers, Italy) uses chondrocytes harvested from the patient and grown in culture *in vitro* then absorbed onto a non-woven pad made of the benzyl ester of hyaluronic acid. The implanted scaffold results in approximately 4 million seeded cells / cm^2 per graft (Marcacci et al., 2005). After the 2 weeks, the graft is arthroscopically implanted into the knee and kept in place by simple adhesion onto the donor site. The results from 216 chondral knee defects in 175 patients, with a minimum 2 year follow up using the previous open knee surgery, were impressive. Eighty eight percent of patients were rated as having normal or nearly normal knees on IKDC rating. The average surface area implanted was 3.5 cm^2 with a maximum of 19 cm^2 (Marcacci et al., 2005).

Table 13.4. Chemical Classes of Matrix (from Hunziker, 2001, pg. 440).

1. Protein-based polymers
   Fibrin
   Collagen
   Gelatine
2. Carbohydrate-based polymers
   Polylactic acid
   Polygycolic acid
   Hyaluronan
   Agarose
   Alginate
   Chitosan
3. Artificial polymers
   Dacron (polyethylene terephthalates)
   Teflon (polytetrafluoroethylene)
   Carbon fibers
   Polyesterurethane
   Polybutyric acid
   Polyethylmethacrylate
   Hydroxyapatite
4. Within/between classes
   Crosslinkage
   Chemical modifications
   Geometrical modifications (to produce fibrillar forms or foams)
   Matrix combinations

Extracellular matrix (ECM) "patches" are considered devices by the FDA, and their practical application is still to be realized in the future. These constructs can be used for tissue augmentation. The ECM patches provide a three-dimensional matrix to attract host cells. Growth factors and cytokines can be added. Examples of these include fascia lata patches, rotator cuff patches, and graft jackets which are all tissue constructs to help healing tissue mend. Neocart ®, which can be considered a third generation extension of ACI, requires cell biopsy, culture and growth in vitro. A major difference is that the cells are placed in a collagen scaffold and pressurized in vitro, which causes the cells to produce extracellular matrix and type II collagen. The construct is then implanted into the knee as a solid sheet that can be shaped to fit the lesion (Kim et al., 2006). Preliminary animal studies demonstrated "hyaline-like" cartilage at the implant site with border-less cellular integration between the porcine-based NeoCart™ and the host cartilage (unpublished data). However, work is also being done looking at these extracellular matrixes as a means to introduce factors to stimulate in situ cartilage growth.

13.4.2 *Growth factors and cytokines*

Cytokines are proteins that are released by cells to trigger biological activities of specific local target cells via receptor binding (Evans, 1999). They have been found to be involved in the regulation of the healing responses including angiogenesis, cell migration and division, matrix synthesis, differentiation of cells, and inflammation (Evans, 1999).

Several growth factors and cytokines have been shown to play an important role in the development of knee osteoarthritis as well as cartilage and joint healing (Table 13.3). Interleukin-1 (IL-1) is one of the important inflammatory mediators in osteoarthritis. It strongly inhibits matrix synthesis by cartilage, and leads to matrix breakdown in high concentrations (Evans et al., 2004; Smith et al., 2000). Insulin-like growth factor-1 (IGF-1) helps preserve cartilage homeostasis, through the synthesis of matrix macromolecules such as proteoglycans and collagen, and decreasing the catabolism of the macromolecules. IGF-1 helps promote the expression of the cartilaginous phenotype and helps the cartilage survive. Tranforming Growth Factor-b (TGF-β), bone morphogenetic protein (BMP), and fibroblast growth factor are molecules that enhance matrix synthesis by chondrocytes. Mesenchymal Stem Cells growing in the presence of TGF-β within a 3-dimentional matrix have shown differentiation into chondrocytes (Kim et al., 2006). Combinations of growth factors may further improve chondrogenesis. Fukumoto et al. (2003) demonstrated that continuous IGF-1, in addition to TGF-β1 for the first 2 days, further enhanced overall total cartilage growth from rabbit mesenchymal stem cells in vitro (Fukumoto et al., 2003). Specifically BMP -12 induce tendon-like and fibrocartilage tissue formation.

13.4.3 *Gene therapy*

Genes are sequences of deoxyribonucleic acid (DNA), which are the genetic blueprints commonly for the synthesis of cell proteins. These sequences are located on specific areas on the chromosomes found in the nucleus of cells. The codes are transcribed into messenger RNA (mRNA) and transferred outside the nucleus into the cell. Ribosome proteins translate the mRNA into the desired proteins, which can perform specific cellular functions and roles in the human body (Evans et al., 2000).

The treatments of many diseases in the future will most likely involve gene therapy. Musculoskeletal problems will be no exception, and early studies have demonstrated successful gene transfer to bone, articular and meniscal cartilage, ligament and tendon (Evans et al., 2000). By transferring new genetic information to cells that contribute to the healing process, the repair or growth process at the cellular and molecular level may be enhanced. A major area of possible gene therapy involves regulating the expression of cytokines and growth factors (Table 13.5). Therefore, gene therapy may enhance the results of cartilage repair and replacement treatments, as well as, stimulate new articular cartilage growth.

Table 13.5. Categories of candidate genes for use in gene therapy for Osteoarthritis.

I

Category Examples	Candidates genes
Growth factor	GF-1, TGF-b, BMP-2,-7, FGF
Cytokine/cytokine antagonist	IL-4, IL-1Ra, sIL-1R, Stnfr
Proteinase inhibitor	TIMP, PAI, serpin
Free radical antagonist	SOD
Transcription factor/signaling molecule	Sox-5,-6,-9,SMAD
Matrix molecule	Type II collagen, COMP
Enzyme	GFAT
Inhibitor of apoptosis	Bcl-2, PAI (Plasminogen activator inhibitor)

13.4.3.1 *Vectors*

To introduce a desired DNA sequence to encode the gene(s) of interest, for example to produce cartilage, a vector that is physically taken up by the targeted cells must be used to deliver the genetic material. Two major categories of vectors used in gene therapy are "viral" and "non-viral" vectors. Viral infections have served as an ideal vector as they infect cells and deliver their genes to the cell nucleus (transduction). Genetic manipulation of the viral structure has enabled the production of vectors that can efficiently integrate the genes into the host cells DNA, or simply deliver functional genes to nondividing cells (Evans et al., 2000). The leading viral vectors used in clinical trials in humans are oncoretrovirus (usually referred to as a retrovirus), lentivirus (also a retrovirus), adenovirus, adeno-associated virus (AAV), and herpes simplex virus (HSV) (Evans et al., 2006; Kim et al., 2006). Retroviral vectors deliver genes that are expressed long-term by infected cells, since the new genetic information is rewritten by all future generations of "daughter cells". However, retroviruses can only infect dividing cells thus limiting the number of cells initially affected and the efficiency of gene transfer overall (Kim et al., 2006). Risks from gene therapy lead to rare but reported cases of malignancies and even death that are attributable to the vectors themselves (Kaiser, 2003; Kim et al., 2006).

Transfer of nucleic acids into target cells can be accomplished by nonviral (transfection). Non-viral vectors include "Naked" DNA, plasmid DNA and DNA coated particles which are projected into cells using a "gene gun" (Evans et al., 2000). Advantages to use of non-viral vectors include relative simplicity, potentially lower toxicity, and fewer problems with immune reactions. The major concern is the lack of efficiency of gene delivery, which make viral vectors the more popular and effective means for gene therapy (Kim et al., 2006).

Vectors can also be delivered either *in vivo* or *ex vivo* (Martinek et al., 2003; Kim et al., 2006). Methods are performed "ex-vivo" by altering cells genetically, then reintroducing them into the body, or "in-vivo", by delivering the vector directly to the site of interest. *In vivo* delivery involves introduction of a vector directly to the desired site of action within the body, which is direct and avoids the need to harvest tissues and culture cells. However, there are difficulties targeting a specific population of cells. Cartilage in particular appears to be relatively resistant to gene transfer. Therefore, ex vivo delivery can be performed in a more controlled manner and guarantees gene transfer to the cells of interest while preventing unnecessary exposure of other cells to potentially toxic vectors. Other benefits of ex vivo techniques include the abilities to verify the activity of the transferred gene and quantify it prior to re-implantation in order to optimize results. Also, the modified cells can be combined with a matrix to enhance tissue regeneration. The disadvantages include additional surgery to obtain the culture tissue and the costs associated with growing these cells in tissue culture (Kim et al., 2006).

Gene therapy strategies for osteoarthritis involve the transfer of complementary DNA (cDNA) encoding antiarthritis gene products to the individual (Evans et al., 2006; Table 13.5). Proteins can act as cytokine antagonists, immunomodulators, growth factors, transcription regulators, enzyme inhibitors, antioxidants, antinociceptive agents, and other functioning agents. Gene transfer enables the body to naturally synthesize the desired products in a continuous, and more regulated manner. Proteins synthesized endogenously as a result of gene transfer have also shown greater biologic activity than their recombinant counterparts (Evans et al., 2006; Kim et al., 2006). For the delivery of the vectors, local, intraarticular delivery to individual diseased joints seems most effective so far (Evans et al., 2005). Systemic delivery, where the vector is delivered into the circulation (Evans et al., 2006), which may result in more widespread side effects. Intra-articular injections are advantageous since they affect the disease more directly with less side effects. The negative aspect is that multi-joint disease requires multiple injections. At the present time, intraarticular gene transfer seems more effective for arthritis conditions (Evans et al., 2006).

13.5 Summary and Conclusions

The Masters athlete represents a growing population that the medical care system must understand and be prepared for. In light of the continuing battle against cardiovascular disease, obesity and poor sedentary lifestyle habits, individuals will be strongly encouraged to exercise for fitness as well as sport throughout one's lifetime. Age and previous injuries unfortunately lead to degenerative changes that in many cases lead to irreversible problems. The aging population will present new demands for treatments that help preserve function.

Treating problems such as the degeneration of the knee's articular cartilage and subsequent development of osteoarthritis will represent a large challenge for physicians and a great burden for the health care system. Early management of articular cartilage problems will include patient education, activity modification and reduction of risk factors to reduce the progression of degenerative changes. Weight loss, exercise, pain control with medications and injections are current mainstays in the treatment of knee osteoarthritis. Medicine continues to investigate ways of altering the chemical pathways resulting in pain, inflammation and tissue breakdown to minimize symptoms and disease, for examples non-steroidal anti-inflammatory drugs and viscosuppplementation injections. Assistive devices such as canes, footwear and braces look at the physics and mechanical stresses affecting the joint to reduce stress and pressure.

Orthopaedic surgery is presently the most definitive treatment for the osteoarthritis of the knee. Procedures range from arthroscopic debridement to realignment surgery to total knee replacement. By mechanically altering the internal derangements and/or stresses affecting the knee, a patient's symptoms and function can be improved for some time. However, as the disease progresses to the end-stage, resurfacing the joint with an implant is the current state of the art, yielding some of the most impressive results for a surgical procedure.

Research often leads to better understanding of pathophysiology and aging is no exception. The future of treatment of osteoarthritis will involve new techniques in the fields of tissue engineering and genetics. Presently, investigations are underway on the uses of matrix scaffolds, stem or precursor cells, and signaling molecules to grow articular cartilage and replace the protective surfaces lost due to age or trauma. Gene therapy explores ways to introduce genetic material into the body's existing cells to produce the desired physiological effects to heal tissues. Continued studies are needed on new technologies in order to advance the field and to pursue the ideal goal of regenerative healing. The new direction of science for the Masters Athlete strives to understand function on a cellular level, in order to develop treatments that can alter disease before it progresses. With this in mind, the goal for management emphasizes quality of life, optimizes the individual's function as a whole and maximizes one's sense of health and well-being.

13.6 References

Adapt Research Groups (2006). Cardiovascular and Cerebrovascular Events in the Randomized, Controlled Alzheimer's Disease Anti-Inflammatory Prevention Trial (ADAPT). *PLoS Clin. Trials,* 1, pg. 33.

Altman, R. D. and Moskowitz, R. (1998), Intraarticular sodium hyaluronate (Hyalgan) in the treatment of patients with osteoarthritis of the knee: a randomized clinical trial. Hyalgan Study Group, *J. Rheumato.,* 25, pp. 2203-2212.

Archibeck M. J., Ayres, D. C., Berger, R. A., Buly, R. L., Garvin K. L., Otterberg, E. T., Stuart, M. J., and Windsor RE (2002). Knee reconstruction. In: K. J. Koval, ed., *Orthopaedic Knowledge Update 7: Home Study Syllabus.* Rosemont, IL, American Academy of Orthopaedic Surgeons.

Baratz, M. E., Fu, F. H. and Mengato, R. (1986). Meniscal tears: the effect of meniscectomy and of repair on intraarticular contact areas and stress in the human knee. A preliminary report, *Am. J. Sports Med.,* 14, pp. 270-275.

Bellamy, N., Campbell, J., Robinson, V., Gee, T., Bourne, R. and Wells, G. (2006a). Intraarticular corticosteroid for treatment of osteoarthritis of the knee, *Cochrane Database Syst. Rev.,* CD005328.

Bellamy, N., Campbell, J., Robinson, V., Gee, T., Bourne, R. and Wells, G. (2006b). Viscosupplementation for the treatment of osteoarthritis of the knee, *Cochrane Database Syst. Rev.,* CD005321.

Booth, F. W., Weeden, S. H. and Tseng, B. S. (1994). Effect of aging on human skeletal muscle and motor function, *Med. Sci. Sports Exerc.,* 26, pp. 556-560.

Bradbury, N., Borton, D., Spoo, G. and Cross, M. J. (1998). Participation in sports after total knee replacement, *Am. J. Sports Med.,* 26, pp. 530-535.

Bresalier, R. S., Sandler, R. S., Quan, H., Bolognese, J. A., Oxenius, B., Horgan, K., Lines, C., Riddell, R., Morton, D., Lanas, A., Konstam, M. A. and Baron, J. A. (2005). Cardiovascular events associated with rofecoxib in a colorectal adenoma chemoprevention trial, *N. Engl. J. Med.,* 352, pp. 1092-1102.

Buckwalter, J. A. and Mankin, H. J. (1998). Articular cartilage: tissue design and chondrocyte-matrix interactions, *Instr. Course Lect.,* 47, pp. 477-486.

Caplan, A. I. (2000). Mesenchymal stem cells and gene therapy. *Clin. Orthop. Relat. Res.,* pp. S67-70.

Caplan, A. I. (2005). Review: mesenchymal stem cells: cell-based reconstructive therapy in orthopedics. *Tissue Eng.,* 11, pp. 1198-1211.

Cautilli, R., JR. (1997). Introduction to the basics of arthroscopy of the knee, *Clin. Sports Med.,* 16, pp. 1-16.

Clegg, D. O., Reda, D. J., Harris, C. L., Klein, M. A., O'Dell, J. R., Hooper, M. M., Bradley, J. D., Bingham, C. O., 3RD, Weisman, M. H., Jackson, C. G., Lane, N. E., Cush, J. J., Moreland, L. W., Schumacher, H. R., JR., Oddis, C. V., Wolfe, F., Molitor, J. A., Yocum, D. E., Schnitzer, T. J., Furst, D. E., Sawitzke, A. D., Shi, H.,

Brandt, K. D., Moskowitz, R. W. and Williams, H. J. (2006). Glucosamine, chondroitin sulfate, and the two in combination for painful knee osteoarthritis, *N. Engl. J. Med.*, 354, pp. 795-808.

Deacon, A., Bennell, K., Kiss, Z. S., Crossley, K. and Brukner, P. (1997). Osteoarthritis of the knee in retired, elite Australian Rules footballers, *Med. J. Aust.*, 166, pp.187-190.

DeHaven K. E., Arnoczky, S. P. (1994). Meniscal repair, Part I: Basic Science. Indications for repair and open repair, *J. Bone Joint Surg.*, 76A, pp. 140-152.

Dequeker, J., Aerssens, J. and Luyten, F. P. (2003). Osteoarthritis and osteoporosis: clinical and research evidence of inverse relationship, *Aging Clin. Exp. Res.*, 15, pp. 426-439.

Dibenedetto, M., Innes, K. E., Taylor, A. G., Rodeheaver, P. F., Boxer, J. A., Wright, H. J. and Kerrigan, D. C. (2005). Effect of a gentle Iyengar yoga program on gait in the elderly: an exploratory study, *Arch. Phys. Med. Rehabil.*, 86, pp. 1830-1837.

Drawer, S. and Fuller, C. W. (2001). Propensity for osteoarthritis and lower limb joint pain in retired professional soccer players, *Br. J. Sports Med.*, 35, pp. 402-408.

Elders, M. J. (2000). The increasing impact of arthritis on public health, *J. Rheumatol. Suppl.*, 60, pp. 6-8.

Evans, C. H. (1999). Cytokines and the role they play in the healing of ligaments and tendons, *Sports Med.*, 28, pp. 71-76.

Evans, C. H., Ghivizzani, S. C., Herndon, J. H. and Robbins, P. D. (2005). Gene therapy for the treatment of musculoskeletal diseases, *J. Am. Acad. Orthop. Surg.*, 13, pp. 230-242.

EvanS, C. H., Ghivizzani, S. C. and Robbins, P. D. (2006). Gene therapy for arthritis: what next?, *Arthritis Rheum.*, 54, pp. 1714-1729.

Evans, C. H., Ghivizzani, S. C., Smith, P., Shuler, F. D., Mi, Z. and Robbins, P. D. (2000). Using gene therapy to protect and restore cartilage, *Clin. Orthop. Relat. Res.*, pp. S214-219.

Evans, C. H., Gouze, J. N., Gouze, E., Robbins, P. D. and Ghivizzani, S. C. (2004). Osteoarthritis gene therapy, *Gene Ther.*, 11, pp. 379-389.

Fraser, J. K., Wulur, I., Alfonso, Z. and Hedrick, M. H. (2006). Fat tissue: an underappreciated source of stem cells for biotechnology, *Trends Biotechnol.*, 24, pp. 150-154.

Fukumoto, T., Sperling, J. W., Sanyal, A., Fitzsimmons, J. S., Reinholz, G. G., Conover, C. A. and O'Driscoll, S. W. (2003). Combined effects of insulin-like growth factor-1 and transforming growth factor-beta1 on periosteal mesenchymal cells during chondrogenesis in vitro, *Osteoarthritis Cartilage,* 11, pp. 55-64.

Galloway, M. T. and Jokl, P. (2000). Aging successfully: the importance of physical activity in maintaining health and function, *J. Am. Acad. Orthop. Surg.*, 8, pp. 37-44.

Ghivizzani, S. C. and Evans, C. H. (2000). Gene therapy for rheumatoid arthritis, *Clin. Orthop. Relat. Res.*, pp. S308-310.

Ghivizzani, S. C., Oligino, T. J., Robbins, P. D. and Evans, C. H. (2000). Cartilage injury and repair, *Phys. Med. Rehabil. Clin. N. Am.,* 11, pp. 289-307, vi.

Glaser, D. L. and Kaplan, F. S. (1997). Osteoporosis. Definition and clinical presentation, *Spine,* 22, pp. 12S-16S.

Heath, G. W., Hagberg, J. M., EhsanI, A. A. and Holloszy, J. O. (1981). A physiological comparison of young and older endurance athletes, *J. Appl. Physiol.,* 51, pp. 634-640.

Hui, J. H., Ouyang, H. W., Hutmacher, D. W., Goh, J. C. and Lee, E. H. (2005). Mesenchymal stem cells in musculoskeletal tissue engineering: a review of recent advances in National University of Singapore, *Ann. Acad. Med. Singapore,* 34, pp. 206-212.

Hunziker, E. B. (2001). Articular cartilage repair: basic science and clinical progress. A review of the current status and prospects, *Osteoarthritis Cartilage,* 10, pp. 432-463.

Jazrawi, L. M., Kummer, F. J. and Dicesare, P. E. (1998). Alternative bearing surfaces for total joint arthroplasty, *J. Am. Acad. Orthop. Surg.,* 6, pp. 198-203.

Jokl, P., Sethi, P. M. and Cooper, A. J. (2004). Master's performance in the New York City Marathon 1983-1999, *Br. J. Sports Med.,* 38, pp. 408-412.

Kaiser, J. (2003). Gene therapy. Seeking the cause of induced leukemias in X-SCID trial, *Science,* 299, p. 495.

Kavanagh, T. and Shephard, R. J. (1977). The effects of continued training on the aging process, *Ann. N. Y. Acad. Sci.,* 301, pp. 656-670.

Kerrigan, D. C., Lelas, J. L., Goggins, J., Merriman, G. J., Kaplan, R. J. and Felson, D. T. (2002). Effectiveness of a lateral-wedge insole on knee varus torque in patients with knee osteoarthritis, *Arch. Phys. Med. Rehabil.,* 83, pp. 889-893.

Khademhosseini, A., Langer, R., Borenstein, J. and Vacanti, J. P. (2006). Microscale technologies for tissue engineering and biology, *Proc. Natl. Acad. Sci. U. S. A.,* 103, pp. 2480-2487.

Kim H. T., Zaffagnini, S., Mizuno S, Abelow S, Safran M. R. (2006). A peek into the possible future of management of articular cartilage injuries: gene therapy and scaffolds for cartilage repair, *J. Orthop. Sports Phys. Ther.,* 36, pp. 765-773

Kirkendall, D. T. and Garrett, W. E., JR. (1998). The effects of aging and training on skeletal muscle, *Am. J. Sports Med.,* 26, pp. 598-602.

Kirkley, A., Webster-Bogaert, S., Litchfield, R., Amendola, A., MacDonald, S., McCalden, R. and FOWLER, P. (1999). The effect of bracing on varus gonarthrosis, *J. Bone Joint Surg. Am.,* 81, pp. 539-548.

Knutsen, G., Engebretsen, L., Ludvigsen, T. C., Drogset, J. O., Grontvedt, T., Solheim, E., Strand, T., Roberts, S., Isaksen, V. and Johansen, O. (2004). Autologous chondrocyte implantation compared with microfracture in the knee. A randomized trial, *J. Bone Joint Surg. Am.,* 86-A, pp. 455-464.

Kujala, U. M., Kettunen, J., Paananen, H., Aalto, T., Battie, M. C., Impivaara, O., Videman, T. and Sarna, S. (1995). Knee osteoarthritis in former runners, soccer players, weight lifters, and shooters, *Arthritis Rheum.*, 38, pp. 539-546.

Langer, R. and Vacanti, J. P. (1993). Tissue engineering, *Science*, 260, pp. 920-926.

Lee, L. W., Zavarei, K., Evans, J., Lelas, J. J., Riley, P. O. and Kerrigan, D. C. (2005). Reduced hip extension in the elderly: dynamic or postural?, *Arch. Phys. Med. Rehabil.*, 86, pp. 1851-1854.

Lexell, J., Taylor, C. C. and Sjostrom, M. (1988). What is the cause of the ageing atrophy? Total number, size and proportion of different fiber types studied in whole vastus lateralis muscle from 15- to 83-year-old men, *J. Neurol. Sci.*, 84, pp. 275-294.

Liu, W., Cui, L. and Cao, Y. (2004). Recent advances in tissue engineering of cartilage, bone, and tendon, *Curr. Opin. Orthop.*, 15, pp. 364-368.

Lussier, A., Cividino, A. A., McFarlane, C. A., Olszynski, W. P., Potashner, W. J. and De Medicis, R. (1996). Viscosupplementation with hylan for the treatment of osteoarthritis: findings from clinical practice in Canada, *J. Rheumatol,* 23, pp. 1579-1585.

Marcacci, M., Berruto, M., Brocchetta, D., DeLcogliano, A., Ghinelli, D., Gobbi, A., Kon, E., Pederzini, L., Rosa, D., Sacchetti, G. L., Stefani, G. and Zanasi, S. (2005). Articular cartilage engineering with Hyalograft C: 3-year clinical results, *Clin. Orthop. Relat. Res.*, pp. 96-105.

Martinek, V., Ueblacker, P. and Imhoff, A. B. (2003). Current concepts of gene therapy and cartilage repair, *J. Bone Joint Surg. Br.*, 85, pp. 782-788.

Moseley, J. B., O'Malley, K., Petersen, N. J., Menke, T. J., Brody, B. A., Kuykendall, D. H., Hollingsworth, J. C., Ashton, C. M. and Wray, N. P. (2002). A controlled trial of arthroscopic surgery for osteoarthritis of the knee, *N. Engl. J. Med.*, 347, pp. 81-88.

Nicklas, B. J., Mychaleckyj, J., Kritchevsky, S., Palla, S., Lange, L. A., Lange, E. M., Messier, S. P., Bowden, D. and Pahor, M. (2005). Physical function and its response to exercise: associations with cytokine gene variation in older adults with knee osteoarthritis, *J. Gerontol. A Biol. Sci. Med. Sci.*, 60, pp. 1292-1298.

Nigg, B. (1998). Biomechanics as applied to sports (Ch 1.3.1). IN Harries M, W. C., Stanish DW, Micheli LJ (Ed.) *Oxford Textbook of Sports Medicine*, Oxford, U.K., Oxford University Press.

Pavelka, K., Gatterova, J., Olejarova, M., MacHacek, S., Giacovelli, G. and Rovati, L. C. (2002). Glucosamine sulfate use and delay of progression of knee osteoarthritis: a 3-year, randomized, placebo-controlled, double-blind study, *Arch. Intern. Med.*, 162, pp. 2113-2123.

Peterson, L., BrittberG, M., Kiviranta, I., Akerlund, E. L. and Lindahl, A. (2002). Autologous chondrocyte transplantation. Biomechanics and long-term durability, *Am. J. Sport. Med.*, 30, pp. 2-12.

Pollo, F. E. and Jackson, R. W. (2006). Knee bracing for unicompartmental osteoarthritis, *J. Am. Acad. Orthop. Surg.*, 14, pp. 5-11.

Pollo, F. E., Otis, J. C., Backus, S. I., Warren, R. F. and Wickiewicz, T. L. (2002). Reduction of medial compartment loads with valgus bracing of the osteoarthritic knee, *Am. J. Sports Med.,* 30, pp. 414-421.

Powell, A. P. (2005). Issues unique to the masters athlete, *Curr. Sports Med. Rep.,* 4, pp. 335-340.

Reginster, J. Y., Deroisy, R., Rovati, L. C., Lee, R. L., LeJeune, E., Bruyere, O., Giacovelli, G., Henrotin, Y., Dacre, J. E. and Gossett, C. (2001). Long-term effects of glucosamine sulphate on osteoarthritis progression: a randomised, placebo-controlled clinical trial, *Lancet,* 357, pp. 251-256.

Richy, F., Bruyere, O., Ethgen, O., Cucherat, M., Henrotin, Y. and Reginster, J. Y. (2003). Structural and symptomatic efficacy of glucosamine and chondroitin in knee osteoarthritis: a comprehensive meta-analysis, *Arch. Intern. Med.,* 163, pp. 1514-1522.

Rogers, M. A., Hagberg, J. M., Martin, W. H., 3RD, Ehsani, A. A. and Holloszy, J. O. (1990). Decline in VO2max with aging in master athletes and sedentary men, *J. Appl. Physiol.,* 68, pp. 2195-2199.

Smith, P., Shuler, F. D., Georgescu, H. I., Ghivizzani, S. C., Johnstone, B., Niyibizi, C., Robbins, P. D. and Evans, C. H. (2000). Genetic enhancement of matrix synthesis by articular chondrocytes: comparison of different growth factor genes in the presence and absence of interleukin-1, *Arthritis Rheum.,* 43, pp. 1156-1164.

Thelin, N., Holmberg, S. and Thelin, A. (2006). Knee injuries account for the sports-related increased risk of knee osteoarthritis, *Scand. J. Med. Sci. Sports,* 16, pp. 329-333.

Wang, C. T., Lin, J., Chang, C. J., Lin, Y. T. and Hou, S. M. (2004). Therapeutic effects of hyaluronic acid on osteoarthritis of the knee. A meta-analysis of randomized controlled trials, *J. Bone Joint Surg. Am.,* 86-A, pp. 538-545.

Wolfe, M. M., Lichtenstein, D. R. and Singh, G. (1999). Gastrointestinal toxicity of nonsteroidal antiinflammatory drugs, *N. Engl. J. Med.,* 340, pp. 1888-1899.

13.7 Review Questions

Q13.1 What treatment provides the best definitive results for pain of knee osteoarthritis:

    A. total knee replacement surgery (arthroplasty)

    B. steroid injections

    C. oral narcotic medications

    D. gene therapy

    E. physical therapy

Q13.2 Non Steroidal Anti-Inflammatory Drugs (NSAIDs) such as Ibuprofen act by inhibiting:

    A. interleukin-10

    B. lipase

    C. cyclo-oxygenase

    D. glucose dehydrogenase

    E. glycosaminoglycans

Q13.3 The following have proven positive clinical results for treating patients with advanced, end-stage osteoarthritis of the knee EXCEPT:

    A. arthroscopy

    B. total knee replacement

    C. high tibial osteotomy

    D. femoral osteotomy

    E. unicondylar arthroplasty

Q13.4 The following are "mechanical" symptoms and signs of knee osteoarthritis suggesting an internal derangement of the knee EXCEPT:

    A. swelling

    B. catching

    C. pain

    D. locking

    E. loose body sensation

Q13.5 Indications to perform arthroscopic surgery for a patient with mild osteoarthritis, knee pain and swelling include:

A. removal of loose bodies / bone chips

B. perform microfracture surgery to stimulate fibrocartilage growth

C. perform a meniscectomy on a symptomatic meniscus tear

D. perform a temporary surgery until the osteoarthritis gets to be more advanced

E. all of the above

Q13.6 Gene therapy involves:

A. transfer of gene chromosomes into the cell nucleus

B. infection of the cell with a retroviral vector containing specific gene sequences

C. injection of proteins that rewrite the cell's genetic materials

D. transplantation of whole cells to create a more viable, functional cell population

E. Use of external modalities to stimulate the cell to produce more DNA

Q13.7 With age, the typical masters athlete experiences the following physiological effects:

A. increased tissue flexibility

B. inability to gain strength with training

C. degeneration of the articular cartilage

D. improvement in cardiorespiratory function and efficiency

E. increased number of muscle cells

Q13.8 Risk factors for degenerative changes at the knee in the older athlete include:

A. previous fracture involving the joint

B. family history

C. history of playing football in high school

D. A and B

E. all of the above

Q13.9 The following are important components for tissue engineering for articular cartilage growth in the knee <u>EXCEPT</u>:

A. stem cells
B. a matrix scaffold
C. growth factors
D. absence of mechanical stimulation
E. adequate blood flow

ANSWERS TO REVIEW QUESTIONS

Chapter 1

A1.1 Muscles can be stimulated externally with surface electrodes, such as used in AFOs, or internally with wires, or Bions™, such as used in treatment for weak shoulder muscles, or for grasping.

A1.2 Passive approaches means that an external machine moves the limb, whereas active approaches require the user to activate his/her residual muscles. There is evidence that the latter is more effective for neurorehabilitation.

A1.3 FItts' law states that accuracy of reaching a target will diminish with difficulty of movement. It is tested by a game in which the player must alternately hit 2 tagets of width, W, spaced a distance of A apart, as quickly as possible. It is formulated such that an index of difficulty is represented by the binary logarithm of 2*A/W. A plot of movement time versus the ID represents Fitts' behavior, and the slope indicates the information processing capability of the task, in bits/sec.

A1.4 Intrinsic and reflex stiffness.

A1.5 Jerk and degree of spontaneous accelerations.

A1.6 It is the ability of the robot to back off active force when it feels resistance (pushing), or active pulling by the user.

Chapter 2

A2.1 D. all of the above

A2.2 A. excimer laser

A2.3 D. presbyopia

A2.4 E. eye needing laser enhancements following initial laser vision correction surgery

A2.5 D. 55 years

A2.6   D. all of the above

A2.7   A. conductive keratoplasty

A2.8   D. A and C

Chapter 3

A3.1   AMD is more prevalent, but RP is more likely to lead to total blindness. Because patients with AMD typically retain their peripheral vision, there would be some risk of further loss of vision with implantation of a retinal prosthesis device.

A3.2   As the population of elderly patients with AMD increases, this may create a large demand for retinal prosthesis among patients with very severe cases of AMD. Regarding patients with RP, many do not become legally <u>blind</u> until their 40s or 50s and retain some central vision all their life while others go completely blind from RP. In some cases, severe RP can occur in early childhood – these patients would be good candidates for retinal prosthesis because their visual system is still developing and could more easily adapt than older adults.

A3.3   C. in advanced stages of retinal diseases, the inner retinal layers of the retina remain viable for long periods of time - by stimulating these remaining functional retinal layers, it may

A3.4   True.

A3.5   C. the minimum level of electrical charge needed to stimulate retinal cells and the maximum level of electrical charge that can cause cell damage differ by four orders of magnitude.

A3.6   C. the lack of knowledge of how the human eye-brain system will adapt to artificial electrical stimulation.

Chapter 4

A4.1   C. Ganglion cell layer

A4.2   B. Hyperopic; elongation; myopia

A4.3   The change in local retinal defocus modulates the rate of neurotransmitter release from inner plexiform cells, causing synaptic changes that alter the local baseline proteoglycan synthesis rate. An increase in proteoglycan synthesis causes the scleral matrix to stiffen, increasing resistance to the expansive force of intraocular pressure and reducing the eyeball's axial growth rate (and vice versa).

A4.4 A. control over emmetropization from higher neural centers

A4.5 There are three forces acting on each node:
- *Two forces caused by spring tension in the node's two attached springs*
- *An internal ocular pressure force acting outwards*

A4.6 C. both hyperopic and myopic defocus can cause equal–size blur circles

A4.7
- *Calculate the spring tension in each spring and sum with the pressure force to determine the total force acting on each node*
- *Use Euler's approximation twice to determine the change in node position*
- *Calculate the new blur circle size at each node and compare it to the previous frame's baseline*
- *Use the change in blur circle to adjust the spring constants in the two nearby springs.*

A4.8 B. The sclera has elastic but not viscoelastic properties

Chapter 5

A5.1 The conduction of sound vibrations through the outer and middle ear is a fairly linear process, and consequently linear gain supplied by a hearing aid does a satisfactory job of compensating for any conductive hearing losses. In contrast, the cochlear performs a nonlinear time-frequency analysis of the sound waves, and therefore cochlear impairment can give rise to distortion or loss of information about the acoustic signal in the auditory nerve activity. More sophisticated amplification schemes are thus required to compensate for sensorineural losses.

A5.2   A. the inner hair cells

A5.3   Young adults can normally hear sounds with frequencies between 20 Hz and around 20 kHz. With aging, the higher frequencies tend to be progressively lost (presbycusis). The most important frequencies for speech are between around 100 Hz and 8 kHz, and consequently the audiogram is usually only measured for frequencies within this range. In addition, the frequency-response of conventional hearing aid receivers (loudspeakers) falls off above 5 kHz, so useful gain above this frequency cannot be achieved.

A5.4   A threshold shift of 15 dB corresponds to the threshold sound pressure increasing by a factor of $10^{15/20} = 5.62$. Note that the sound *intensity* (i.e., sound power per unit area, which has units of W/m^2 in the SI system) is proportional to the squared pressure, so a 15 dB HL corresponds to the threshold sound *intensity* increasing by a factor of $10^{15/10} = 31.62$.

A5.5   Audiogram #1 has a PTA of $\frac{1}{3}(59+73+81) = 71\,dB$ HL and is thus classified as a severe loss, although there is a profound loss (> 90 dB HL) at the higher frequencies. Audiogram #2 has a PTA of 17.33 dB HL, and consequently it would be classified as being within the range of "normal" hearing. However, an individual with such a hearing loss may still benefit from the use of a hearing aid. Audiogram #3 has a PTA of 47 dB HL and is consequently classified as a moderate loss.

A5.6   The PTAs for these three audiograms were calculated in Q5 above. The X values for (5.1) are 0.15 times the respective PTAs. The resulting gains prescribed at each audiogram frequency are given in the table below. Note that the negative gains for 250 and 500 Hz in the prescription for audiogram #2 would be set to zero in fitting most hearing aids.

F (kHz)	0.25	0.5	1	2	3	4	6
G_i #1 (dB)	12.9	20.9	34.3	34.8	39.0	43.1	40.9
G_i #2 (dB)	−9.8	−2.3	9.8	8.4	8.3	10.2	9.6
G_i #3 (dB)	3.1	12.4	22.6	21.9	25.8	25.5	27.1

A5.7 The primary motivation for compression algorithms is to fit the range of sound intensities experienced by a hear aid users into the range of intensities that are both audible and comfortable for that individual. That is, compression is primarily aimed at dealing with the loudness recruitment phenomenon. Additional uses for compression include avoiding distortion in the hearing aid circuitry, providing automatic volume control, and reducing background noise.

A5.8 Damage of the outer hair cells leads to both an elevation and a broadening of threshold tuning curves of auditory nerve fibers, whereas inner hair cell impairment results primarily in elevation of the tuning curve.

A5.9 From the definition of Q_{10} given in Fig. 5.11, the normal bandwidth is:

$$\text{BW} = \frac{\text{BF}}{Q_{10}} = \frac{3\,\text{kHz}}{5} = 600\,\text{Hz} .$$

A half-octave downward shift in the BF corresponds to:

$$\text{impaired BF} = 2^{-\frac{1}{2}} \times \text{normal BF} = 2^{-\frac{1}{2}} \times 3\,\text{kHz} = 2.12\,\text{kHz} .$$

The impaired bandwidth is 3.5×600 Hz = 2100 Hz, and consequently:

$$\text{impaired } Q_{10} = \frac{\text{impaired BF}}{\text{impaired BW}} = \frac{2.12\,\text{kHz}}{2.1\,\text{kHz}} = 1.01 .$$

A5.10 Miniaturization of hearing aids has been driven primarily by the desire to have a more comfortable hearing aid and one that is more cosmetically appealing, i.e., less visible. The main disadvantages of smaller hearing aids are the difficulty of fitting all the components into a smaller package, an increase in occurrence of acoustic feedback resulting from having the microphone and receiver closer together, and users having difficultly manipulating smaller control buttons, switches and dials on the hearing aid.

A5.11 C. A moderate, high-frequency sensorineural hearing loss. Large gains cannot be obtained in open fittings without acoustic feedback, so they are most suitable for mild or moderate high-frequency losses. Receiver-in-the-ear hearing aids can achieve somewhat higher gains at lower frequencies than a standard open fitting.

A5.12 The main advantage of implantable components is that they are not exposed to damaging environmental conditions. For example, non-implantable hearing aids need to be removed when swimming or showering, whereas fully-implantable hearing aids can be used during such activities. The principal disadvantages are the surgical procedures required to implant the device and the possible complications that arise from surgery, the difficulties in powering the device, the biocompatibility requirements for implantable materials and devices, difficulties in repairing or upgrading the device, and the higher cost.

Chapter 6

A6.1 False. A cochlear implant restores hearing to some degree but it is not perfect hearing. Most people with a cochlear implant do not enjoy music.

A6.2 True. People with cochlear implant can understand more than 90% of speech in sentences in quiet. However, speech understanding is much poorer in background noise.

A6.3 False. Most ABI listeners have much poorer speech recognition than the average CI listener. Only a small number of ABI listeners who did not have VIII nerve tumors can achieve speech recognition at a level similar to cochlear implants.

A6.4 F. The auditory cortex has been implanted in animals but not yet in humans.

A6.5 False. Early implant signal processing did this and achieved only limited speech recognition. Performance improved dramatically when signal processing presented the unprocessed signal from each frequency band to the electrodes.)

A6.6 False. Cochlear implants are now being implanted in people with substantial residual acoustic hearing. People appear to be able to integrate acoustic hearing at low frequencies with electric hearing at high frequencies.

A6.7 False. In a deaf ear there are no biological mechanisms for parsing an electric signal into its frequency-specific parts. Only a multichannel device can achieve good speech recognition by splitting the signal into its spectral components and delivering spectrally selective information to different groups of frequency-specific neurons.

Chapter 7

A7.1   C. diameter

A7.2   C. nylon stents

A7.3   Compliance mismatch

A7.4   D. blood pressure flow

A7.5   A. normal vascular physiology

A7.6   E. length

A7.7   True.

Chapter 8

A8.1   C. 7 L/min

A8.2   A. 1 KHz

A8.3   D. 2.0

A8.4   D. pressure gradient

A8.5   D. cardiac output

A8.6   B. 0.70

A8.7   A. catheter lumen diameter

A8.8   C. a stiff catheter and a stiff transducer

A8.9   D. tonometer

A8.10 A. reflected pressure is significantly increased

Chapter 9

A9.1   CHF is the progressive inability of the heart to contract. It afflicts more than 5 million people in the United States and has become the most common admitting diagnosis for patients older than 65.

A9.2   While there have been great advances in the medical and surgical management of CHF, including surgical ventricular restoration, ventricular assist device support, and the gold standard of heart transplantation, over 100,000 people with CHF are classified as having 'no-option' annually.

A9.3   False.

A9.4   C. 4-5 years

A9.5   F. all of the above

A9.6   CSCs are multipotent, clonogenic cells found in niches throughout the heart, most commonly in the apex and atrial tissue, characterized by the presence of surface stem cell antigens c-kit, Sca-1, and MDR1, but lacking transcription factors and surface proteins of cardiomyocytes and endothelial cells. These cells give rise to cardiomyocytes, smooth muscle cells, and endothelial cells.

A9.7   CSCs are subject to the same ischemic insults that plague other myocardial tissue and decrease in number with age decreasing their potential. However, CSCs have been successfully isolated and expanded in vitro from percutaneous endomyocardial biopsy. A large population of CSCs can be grown in a relatively short period of time and be used for cell based therapy.

A9.8   Cells can be delivered to the myocardium by either intravascular or intramuscular injection. Intravascular injection can take place directly into the coronary arteries during coronary angiography. Intramuscular injection can be undertaken percutaneously with catheter based needles or via surgical approaches during open operations or using a minimally invasive procedures.

A9.9   F. All of the above

Chapter 10

A10.1   C. coronary artery disease

A10.2   False.

A10.3   True.

A10.4   D. 1 and 3 are correct

A10.5 False.

A10.6 E. 1-3 are correct

A10.7 C. accelerated atherosclerosis

A10.8 D. none of the above

A10.9 False.

Chapter 11

A11.1 The heart is composed primarily of cardiac muscle. The cardiac muscle receives an abundant blood supply through the coronary arteries. Occlusion of a coronary artery can restrict the blood supply to the myocardium, and result in injury of these muscle cells (cardiomyocytes) and eventual cardiomyocyte death; this process is termed myocardial infarction (heart attack).

A11.2 Stem cells are defined as undifferentiated cells that have the ability to self-renew and the potential to differentiate into various cell types that make up the body. Stem cells can be isolated from embryo, or various adult somatic tissues.

A11.3 A and C are true.

A11.4 A, B, C and D.

A11.5 Stem cells derived from adult somatic tissue can develop into mature cell phenotypes different from their original lineage in response to microenvironmental cues and this phenomenon is termed transdifferentiation. For example, hematopoietic stem cells from bone marrow turning into cardiac muscle cells would be termed transdifferentiation.

A11.6 There are two basic approaches: one is direct injection. Direct injection of stem cells into infarcted myocardium can be performed during open-heart surgery, by minimally invasive thoracoscopic procedures or percutaneously by injecting cells via a catheter. Catheter injection includes catheter-based needle injection from the left ventricular cavity, ultrasound-directed intramyocardial injection through the coronary sinus or the great cardiac vein. Another approach to delivering cells is through the systemic vasculature. The site of introducing stem cells into the circulatory system includes intravenous injection, intracoronary injection, intra- aortic root administration and retrograde venous infusion. The stem cells "home" to the injured heart from the systemic vasculature after administration.

A11.7 Stem cell "homing" is a multistep process whereby the cells seek out injured myocardium, traveling to an area that is in need of such cells. Homing includes adhesion of the cells to the endothelium, transmigration through the blood vessel wall and migration within the target tissue. Stem cell "homing" through the systemic vasculature is a potential approach for stem cell delivery.

A11.8 A and C.

Chapter 12

A12.1 C. Great strides have been made in fashioning knee replacement components that mimic the normal knee and thus improve its function. With better surgical techniques, recovery is faster and the prostheses can last longer. Unfortunately, these prostheses still have limitations and patients should not jog or run excessively after undergoing knee replacement surgery.

A12.2 True. Because a unicompartmental knee replacement resurfaces only a single compartment, the arthritis must be confined to that compartment. If the arthritis involves <u>more</u> than the single compartment, then total knee replacement should be done.

A12.3 D. Approximately 90% of patients who undergo successful knee replacement surgery – and do not abuse their implant – can expect between 15 and 20 years of excellent function.

A12.4 E. All these answers are correct and are well-known potential risks when undergoing a total knee replacement.

A12.5 A, C, E. Moderate activities are encouraged following knee replacement and include swimming, doubles tennis, and bowling. Activities which involve heavy loads with jumping and running, vigorous twisting and cutting such as basketball, running, singles tennis are discouraged.

Chapter 13

A13.1 A. total knee replacement surgery (arthroplasty)

A13.2 C. cyclo-oxygenase

A13.3 A. arthroscopy

A13.4 C. pain

A13.5 E. all of the above

A13.6 B. infection of the cell with a retroviral vector containing specific gene sequences

A13.7 C. degeneration of the articular cartilage

A13.8 D. A and B

A13.9 D. absence of mechanical stimulation

SUBJECT INDEX